ADVANCE PRAISE FOR CONVICT CONDITIONING

In *Convict Conditioning* Paul Wade has laid out a logical and effective "zero to hero" progression in key bodyweight strength exercises and presented a solid training philosophy. Get this book.
—Pavel Tsatsouline, author of *The Naked Warrior*

Convict Conditioning gives honor and respect to body-weight training. This book is an old step in a new direction and I welcome it. I feel *Convict Conditioning* provides the progression, precision and clarity that is necessary to combat our cultural decline in simple body knowledge.
—Gray Cook, MSPT, OCS, CSCS, Functional Movement Systems, author of *Body in Balance*

Convict Conditioning is a fantastic text crammed with solid information, and tons of vital nuggets and powerful insights that when followed will pack your frame with rock-hard, functional muscle. Like a hard thrust with a razor-sharp shank, ex-con Paul Wade's writing style rips through all the nonsense that fill the glossy muscle mags, to get to what's real: You don't need free weights, fancy machines, spray-on tan and carefully torn T-shirts to build powerful muscle. All you really need is your own body, a few simple exercises and a plan. You provide the body, *Convict Conditioning* gives you the rest in a highly readable, easy-to-understand format that teaches you *what* to do and *how* to do it. As a guy who has written extensively on exercise, I highly recommend this book.
—Loren Christensen, author of *Solo Training* and *The Fighter's Body*.

To paraphrase a famous political quote: "It's the progressions stupid." Coach Wade has laid out a set of progressions in *Convict Conditioning* that can lead to mastery of the big 6 bodyweight exercises and you would be wise to listen. This is knowledge proven in "extreme" conditions. So respect the progressions and put in your time—you'll be stronger for it.
—Brett Jones, Master RKC, CSCS, CK-FMS

Outstanding! By far the most innovative fitness book in years. Many talk about "mastering your body weight" yet *Convict Conditioning* actually delivers a blueprint for anyone, regardless of your current fitness. The training "progressions" are genius. I had illusions I was able to do some Master Steps right away but was unable to CORRECTLY get past step 6 in one of the big six and was at steps 3-5 on most. This program will give me the tendon strength to blast past my previous body weight abilities and real usable strength and speed for hand-to-hand training! I've already pre-ordered a case of books for my friends and associates. Don't hesitate—just get it and start getting real, usable, strength and power to move your human machine!
—Tim Larkin, Master Close Combat Instructor, targetfocustraining.com

Convict Conditioning by El Entrenador is a remarkable book on how to take your bodyweight training to extreme levels. *Convict Conditioning* deserves a place on the bookshelf next to *The Naked Warrior*.
—Kenneth Jay, Master RKC, author of *Viking Warrior Conditioning*

Convict Conditioning is a refreshing book on strength. While there are many books on the topic of body weight conditioning, very few focus on true strength through body weight movements. This is not another book on how to do 50 pushups; this is a book to learn how to do *One Arm Handstand Pushups, One-legged Squats,* or how about *One Arm Pull Ups?* Truly the stuff of comic books, but completely attainable with a crystal clear progression plan.

Paul Wade is highly entertaining and motivating in his delivery, I guarantee you will find this a pager burner. This program is completely scalable to challenge any person, from your Mom, to any weekend warrior, to an elite level athlete in the off-season.

I have implemented several of the drills in to my training, the progressions for the bridge and core drills are particularly helpful to every person's power program. I believe *Convict Conditioning* would be exceptionally valuable to military preparation programs, wrestling coaches, and martial arts instructors. The drills will quickly develop body mastery and skill, with simple modifications to movements already heavily employed in those areas. With its focus on strength development, it will yield high dividends in short order.

Convict Conditioning should definitely be on your watch list. I think this program combined with Pavel's *Naked Warrior* would allow someone to build strength that would cause Spiderman to look over his shoulder.
—Adam T Glass, RKC II, Professional Performing Strongman

Coach Wade's book comes along at a critical time for me, both personally and professionally. (And no, I'm not going to jail!). His bodyweight training progressions will help me create better, more efficient workouts for both myself and my members. If you are a serious student of bodyweight exercise and physical culture, you must get this book. And if you enjoy a little bit of the dark side, the origin story of Coach Wade's knowledge will help you tear through this book in one sitting.
—Craig Ballantyne, Turbulence Training

I DID NOT want to like this book. In fact, I did not even want to read it because of the title. BUT not only do I like this book, I LOVE IT. It is probably the best compilation of callisthenic exercises and training progressions I have seen; reaching all the back to the beginnings of organized bodyweight exercise.

As an ex elite gymnast and gymnastics coach, using the body as the resistance to strengthen oneself is near and dear to my heart and is the base for any truly functional training regimen. After all, if you can't use your own weight what do you need added resistance for? Coach Wade understands this completely and has crafted programs that will make anyone who uses them a complete physical animal in no time flat.

Easy to read, so well organized and thought out I had no choice but to embrace it wholeheartedly. The progressions of the exercises are brilliant and make even the most difficult of these movements accessible to all who have the heart and stamina to stay the course.

Coach Wade goes to the heart of true training with correct biomechanics, kinesiology and training progressions that so many in the word of physical training just seem to miss these days. Bravo Coach, bravo, an epic book that deserves to be in the library of all who love the world of strength as well as a historical understanding of the foundation of all modern resistance training.
—Mark Reifkind, Master RKC Instructor, Girya Kettlebell Training

Convict Conditioning is jam packed with the most powerful bodyweight training information I have ever come across. It's the book I WISH I had in my hands when I was a competitive wrestler, BUT, even more important to me is that I can pass on this knowledge to my clients AND my son and daughter when they grow up. That's how impressed with and trustful I am of the information in this book.
—Zach Even-Esh, author *The Ultimate Underground Strength System*

CONVICT CONDITIONING

How to Bust Free of All Weakness—
Using the Lost Secrets
of Supreme Survival Strength

BY PAUL "COACH" WADE

CONVICT CONDITIONING

How to Bust Free of All Weakness— Using the Lost Secrets of Supreme Survival Strength

BY PAUL "COACH" WADE

Published in the United States by:
Dragon Door Publications, Inc
P.O. Box 4381, St. Paul, MN 55104
Tel: (651) 487-2180 • Fax: (651) 487-3954
Credit card orders: 1-800-899-5111
Email: dragondoor@aol.com • Website: www.dragondoor.com

ISBN 10: 0-938045-76-8   ISBN 13: 978-0-938045-76-2

This edition first published in January, 2010

Printed in the United States of America

Book design, and cover by Derek Brigham
Website http//www.dbrigham.com • Tel/Fax: (763) 208-3069 • Email: bigd@dbrigham.com

DISCLAIMER
The author and publisher of this material are not responsible in any manner whatsoever for any injury that may occur through following the instructions contained in this material. The activities, physical and otherwise, described herein for informational purposes only, may be too strenuous or dangerous for some people and the reader(s) should consult a physician before engaging in them.

To Melanie Shoshana Ault

A dame worth busting out
of high security for.

—DISCLAIMER!—

Fitness and strength are meaningless qualities without *health*. With correct training, these three benefits should naturally proceed hand-in-hand. In this book, every effort has been made to convey the importance of safe training technique, but despite this all individual trainees are different and needs will vary. Proceed with caution, and at your own risk. Your body is your own responsibility—look after it. All medical experts agree that you should consult your physician before initiating a training program. Be safe!

This book is intended for entertainment purposes only. This book is not biography. The names, histories and circumstances of the individuals featured in this book have accordingly been changed either partially or completely. Despite this, the author maintains that all the exercise principles within this volume—techniques, methods and ideology—are valid. Use them, and become the best.

—TABLE OF CONTENTS—

FOREWORD

Some time in 1969. A brash Cambridge undergraduate sat hunched in the reverent silence, as two saffron-clad Tibetan Buddhist monks lectured on the mysteries of meditation and enlightenment.

The monks radiated gentle peace and ease. Their eyes crinkled with humor, as if sharing a perpetual inside joke. "Everything is beautiful, nothing matters," they seemed to hint. Their words washed over the young man's head—mostly wasted—as his mind darted from restless thought to restless thought.

One monk began to speak of the inner freedom that arises from the practice of deep meditation. The monk used an analogy: "You can be locked in a prison cell—apparently in bondage—and yet you remain free inside. Nobody can take that inner freedom from you."

The undergrad exploded out of his seat with an angry rebuttal. "How can you say that? Prison is prison. Bondage is bondage. There can be no real freedom when you are being held against your will!" A deep button had been pushed, the knee-jerk response out of all proportion to the monk's analogy.

The fellow monk smiled beatifically at the angry young man. "It is good to question your teachers," he said with absolute sincerity and no hint of irony. And the monks continued with their talk, flowing like a river round the jagged boulder in their midst.

Forty years later. Some time in 2009. The volatile young Cambridge undergrad is now a somewhat wiser and a whole lot more mellow fellow. He's running a dynamic and rapidly expanding venture called Dragon Door Publications—a vehicle for those with a passion for the cultivation of physical excellence.

And I'm about to introduce the world to one of the most exciting books I have ever read. It's a book about prison. It's a book about freedom. It's a book about survival. It's a book about humanity. It's a book about strength and power. It's a book that belongs in the hands of our military, our police, our firefighters, and all who protect our country from harm. It's a book to circulate in our high schools and colleges. It's a book for the professional athlete and for the out-of-shape desk jockey. It's a book for stay-at-home moms. It's a book for boomers seeking to reverse the sands of time. It's a book for anyone seeking the secrets of supreme survival strength.

It's a book by an ex-con—a man stripped of his freedom over a twenty-year period; a man confined in some of the harshest prisons in America. Forced into strength by the brute needs of base survival. A man stripped of all but his body and mind—who chose to cultivate himself against all odds and create a private freedom no one would be able to prize from him. The freedom of a strong body and a strong mind.

It's a book called *Convict Conditioning*.

Convict Conditioning?! How and why would a company of Dragon Door's stature dare publish a book with such a title? Surely, this has to be some glib celebration of the criminal—hardly deserving of one of the world's premier fitness publishing companies?

Many of our country's leading fitness experts have read preview copies of *Convict Conditioning*—and loved the contents. In fact, in many cases, raved about the contents. But in many cases, they balked and winced at the title. Convict Conditioning?! "John, the contents are superb, but they deserve a better title. This book belongs with every member of the military, every law enforcement officer, it should be given to every child by their parents…but how many of them are going to read it, with a title like this?"

I did waver, I admit. Not about the book, but the title. Would I be selling America—and even the author, Paul Wade—short by such a title? Would those two words, "Convict Conditioning," somehow turn away the hundreds of thousands who stand to benefit from the strength strategies within its pages? Would the title relegate these wonderful secrets to just a small band of enthusiasts who grasp the brilliance of Paul's Big Six progressions—and could care less about the title?

But the more I thought about it, the more absolutely convinced I was that the title had to stand. Because *Convict Conditioning* is about exactly that: a strength-survival system born from one of the most daily-dangerous environments any man can be placed in. *Convict Conditioning* is about taking your strength and power to a level where no predator would remotely consider attacking you. *Convict Conditioning* is about achieving an aura of strength and power that sends a dramatic and entirely unambiguous message to other limbic systems: "Don't even think about it!"

To call this reservoir of knowledge by any other name would be to do it a great disservice. It would be akin to taking a rare, rich Roquefort—bleeding with potency—and calling it Cheddar Mild. Sorry, can't do it.

And the central message needs to stand: there IS a freedom that cannot be taken from you—whatever little box you may be stuck in. And that's the freedom to cultivate the magnificence of your own body and mind, regardless of external environment. Paul Wade has created both a stunning testament to that truth—and a master-plan on how you can achieve that magnificence yourself.

Dive into the pages of *Convict Conditioning* and you will quickly realize that this is no celebration of "convictness"—no literary equivalent of gangsta rap. In fact, it's a book that will make you fervently wish you never, ever end up where Paul had to tread for so many years. But it's also a book to inspire you to achieve heights of physical excellence you may have once considered impossible.

And then comes another consideration: because this wisdom has been passed to us by an ex-convict, is this wisdom somehow tainted? If a police officer or a high school coach—for instance—use Paul's system and achieve unprecedented new levels of strength and power, have they somehow sullied themselves, betrayed their profession, because the wisdom came from an ex-con? Hardly, I would say. Because that would deny one of the great spiritual truths embodied in *Convict Conditioning*: "Judge not, that ye be not judged." And deny the central message of hope within this book—any human being has the potential for redemption, however dark their situation.

I recently tried to turn my 18-year old son, Peter on to one of the rock icons I had revered in my own teenage years—Lou Reed. After listening to a short excerpt of Lou Reed and the Velvet Underground, his response was definitive: "Dad, there can be only one Bob Dylan." While I disagreed with Peter about Lou, he wasn't that far off the mark. Lou Reed had idolized Bob Dylan—and because there was indeed "only one Bob Dylan" had a helluva time making the separation. To my mind, Lou achieved that rare stature. "There is only one Lou Reed," I would say.

In my life as a publisher I have had the good fortune to offer three remarkable authors to the world: Pavel Tsatsouline, Ori Hofmekler and Marty Gallagher. All three have an iconic stature that can be summed up in the phrase "there is only one…" There can be only one Pavel. There can be only one Ori. There can be only one Marty. And now I am equally privileged to add a fourth author to that list. There can be only one Paul Wade.

—John Du Cane
CEO, Dragon Door Publications

– Part I –
Preliminaries

The modern fitness scene is largely defined by the presence of pumped up, muscle-bound bodybuilders, expensive exercise machines, and steroids.

It wasn't always this way.

There was a time when men trained to become *inhumanly strong* using nothing but their own bodyweight. No weights. No machines. No drugs. Nothing.

If you want to know more about the *real* old school arts of power, read on...

1: INTRODUCTION

A JOURNEY OF STRENGTH

Walk into virtually any gym in the world and you will find any number of pumped up steroid users who think that they are "strong" men because they have eighteen-inch arms, can bench press a heavy bar, or look big in a tank top or T-shirt.

But how many of them are *truly* powerful?

- How many of them have genuine athletic strength they can *use*?
- How many of them could drop and give you twenty perfect one-arm pushups?
- How many of them have spines that are strong enough, flexible enough and healthy enough that they can bend over backwards and touch the floor?
- How many have the pure knee and hip power to squat right down to the ground and stand up again—on one leg?
- How many of them could grab hold of an overhead bar and execute a flawless *one-arm* pullup?

The answer is:

Almost none.

You will find almost no bodybuilder in any gym today who can perform these simple body-weight feats. And yet the kind of bloated poser you see strutting the average gym floor is viewed by the media and the modern public as the epitome of strength and fitness.

The bodybuilder-type has become the accepted status quo of ultimate conditioning. This seems like total insanity to me. What does it matter how much weight you claim to be able to lift in a gym or on a special machine? How can somebody be considered to be "strong" if he can't even move *his own body* around as nature intended?

Becoming Strong

The average gym junkie today is all about *appearance*, not *ability*. Flash, not function. These men may have big, artificially pumped up limbs, but all that the size is in the muscle tissue; their tendons and joints are weak. Ask the average muscleman to do a deep one-leg squat—ass-to-floor-style—and his knee ligaments would probably snap in two. What strength most bodybuilders do have, they cannot use in a coordinated way; if you asked them to walk on their hands they'd fall flat on their faces.

I don't know whether to laugh or cry when see the current generation of men duped into handing over a fortune in overpriced gym memberships and for weights and other exercise gadgets, all in the hope of becoming strong and powerful. I want to *laugh* because I admire the con trick for what it is—a perfect grift. The fitness industry has duped the whole world into thinking it can't get by without all this equipment; equipment it then sells to the mark, or rents out at exorbitant prices (in the case of gym membership). I want to *cry* because it's a tragedy; the average modern trainee—who is not on steroids—makes little gain in size from year to year, and even less progress in true athletic ability.

To become hugely powerful, you don't need weights, cables, fancy machines, or any other crap that the industry or the informercials are brainwashing you into thinking you can't do without. You can gain Herculean strength—genuine brawn and vitality—with no special equipment at all. But to unlock this power—the power of your own body—you need to know how. You need the right method, the *art*.

Such a method does in fact exist. It's based on traditional, ancient forms of training, techniques which are as old as training itself. This method has evolved by trial-and-error over the centuries, and has proved its superior ability to transform flimsy men into steel-forged warriors time and time again. This method is *progressive calisthenics*—the art of using the human body to maximize its own development. Calisthenics today is seen as a method of aerobics, circuit training or muscle endurance. It isn't taken seriously. But in the past—before the second half of the twentieth century—all of the world's strongest athletes earned the bulk of their power through performing calisthenics *progressively*—to become stronger and stronger, day by day, week by week, year after year.

The Forgotten Art of Bodyweight Training

Unfortunately you will not be able to learn this art in any gym in the world. It has become lost to the vast majority of athletes during the modern era—quite recently in fact. It has been mercilessly pushed out of the light of day by a childish fascination with the plethora of new training technologies that have sprung up over the last century or so; everything from plated barbells and dumbbells to cable machines and hundreds of other novelties. The knowledge of how to perform calisthenics properly has been choked, nearly strangled to death by the propaganda of fitness manufacturers who want to sell you your right to train your own body and mind.

Because of this assault, the traditional arts of calisthenics have become degraded, relegated to high school fitness methods for children. "Calisthenics" currently involves pushups, pullups and squats; all fine exercises, but done for high repetitions which will build stamina though develop little in the way of strength. A *real* master of progressive calisthenics—"old school" calisthenics— also knows how to build *maximum raw strength*. Much more than the average trainee could possibly hope to develop with a barbell or a resistance machine. I've seen men trained in old school calisthenics who were powerful enough to break steel handcuffs, tear apart a chain-link fence, and punch a wall hard enough to take big chunks out of it, splitting the bricks in the process.

How would you like that kind of awesome bodily strength?

I can teach you how to develop it in the pages of this book, but you won't get it from going to a gym or doing high-rep pushups. That kind of raw, animal ability to unleash your body's own powers only comes from knowing how to do *old school* calisthenics.

How I Learned My Craft: Doing Time

Luckily, the hidden system of old school calisthenics *has* survived. But it was only able to survive in those dark places where men need maximum strength and power just to stay alive; places where, for prolonged periods, barbells, dumbbells and other forms of modern training equipment may not be available, if ever. Those places are called penitentiaries, jails, correctional institutes and all the other names civilized men give to the cages where they keep less civilized men safely behind bars.

My name is Paul Wade, and sadly I know all about life behind bars. I entered San Quentin State Prison for my first offense in 1979, and went on to spend nineteen of the following twenty-three years inside some of the toughest prisons in America, including Angola Penitentiary (a.k.a. "The Farm") and Marion—the hellhole they built to replace Alcatraz.

I also know about old school calisthenics; maybe more than anybody else alive. During my last stretch inside, I became known by the nickname *Entrenador*, which is a Spanish word for "coach," because all the greenhorns and new fish came to me for my knowledge on how to get incredibly powerful in super-fast time. I garnered a helluva lot of favors and benefits that way, and I earned it, too—my techniques work. I myself got to a level where I could do more than a dozen one-arm handstand pushups without support—a feat I have never seen replicated, even by Olympic gymnasts. I won the annual Angola pushup/pullup championship held by the inmates for six years in a row, even though I was subject to full daily shifts of manual labor in the working farm. (This was a technique used in the Pen to reduce trouble—inmates put to work on the farm were generally too exhausted by the end of the day to mess with the guards.) I even came third in the 1987 Californian Institutional powerlifting championship—*despite the fact that I have never trained with weights.* (I only entered on a bet.) For more years than I care to count, my training system has kept me physically tougher and head-and-shoulders stronger than the vast majority of psychos, veteranos and other vicious nutjobs I've been forced to rub shoulders with for two decades. And most of these guys worked out—*hard.* You might not read about their training methods or accomplishments in fitness magazines, but some of the world's most impressive athletes are convicts.

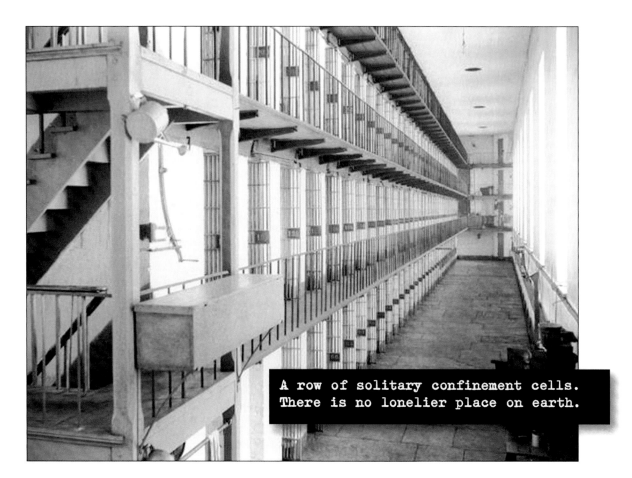

A row of solitary confinement cells. There is no lonelier place on earth.

Throughout my time in prison, getting and staying as strong, fit and overall tough as possible has been my trade. But I didn't learn that trade in a comfortable chrome-covered gym, surrounded by tanned posers and spandex vixens. I didn't qualify as the result of a three-week correspondence course, like most of the personal trainers around today. And I sure as hell ain't some fatass writer who never sweated a day in his life, like a lot of the guys who churn out "fitness" or "bodybuilding" books. Nor was I born a "natural athlete." When I first would up in the joint—only three weeks after my twenty-second birthday—I weighed a hundred and fifty pounds soaking wet. At 6'1 my long, gangly arms looked like pipe cleaners and were about half as strong. Following some nasty experiences early on, I learned pretty quickly that other prisoners exploit weaknesses like they breathe air; intimidation is the daily currency in the holes I've wound up in. And as I wasn't planning on being anyone's bitch, I realized that the safest way to stop being a target was to build myself up, fast.

Luckily after a few weeks in San Quentin, I was placed in a cell with an ex-Navy SEAL. He was in great shape from his military training, and taught me how to do the basic calisthenics exercises; pushups, pullups, deep knee-bends. I learned good form early on, and training with him over the months put some size on me. Working out in the cell every day gave me great stamina, and soon I was able to do hundreds of reps in some exercises. I still wanted to get bigger and stronger however, and did all the research I could to learn how to get where I wanted to be. I learned from everyone I could find—and you'd be surprised at the cross-section of people who wind up in the joint. Gymnasts, soldiers, Olympic weightlifters, martial artists, yoga guys, wrestlers; even a couple of doctors.

At the time I did not have access to a gym—I trained alone in my cell, with nothing. So I had to find ways of making my own body my gymnasium. Training became my therapy, my obsession. In six months I had gained a ton of size and power, and within a year I was one of the most physically capable guys in the hole. This was entirely thanks to old school, traditional calisthenics. These forms of exercise are all but dead on the outside, but in the prisons knowledge of them has been passed on in pockets, from generation to generation. This knowledge only survived in the prison environment because there are very few alternative training options to distract people most of the time. No pilates classes, no aerobics. Everybody on the outside now talks about prison gyms, but trust me, these are a relatively new import and where they do exist they're poorly equipped.

One of my mentors was a lifer called Joe Hartigen. Joe was seventy-one years old when I got to know him, and was spending his fourth decade in prison. Despite his age and numerous injuries, Joe still trained in his cell every morning. And he was strong as hell, too; I've seen him do weighted pullups using only his two index fingers for hooks, and one-arm pushups *using only one thumb* were a regular party trick of his. In fact he made them look easy. Joe knew more about real training than most "experts" will ever know. He was built in the old gyms in the first half of the twentieth century, before most people had even heard of adjustable barbells. Those guys relied largely on bodyweight movements—techniques that, today, we would regard as part of gymnastics, not bodybuilding or strength training. When they did lift "weights," they didn't lift seated on comfortable, adjustable machines; they lugged around huge, uneven objects like weighted barrels, anvils, sandbags and other human beings. Lifting like this calls into play qualities that are important for power, qualities that are missing in modern gyms—things like grip stamina, tendon strength, speed, balance, coordination and inhuman grit and discipline.

This kind of training—done properly, with the right know-how—made the old-timers hugely strong. In St. Louis in the 1930s, Joe worked out with The Mighty Atom, one of the most famous strongmen of all time. Standing at just 5'4" and weighing 140 lbs., The Atom was a phenomenon. He performed feats on a daily basis that would make modern bodybuilders cry for their mommies. He broke out of chains, drove spikes into pine planks with his palms, and bit penny nails clean in half. On one occasion in 1928, he prevented an airplane from taking off, by pulling on a rope attached to it. He didn't even bother to use his hands—he tied the rope to his *hair*. Unlike modern gym junkies, The Atom was strong all over, and could prove it *anywhere*. He was famously able to change a car tire with no tools—he unscrewed the bolts bare-handed before lifting the car up and slipping on the spare! In the mid nineteen-thirties he was viciously attacked by six burly longshoreman, and he hurt them so badly that as a result of the brawl *all six* had to be sent to hospital. It was lucky he was never sent to prison for it, because he regularly bent steel bars like hairpins. These were phenomenal feats for a pre-steroid era. Like Joe, The Atom didn't need phony muscle drugs and as a result he was frighteningly strong well into his later years. In fact, he didn't quit performing as a strongman until he was in his eighties. Over many long recreation periods, Joe regaled me with tales of the feats of strength of the depression-era strongmen he knew and trained with, world-class power-men whose names are now lost in the mists of history.

I was lucky enough to learn a huge amount about their training philosophies, too. For example, Joe emphasized the fact that a lot of the old-timers focused on bodyweight training to get really strong. They might have *demonstrated* their power by unleashing it on external objects like nails and barrels, but in many cases they actually *built* that basic strength through control of the body. In fact, Joe *hated* barbells and dumbbells. "Kids today are so dumb, trying to get big with their barbells and dumbbells!" he'd often tell me as we ate in the cafeteria. "You can get the most impressive physique using your own body. That's the way the ancient Greek and Roman athletes trained—and look at the muscles on the classical sculptures from that era. The guys in those statues were bigger *and* more impressive than all these drugged-up jerks you get these days!" And this is true; just take a look at a sculpture like the *Farnese Hercules*, or the copy of *Laocoön* now in the Vatican. The model athletes who posed for those sculptures were clearly hugely muscular, and would easily win natural bodybuilding contests today. And the adjustable barbell wasn't invented until the nineteenth century. If you still don't agree, check out a modern male gymnast. These guys almost exclusively use their bodyweight in training, and many have physiques which would put bodybuilders to shame.

Joe is no longer with us, but I promised him that the best of his training wisdom wouldn't die out. A lot of it is in this book. Rest in peace, Joey.

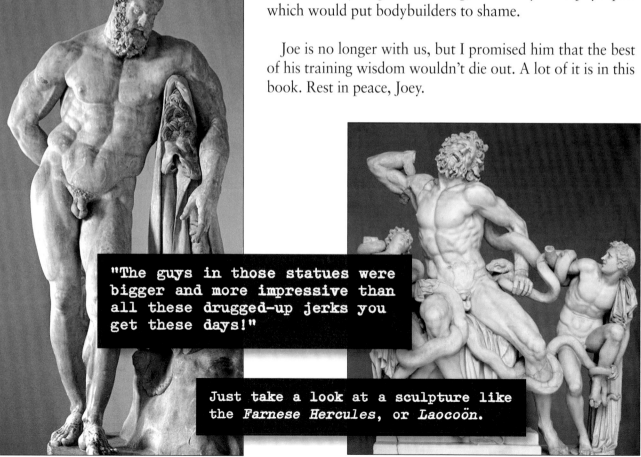

"The guys in those statues were bigger and more impressive than all these drugged-up jerks you get these days!"

Just take a look at a sculpture like the *Farnese Hercules*, or *Laocoön*.

From Apprentice to Teacher

It's safe to say that over the years I've had the opportunity to see how literally thousands of prisoners work out, both in the weights pit in the yard (if a prison had one) and in their cell, with nothing. I've talked with a vast number of real veterans—many of them elite-level athletes—for whom training is a religion, a way of life. Over the years I've picked up a great number of advanced tips and techniques which I've slowly incorporated into my system. It's fair to say that I've gleaned as much conditioning acumen from prison life as anybody has. But prison life is rarely easy or safe. I never rested for a single day; I always translated my knowledge into pain and sweat, experimenting on myself. As a result, I was always known as being in superb condition, the guy who was nuts about training. Any incident I got involved in with was over quick, because I was so explosive, in such good shape. All this gave me a mystique over time which ensured I got much more respect than I would have done without my training. I even got some admiration from the hacks (guards) for my lifestyle and ability. In the nineties, I was in Marion Penitentiary, which was in permanent lockdown following the murder of two guards. (By "permanent lockdown," I mean that all inmates were left in solitary confinement for twenty-three hours per day, every day.) To crush any potential trouble, the hacks did the rounds checking out the inmates every forty minutes. There was a running joke in Marion that the hacks would see me doing pushups, and return forty minutes later, and I'd still be doing them—the same set.

In my last few years in prison this reputation as an athlete got me a lot of daily requests for coaching, mainly from fresh inmates. They had all heard that I could teach them how to get prison tough in no time, and for a modest fee. They wanted to know the lost art (lost on the outside!) of gaining impressive muscles and stamina combined with real, raw animal power and strength—all with no equipment, because most of them were too low in the pecking order to get by in the weights pit in the yard.

I've seriously coached many hundreds of convicts in my time, and this gave me a lot of experience I couldn't have gained from just training alone. It allowed me to see how my techniques applied to different body-types, different metabolisms. I learned a lot about the mental aspects of training, about motivation and the distinct approaches that separate one student from another. I developed principles that allowed me to quickly tailor my methods to any individual's needs. By doing this I was able to fine-tune my system, and break all my knowledge down in a way that was easy to pick up by anybody, whatever their level of development.

The book you are holding now—which is mostly my secret "training manual" which I wrote while on the inside—represents the fruits of those countless hours of teaching. It's my baby. And it works. My system *had* to work! If I failed to train anybody to their maximum toughness, the consequences would not be a missed lift at a tournament, or second place in a bodybuilding competition. Prison is rough. The goal of being strong and in peak shape is *survival*. To be weak, or perceived as weak, in the joint can literally mean *death*. And all my trainees are alive and thrivin', thank ya very much.

Lights Out!

I could write a whole book on how important strength and the aura given off by a male in true hardcore condition can be in prison. One day, maybe I will. But this is not a book about prison life, it's a book about physical training. I've discussed some prison experiences only to try and demonstrate the kind of brutal, isolated, strangely traditional environment in which many of the old school training techniques have survived. You don't need to get yourself incarcerated to use the system in this book. Far from it. But it's a safe bet that if my method of conditioning works for athletes in the harshest, most vicious environment known to man—lockup—then it can work for you.

It *will* work for you!

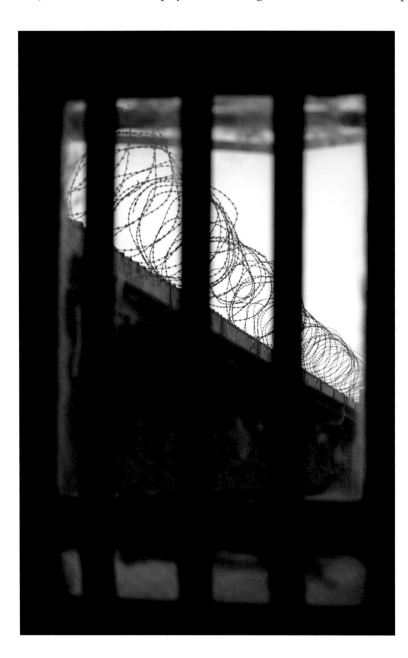

2: OLD SCHOOL CALISTHENICS

THE LOST ART OF POWER

Calisthenics is not a word commonly heard much in strength circles anymore; indeed, most personal trainers would have trouble even spelling it. The word itself has been used in the English language since at least the nineteenth century, but the term has very ancient origins. It comes from the ancient Greek *kallos* meaning "beauty," and *sthénos*, which means "strength."

Calisthenics is basically the art of using the body's own weight and qualities of inertia as a means of physical development. *Convict Conditioning* is, essentially, an advanced form of calisthenics designed to maximize power and athletic ability. Unfortunately modern calisthenics is not really understood as a hardcore strength training technology. If you mention calisthenics today, most people would think only of high repetition pushups, crunches, and less taxing exercises like jumping jacks or running on the spot. Calisthenics has become a secondary option, a cheap form of circuit training more like an aerobic exercise. But it wasn't always this way.

The Ancient Art of Bodyweight Training

It has long been known that the correct practice of bodyweight exercise both perfects the physique and develops great strength. Ever since prehistory, when the first men wished to develop and display their power they did so by demonstrating their control over their body; lifting the body up, bending the knees and jumping, and pressing the body away from the surface of the earth using the strength of the limbs. These actions eventually evolved into what we would recognize today as the art of calisthenics.

Calisthenics was *never* seen as an endurance training method by the ancients—it was primarily understood as a strength training system. It was the art used by the finest soldiers to develop maximum fighting power and an intimidating musculature.

One of the earliest records of calisthenics training was handed down to us by the historian Herodotus, who recounts that prior to the Battle of Thermopolylae (c.480 BC) the god-king Xerxes sent a party of scouts to look down over the valley at his hopelessly outnumbered Spartan enemies, led by their king, Leonidas. To the amazement of Xerxes, the scouts reported back that the Spartan warriors were busy training their bodies with calisthenics. Xerxes had no idea what to make of this, since it looked as though they were limbering up for battle. The idea was laughable, because beyond the valley lay Xerxes' Persian army, numbering over one hundred and twenty thousand men. There were only *three hundred* Spartans. Xerxes sent messages to the Spartans telling them to move or be destroyed. The Spartans refused and during the ensuing battle the tiny Spartan force succeeded in holding Xerxes' massive army at bay until the other Greek forces coalesced. You might have seen a dramatization of this battle in Zac Snyder's epic movie *300* (2007).

The Spartans are still widely regarded to have been the toughest warrior race to have ever existed.

The Spartans are still widely regarded to have been the toughest warrior race to have ever existed, and they were not too proud to focus their training on calisthenics. In fact, their ancient style of calisthenics training was a major reason why they were such impressive warriors. And the Spartans weren't the only ancient Greeks who had faith in calisthenics. It was documented by Pausanius that all the great athletes of the original Olympic Games were trained in calisthenics; including the finest boxers, wrestlers and strongmen of the ancient world. Surviving images from Attic pottery, mosaics and architectural reliefs contain a great many scenes which unmistakably illustrate serious calisthenics training. The physical ideal we know today as the "Greek god" comes from these images, which were originally modeled on the athletes of the Games—athletes who would have reached their level of development via training in calisthenics. The Greeks understood that the practice of calisthenics developed the physique to its maximum natural potential; not in an ugly, bloated way like today's bodybuilders, but in perfect proportion with the harmony of natural aesthetics. It achieves this harmony effortlessly, because the resistance used by the body is the body itself—not too light, not too heavy. Mother nature's perfect level of resistance. The Greeks knew that that calisthenics produced not only great power and athleticism but also grace in movement and beauty of the physical form. This, of course, is the source of the term calisthenics, which combines the Greek words for *beauty* and *strength*.

The arts of calisthenics training—as with so many things—were passed from the Greeks to their antecedents, the Romans. While the Roman army represented the pinnacle of martial organization, the cream of the athletic arts was reserved for the *gladiators*—the fighters competing at the public amphitheaters. The Roman historian Livy described how these "super warriors" of their time worked in the *ludi* (training camp) day in, day out using bodyweight exercises that we would today class as advanced calisthenics. Through the constant repetition of their techniques, the gladiators reportedly became so strong that the crowd passed around hushed stories that these powerhouses were the illegitimate offspring of mortal women and Titans—the mighty giants who warred with the gods before humanity came to be. The enormous physical toughness bestowed on the gladiators by calisthenics combined with their combat training nearly undid the Empire in the first century BC, when Spartacus and his gladiators rose up and challenged the order of the Emperor. The hardcore warriors of the gladiator army were so physically powerful that they laid waste to numerous Roman legions, despite being ill-equipped and horribly outnumbered.

There were doubtless many different systems of calisthenics training used by the ancients. What we do know from the surviving descriptions and images was that the bodyweight training performed by these legendary warriors and athletes bore little resemblance to what is known as "calisthenics" today. Rather than being a relatively soft form of aerobic training, their systems would have looked more like gymnastics, and would definitely have been geared more solidly to the progressive development or power and strength.

The Tradition of Strength

This form of physical training continued long after the fall of the classical civilizations. For most of human history it was simply taken as accepted fact that the ultimate way for an athlete to become stronger was by manipulating bodyweight according to progressive principles.

Centuries passed, and the knowledge of the ancients remained alive in the military training camps of Byzantium and Arabia. It returned more fully to Europe via the crusades, a half-forgotten friend reintroduced to warlike Europeans more hungry than ever for knowledge of power. It is well known that a major part of a squire's schooling to become a knight would have involved physical training, and there is a great deal of evidence that his training would have been based around calisthenics. Illuminated manuscripts and tapestries exist showing squires performing pullups from trees and wooden apparatus, as well as accomplishing inverse feats of strength that look like handstand pushups. The fact that medieval soldiers trained for power—centuries before the invention of the barbell or dumbbell—is beyond dispute. The Western armies of the Middle Ages had *unbelievable* strength; the longbowmen beloved of Henry V were said by contemporary commentators to be so strong that they could pull a tree up by its roots. This may have been propaganda, but later longbows salvaged from Henry VIII's ship *The Mary Rose* have been estimated to have a draw weight of up to 900 Newtons; which is roughly 200 lbs. No archer alive today is capable of handling a bow like that.

Throughout the Renaissance, these old methods lived on through military use, and were further disseminated around Europe by minstrels; traveling acrobats, singers and jugglers who would perform feats of strength and gymnastics at villages, towns and courts for their daily bread. This spread of knowledge continued, as would be expected, through the Enlightenment era, a period when all knowledge on every subject was seen to be a blessing and of value to humanity.

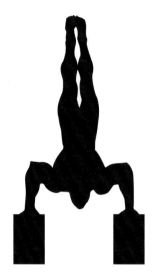

During the nineteenth century, bodyweight training for strength was still alive and well. In fact, if the classical days of ancient Greece were the first Golden Age of physical culture, there can be no doubt that the late nineteenth century represented the second great Golden Age. All over the rapidly changing world, health experts were recognizing and beginning to scientifically document the unsurpassed value of bodyweight training. In Prussia, legendary ex-military commander Friedrich Ludwig Jahn began formalizing the practice of bodyweight training with minimal apparatus; the horizontal and parallel bars, the vaulting horse and the balance beam. The sport of "gymnastics" as we know it today was created. The tradition of the traveling strength show, popularized by the Renaissance minstrels, lived on in the circus, and the era of the *strongman* was born. Scores of phenomenal athletes littered the globe; this period spawned legends such as Arthur Saxon, Rolandow, even Eugen Sandow—the man whose mighty physique informs the Mr. Olympia statue, the highest prize in the sport of modern bodybuilding. These men were as powerful as human beings have ever been—more powerful even, than modern steroid junkies. Saxon could press 385 lbs. overhead with one arm; Rolandow could effortlessly tear three decks of cards at once, a feat that should be impossible; and Sandow broke steel chains wrapped around his torso, merely by flexing. Calisthenics played a significant role in building up all these men. Remember, plate-loading barbells and dumbbells weren't even *invented* until the twentieth century. Before this innovation, the vast majority of the world's most muscular upper bodies were developed by hand-balancing and work on the horizontal bar.

Twentieth Century Greats

Even during the first half of the twentieth century, most of the true legends of strength were built by bodyweight training. In those days you weren't considered "strong" unless you could do one-legged squats and pullups easily, or stand on your hands. Yes, barbells and dumbbells were used, but only *after* bodyweight feats had been mastered.

Back then, even the super-heavyweights were masters of advanced calisthenics. British strongman-turned-wrestler Bert Assirati wowed crowds in the thirties by bending over backwards into a bridge before kicking himself up into a one-arm handstand—and he weighed in excess of 240 lbs. Assirati remains the heaviest athlete in history to perform the incredibly difficult "iron cross" hold on the hanging rings.

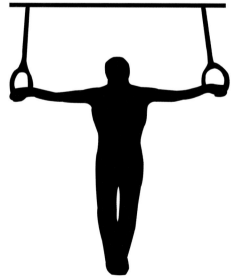

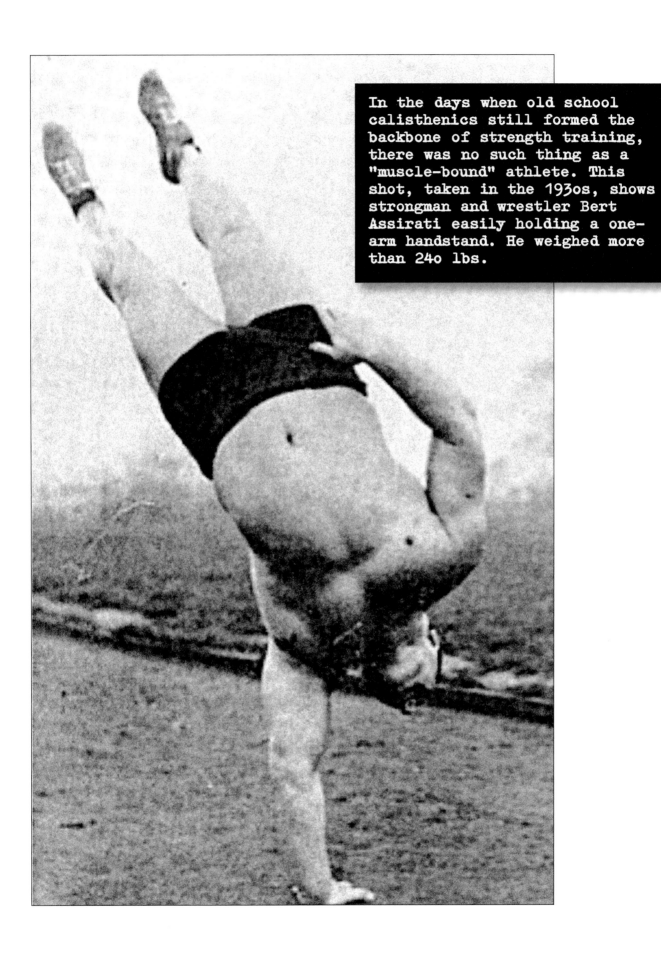

In the days when old school calisthenics still formed the backbone of strength training, there was no such thing as a "muscle-bound" athlete. This shot, taken in the 1930s, shows strongman and wrestler Bert Assirati easily holding a one-arm handstand. He weighed more than 240 lbs.

During the forties and fifties the strongest athlete in the world was probably the Canadian monster Doug Hepburn. Hepburn is considered to be one of the greatest pressers of all time, jerking 500 lbs. off the rack, and strictly pressing 350 lbs. from behind his neck, all back in the days before steroids and performance drugs. Despite practically *crushing* the scales at a weight of nearly 300 lbs., Hepburn made bodyweight training the cornerstone of his strength work, and it showed—his upper body was the size of a Buick, and capped by shoulders wider than the average doorframe. Although he excelled at lifting weights, Hepburn attributed his freakish pressing power to his mastery of handstand pushups. During his workouts, he used to perform handstand pushups without support, and regularly did those pushups on special parallel bars which allowed him to descend deeper than is normally possible. This giant of a man proved once and for all that muscular bodyweight is no barrier to excellence in calisthenics. Despite all his size, Hepburn never became muscle-bound or slow, because he took bodyweight training seriously—an attitude sorely lacking in most modern bodybuilders.

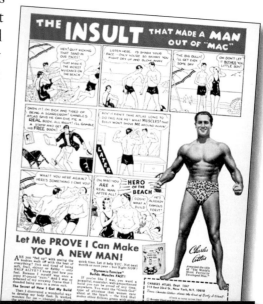

Perhaps the last great champion of bodyweight training was "The World's Most Perfectly Developed Man," Angelo Siciliano—better known as *Charles Atlas*. Siciliano sold hundreds of thousands of mail-order "Dynamic Tension" courses through the fifties and sixties. His method was a hybrid of traditional calisthenics with some isometric techniques. He taught a whole generation of comic-book readers that they didn't need to train with weights to stop getting sand kicked in their faces.

Angelo Siciliano—better known as *Charles Atlas*—sold hundreds of thousands of mail-order "Dynamic Tension" courses through the fifties and sixties.

But he was the last of a dying breed.

The End of an Era

As the second half of the twentieth century moved forwards, a lot of the older arts and training systems were left behind. They began to die out. In many ways, this loss was a direct and inevitable consequence of the Industrial Revolution. Following the Industrial Revolution, human life began to become increasingly dominated by technology. This was as true in the field of exercise and strength development as anywhere else. The twentieth century saw a veritable explosion in new forms of training technology, and our approach to exercise altered accordingly.

At the core of these changes were the good old plate-loading barbell and dumbbell. Barbells and metal free weights have been around for centuries, but the twentieth century approach to fitness was truly ushered in during 1900 when British athlete Thomas Inch invented the plate-loading barbell. Before long, cables and weight stacks were added to the mix, and shortly after their inception weight training machines which bore no resemblance to free weights became all the rage. In the nineteen-seventies, nobody was anybody who didn't train on *Nautilus* machines—resistance devices so named because their primary cam lever was shaped like a *Nautilus* mollusc shell. During this era, Nautilus gyms grew up all over America, and now hardly any gym in the world can be found that isn't mostly populated with complicated and confusing strength machines. Even barbells and dumbbells have had to take a back seat. And as for bodyweight exercises? Despite a handful of advocates—like Charles Atlas—progressive bodyweight training slowly moved towards extinction as the twentieth century wore on.

The Difference Between "Old School" and "New School" Calisthenics

All of these changes have altered the way we exercise very radically in a very short space of time, and we have lost something extremely valuable along the way. For many thousands of years—almost all of human history—men who wanted to get big and strong trained themselves with bodyweight exercises. Great systems of knowledge and sophisticated philosophies regarding training methods and techniques were passed down from generation to generation. Impressive (and supremely effective) methodologies evolved, methodologies which were based largely around strength and power; methodologies which were intelligent and progressive, the product of many centuries of trial and error. These priceless arts were designed to make an athlete stronger and stronger, until he achieved the peak of human ability—not only in strength, but in agility, motive power and toughness. This is what I mean when I talk about *old school* calisthenics.

When the barbells and machines began to really take over in the second half of the twentieth century, all of this hard-earned ancient knowledge became considered redundant. Immaterial to the modern age. Dazzled by the new gadgets and the methods associated with them, fewer and fewer people continued using these ancient old school methods and they began to die out.

Today, bodyweight strength training has been almost totally replaced by weight-training with machines, barbells and dumbbells. Bodyweight training is seen as the feeble sibling of these newer approaches, and has been relegated to the sidelines. The old school skills and systems dwindled through disuse and became lost. All that survived was the basic minimum. Today, when people—even so called strength "experts"—talk about bodyweight training, they only really know the beginners' movements—pushups, deep knee-bends, etc. To this they add a few useless and pathetic modern exercises, like ab crunches. These exercises are given to school children, weaklings, or are done as warm ups or to develop light endurance. Compared to the traditional, strength-based attitude, this approach could be called *new school* calisthenics. Old school calisthenics—which involved bodyweight systems designed to progressively develop inhuman power and strength—have almost died out.

Almost.

The Role of Prisons in Preserving the Older Systems

There was one place that the old school calisthenics never died out; a place where the older systems were perfectly preserved, like an ancient insect trapped in amber—in *prisons*.

The reason for this is obvious. The massive revolution in training technology which killed off old school calisthenics on the outside never occurred in prisons. Either that, or it occurred very late. The barbell and dumbbell-based gyms that became the rage in the fifties and sixties? Not in prisons. Very primitive weight pits didn't start appearing until the late seventies. The "indispensable" strength training machines upon which most gyms became built in the seventies and eighties are still largely absent from prison gyms.

In effect, this means that—while the rest of the strength training world was undergoing a huge "modernization" during the twentieth century—prisons were like a bubble. The traditions that were being killed off in gymnasiums up and down the country stayed alive in prisons, because they weren't choked to death by technology and the money associated with novelty gimmicks. During the eighteenth and nineteenth centuries, the guys who got incarcerated and knew how to do *true* bodyweight training based on strength—the gymnasts, acrobats, circus performers and strongmen—passed their knowledge on to other inmates. This knowledge—old school calisthenics—was *gold* in prisons, where no exercise equipment at all was to be found, with the exception of the bars overhead and the floor below. And being physically strong as well as agile was essential—those days were *tough*.

Life in prisons today is harsh, but going back a century or so, things were even harder. Beatings and cruel treatment were a part of the expected daily grind, and inmates killed and seriously wounded each other as a matter of routine. The handful of guys who trained for strength in their cells did so to literally *stay alive*. They trained furiously and with enormous seriousness—being powerful was a life or death matter! In this sense, those inmates from our past were no different from the Spartans led by Leonidas sixty-eight centuries ago. They all depended on their power to survive, and in order to develop that power they trained in traditional calisthenics.

The Origin of Convict Conditioning

To this day, prisoners all over the world still train using old school calisthenics. During my decades inside the nation's prisons, I've been obsessed with strength and fitness. Over time, this changed into an obsession with bodyweight training—calisthenics. Only after several years inside did I begin to understand the true nature and value of productive bodyweight exercise, and it took years after that until I was able to piece together the "secret history" of old school calisthenics, and the role that prisons have played in preserving these arts.

In my time, I've read everything I can about training and exercise, and ways of developing the body with little or no equipment. I've had the privilege of seeing how hundreds of unbelievably strong and athletic prison-trained men work out, using only their bodyweight. Many of these guys have had phenomenal ability and practically Olympian strength and fitness; but you'll never see them or get to read about their training in magazines due to their personal histories and lowly place on society's ladder. I've seen what these men can do, and spoken to them in depth about their methods. I've been honored to befriend and spend long periods with the *previous* generation of convicts, guys who were old enough to remember the strongmen who were *actually trained* by the strongmen of the second Golden Age of physical culture; guys who met the old strongmen, heard their theories and knew how they exercised. Following their lead, I've trained myself day and night with merciless techniques until my body ached and my hands bled; I've coached hundreds of other athletes, further honing my knowledge of bodyweight exercise.

I've made it my job to find out more about old school calisthenics than any other man alive. Over the years, I've collected dozens of notebooks and taken the finest ideas and techniques from all the systems I've learned on the inside, to develop the *ultimate* form of calisthenics...a method that can be used progressively to develop titanic power, agility and fitness; a method that requires no special equipment, minimal time and minimal complexity in application.

This system represents the best of the best of what I've learned. It is the system which is known today as *Convict Conditioning*, and it's the subject of this book. But despite the name and the origins, *Convict Conditioning* isn't just for prisoners—it has a whole host of benefits to offer *anybody* who wants to become extremely powerful and fit while staying at the peak of health.

Lights Out!

I've found that when I talk to people on the outside about the kind of gritty, hardcore, push-till-you-drop bodyweight exercise programs that are still regularly performed in prisons, I'm, invariably met with a wave of enthusiasm. Guys love to hear about it! After a spirited discussion, lifters and athletes tell me with a serious look in their eye that they'll dedicate themselves to *mastering* bodyweight work. Then I find out—only weeks later—that they never even tried calisthenics. They're back in the gym working exclusively on machines and free weights, on the same unproductive routines everybody else is doing, getting nowhere.

I can't really say I blame them. People find it difficult to commit themselves to a method of training that's so individualistic—something that nobody else on the outside seems to be doing. What most trainees need in order to really psychologically invest some energy in old school calisthenics is a good dose of *reality*. They need to know the differences between the unproductive, costly and damaging new methods of working out and the productive, free and safe arts of progressive bodyweight training—"traditional" arts that will become tomorrow's cutting edge.

I'll discuss the differences between calisthenics and more modern methods in the next chapter.

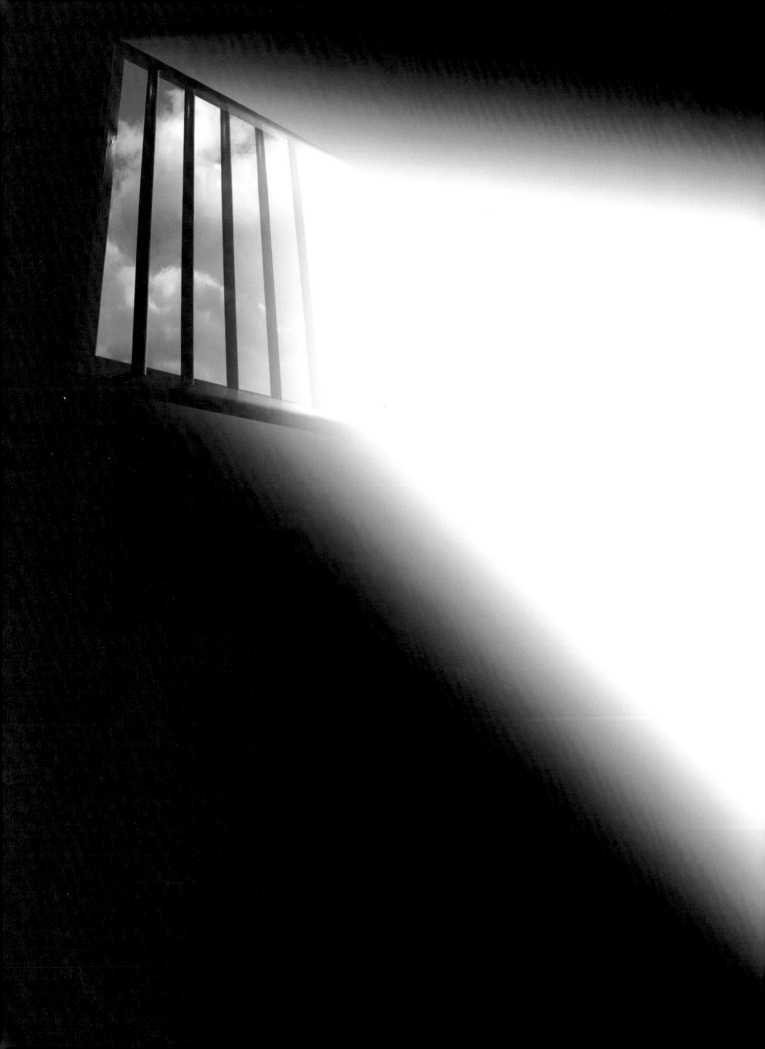

3: The Convict Manifesto

Bodyweight Training vs Modern Methods

I am living proof that you don't need to get to the gym and use modern machines and gimmicks to gain a lot of muscle and power. My many "students" working out in prisons all over the nation are proof too.

But my methods are so far from the status quo now that a lot of trainees will have trouble accepting them. There's a reason for my opinions being so out of step with the "norm." I come from a background were there were no protein shakes, no adjustable barbells, no *Nautilus* machines or *Bowflex*. A harsh, tough environment where men have only their bodies and a hell of a lot of aggression and spare time to build up their muscles and maximize their strength. I, and many others, have achieved these goals—but we did it by looking back, and using our bodies plus traditional, time-tested techniques, *not* by turning to flashy equipment and gadgets.

Some people will never accept that old school calisthenics works, because they've been brainwashed into thinking that they need free weights and modern gym equipment to reach their full potential. If you're going to embrace *Convict Conditioning*, you'll have to be prepared to put any indoctrination and preformed opinions to one side—at least long enough to give my methods a shot. In this chapter I'm going to show you *why* what you might have been taught about modern training is misleading, false, or downright wrong.

Modern Physical Culture— a Bastard Child

I love the world of strength and fitness. But when I take a look at the direction training and athletics are headed in the outside world, it almost makes me want to head to San Quentin and bang on the main gate to go straight back inside. When old school calisthenics began to die out, so did physical culture in general. The world of physical conditioning has never been in such a desperately low, pitiful situation as it is today.

Ever.

Some disagree with this opinion, presenting the elite athletes and world record holders of the modern era as proof that the science of conditioning has never been so highly advanced. But for a moment, forget the modern champions and pro athletes you see playing sports on TV. Thanks to recent media reports and exposés, the general public are finally beginning to grasp the fact that most of the top guys (whether you believe it or not) only achieve their (temporarily) high level of ability due to performance drugs such as anabolic steroids, testosterone variants, growth hormone, insulin and numerous other substances. Even a short way into their career, virtually all of those involved in intense, competitive sports find themselves held together by painkillers, cortisone, tranquilizers and other analgesic and relaxant chemicals which allow their joints to (again, *temporarily*) cope with the unnatural stresses of training and competing. This is not to mention the *recreational* drugs that are now flooding pro sports—drugs like alcohol, cannabis, cocaine, and even crack (!) are now used everywhere in sports by weak-minded athletes who can't adjust to the pressures of their game. And as for training methods? Despite what you may have read or heard, very few pro athletes know how to condition themselves all that well. From the high school level (and even before) the majority of precociously talented future pros are taken on and trained full-time by coaches and trainers who do the thinking for them.

Kill the Gym

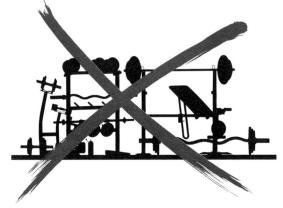

So let's ignore the pros and modern-day Olympians for right now. For a while, let's also ignore convicts and their training methods. What about everyone else?

The rest of us are told—by the magazines, TV shows, fitness gurus and even government health agencies—that if we want to shape up, we need to "get to the gym." What does this entail? Generally speaking, it involves two things these days; cardio machines and weights work—either free weights, or expensive resistance machines.

It's difficult to think of anything more futile, depressing and tedious than the cardio machine section of a modern gym. You've all seen the drill; rows and rows of gym members silently rowing nowhere, spinning their wheels or stepping up non-existent stairs with very little intensity and winning hardly any gains by way of real-world results.

And as for the weights work? There tend to be two types of approaches to this. Firstly, there's the generalized, feminine "toning" attitude—get into a machine on its lowest setting or pick up the teeniest dumbbells you can, and begin the monotonous counting. This charade might look good in a chrome-clad gym if you are covered in spandex but trust me, it does zero for your health and absolutely nothing for your fitness and conditioning levels. Then there's the "macho" school of weight-training; heavy bench presses and plenty of biceps curls are the rule, here. Never mind that these exercises ruin the joints and actually do little for *genuine* functional strength; never mind that modern "bodybuilding" either neglects or damages those muscles which are most crucial for authentic power and athleticism—the spinal erectors, the waist, the hands and feet, the neck, and the deeper tissues of the human system like the *transversus* or *rotator cuff* muscles. As long as you look pumped up in a T-shirt, that's all that matters, right?

Throw in a little bit of silly, non-committal stretching between stations that does about as much good as a dead dog, and there you have something approaching the average gym workout everybody is supposed to be doing.

The Modern Fitness Scam

I applaud *anyone* who gets off the couch to go out and train, but just take a look at the *results* of the average person who goes to the gym. (You might even be such a person yourself.) How much headway towards their fitness goals do they really make? The sad truth is that most people make negligible conditioning gains from the kind of workout described above. The dedicated ones trudge to the gym, week in, week out, but perhaps beyond a minor initial improvement they hardly ever seem to change at all, let alone attain their peak potential.

And these are the trainees who keep at it! Ninety percent of those who join a gym quit within two months due to lack of results. But who can honestly blame people for getting de-motivated with such lackluster results, from methods that—to cap it off—are boring, too?

Back in California in the fifties, there was a chain of gyms offering *lifetime* memberships for a modest fee. By "lifetime," I mean it—people paid an up-front lump sum, and could train at the gym any time, *for life*. Sound like a good deal? It was—for the gym owners. More than 99% of those who took the offer joined and quit after a few months, never to come back. The gym owners, of course, understood the business and knew full well that this would happen. The flunk out rate has always been the same with gyms—astonishingly high.

Is this true for you? Have you ever joined a gym all fired up with enthusiasm and good intentions, only to give up shortly after? The chances are if it's *not* true for you, you will personally know many others this sad story applies to. But if an activity—such as gym training—really is as valuable, and instantly life-enriching as we are told it is, why is there such a massive drop out rate? The answer in part lies in the fact that people *aren't* getting the kind of results they should expect.

Quite aside from the inefficiency of the average gym-based fitness routine, it's incredibly inconvenient. The standard gym session is a pain in the backside. It's not just the training—it's the getting there. Gyms require a lot of floor space, to accommodate all the equipment. For this reason, most gym owners can't afford to rent central locations; they usually lease or buy space outside of town, in industrial or run-down areas. Most trainees have to drive or take public transport to get there. You have to get ready by showering beforehand, you need to wash and launder your gym clothes, get changed, pack your gym bag (towel, water, supplements, membership card), etc. How many people are in the mood for all that after a hard day at work or school?

Then when you get there, even if you have a training routine prepared, the equipment you require is often in use. Evenings are the worst; it's just not fun hanging around in a gym inhabited by heaving, sweaty guys. (Unless you're into that kind of thing.)

Why do people bother putting themselves through this rigmarole in the first place? Because we are told that—to become who we want to be—we *need* to. To get in shape, we *need* gym membership. To get chiseled abs, we *need* the flashy gadgets. To get big pecs, we *need* the expensive, scientifically engineered training machine. To work out safely and in comfort, we *need* the designer training shoes. To get buff, we *need* all these protein pills, shakes and other supplements. Why are we told this? It's all down to money, folks. The "experts" on the infomercials telling you that you *need* this kind of gadget, or that kind of equipment to develop your pecs or abs or whatever—they are the guys *selling* that stuff! The same is true of dietary supplements. The muscle magazines that feature all the pro bodybuilders pushing supplements aren't ultimately financed by the bodybuilding fans. There is no money in pro bodybuilding. The magazines are either sponsored by or (in most cases) published by the companies who make those supplements. The bodybuilders featured in their publications *aren't* built by supplements and protein shakes. They are built by steroids.

Like so many things in our modern, money-driven world, the vision most people have been peddled regarding what they "need" to get in shape, is a big lie. It's a scam. You don't need all these products and extras to reach the pinnacle of strength and fitness.

All you need is your body, the right knowledge, and a big bucketful of determination.

The Basic Benefits of Bodyweight Training

I could pretty much write a thesis on why old school calisthenics is in a different league to modern, gym-based training. But since space is short, I'm going to stick to the basics. Here are *six* damn important areas where old school calisthenics scores over other, more modern methods:

1. Bodyweight Training Requires Very Little Equipment

There has never been a system of strength training more perfectly in harmony with the principles of independence and economy, and there never will be. Even the most ardent weightlifter will have to admit this fact.

For the master of calisthenics, his or her body becomes a gymnasium. Most exercises require no equipment, although if you wish the exercises can be enhanced with a few items that can be found lying around in almost any home. The very most you'll need is a place to hang from, and every one of us can locate such a place if we look; stairs, a loft hatch, even the branches of a tree! No gym is required, and very little space—at most, the equivalent to the length of your own body, often even less.

Whereas other strength training systems use metal weights, cables, chains or machines to produce resistance, the vast majority of calisthenics exercises exploit a free form of resistance—*gravity*. With no gym or equipment required, there is nothing to store away; no clutter. Plus, it means that you can train anywhere you happen to find yourself—on holiday, in a different city, at work—anywhere. You aren't tied to specific locations. This factor is precisely why calisthenics has survived and thrived in prisons, where equipment is minimal and a prisoner could be moved anywhere—even solitary confinement—at a moment's notice.

Another big plus is that calisthenics training is *free*. No equipment means no financial investment, and no gym means no membership fee. *Ever*.

2. Bodyweight Training Develops Useful, Functional Athletic Abilities

Calisthenics is the *ultimate* in functional training. This is another one of the reasons it's so popular with convicts—when trouble kicks off, you need to be able to really move in prison. "All show and no go" might be okay in a nightclub, but in the Pen you had better be able to handle yourself.

In nature, the human body doesn't need to move barbells or dumbbells around. Before it can move anything external at all, it has to be able to move *itself* around! The legs need the strength to be able to easily manage the weight of the torso in athletic motions, such as running or in combat; the back and arms require the power to be able to pull or push the body up or away.

It's sad to see that so many modern bodybuilders don't understand this fact. They train, first and foremost, to be able to move external objects. They may become very good at it, but this approach neglects and eventually compromises the prime athletic directive of *self-movement*. I have met hulking trainees who could squat five hundred pounds, but who waddled up a flight of stairs, wheezing like old men. I know one powerlifter who can bench press four hundred pounds, but who can hardly comb his hair due to his uneven, unnatural physical development.

The practice of calisthenics will not cause any of these movement problems, because it is essentially a form of training in movement. Old school calisthenics will make you supremely strong, but no matter how advanced you become in this area, you will only ever become more agile and limber in your movements, never less, because you are training the muscles to move *the body* rather than something external.

3. Bodyweight Training Maximizes Strength

Calisthenics movements are the most efficient exercises possible, because they work the body as it evolved to work; not by using individual muscles, or the portions of a muscle, but as an integrated unit. This means developing the tendons, joints and nervous system as well as the muscles.

This synergy in motion is what causes calisthenics to build such impressive strength. Many weight-trainers—no doubt influenced by bodybuilding philosophy—believe that rippling muscles are the source of strength. In fact, it's the *nervous system* that causes the muscle cells to fire, so your strength and power are largely determined by the efficiency of your nervous system. The nervous component of strength explains why one man can have muscles far, far smaller than another, yet be vastly stronger.

Very strong men will all tell you that tendon strength is probably more important for true power than muscle size. Calisthenics motions work the joints and tendons as they are meant to be worked, resulting in greater levels of power than weight-training movements can develop. (See *reason 4*.)

Another reason why calisthenics are so efficient in developing raw strength is that they train the athlete to work multiple muscle groups at once. A bodyweight squat, for example, works not just the quadriceps at the front of the thighs, but the gluteus maximus and minimus, the spine, the hips, abdomen and waist, and even the muscles of the toes. Proper bridging works over a hundred muscles! This fact overlaps perfectly with *reason 2*, given above, because the body has naturally evolved to move in a compound, holistic fashion. Many bodybuilding motions—particularly those done on machines—artificially isolate muscles, causing uneven development and lopsided functioning. In bodybuilding and a lot of weight-training, you get locked into a simple groove when performing techniques. This means that relatively small areas of the physical system (sometimes only individual muscles) get targeted by an exercise. But when training in calisthenics, you are forced to move your *entire* body; this requires coordination, synergy, balance and even mental focus. All these things develop nervous power, as well as muscular strength.

4. Bodyweight Training Protects the Joints and Makes Them Stronger—for Life

In prison, you need to be all-over strong—no matter how old you are. Being hindered by weak or painful joints would make you very vulnerable, however big your muscles might look. It may surprise you, but this is one important reason why a lot of convicts deliberately avoid weight-training.

One of the major problems with modern forms of strength and resistance training is the damage they do to the joints. The joints of the body are supported by delicate soft tissues—tendons, fascia, ligaments and bursae—which are simply not evolved to take the pounding of heavy weight-training. Weak areas include the wrists, elbows, knees, lower back, hips, the rhomboid-complex, spine, and neck. The shoulders are particularly susceptible to damage from bodybuilding motions. You'll be lucky to find anybody who has been lifting weights for a year or more who hasn't developed some kind of chronic joint pain in one of these areas.

Don't just take my word for it. Go into any hardcore gym and you'll see lifters wrapping their wrists and knees, strapping their backs up with high-tech belts, and applying stabilizing straps around their elbows. The locker room will stink of menthol heat rubs and analgesic liniments, all applied to keep the pain at bay. Joint problems are a bodybuilder's constant companion. When the bodybuilder starts to abuse steroids, these problems become even worse; the muscles begin to develop at an incredibly fast rate—faster than the joints can keep up. By the time most body-builders are in their late thirties, the damage is done and pain is a way of life, whether they stop training or not.

This damage is done because bodybuilding motions are largely *unnatural*. In order to place a great deal of emphasis on the muscles, the body is forced to hoist heavy external loads in motions and at angles not usually found in nature. One side-effect of this punishment is a vast amount of stress on vulnerable joints, joints which are forced to endure this horror repetitively over time. The result is soft tissue tears, tendonitis, arthritis and other maladies. The joints become inflamed and scar tissue or even calcifications begin to build up, making the joints weaker and stiffer. Bodybuilding movements primarily target the muscles, which adapt much faster than the joints; this means that the more muscular and advanced a bodybuilder becomes, the worse the problem gets.

When performed properly and in sequence, the calisthenics motions in this book will not cause joint problems—on the contrary, they progressively strengthen the joints over an athlete's lifetime, and actually heal old joint injuries. This beneficial effect occurs for two reasons. The first reason is basic physics; the resistance used is never heavier than the lifter's own bodyweight. The ridiculous, excessively heavy loads so admired in bodybuilding do not occur. The second reason is down to *kinesiology*—which is the science of movement. Simply put, the body has evolved over millions of years to be able to move itself, first and foremost; it was never "designed" to lift progressively heavier external loads on a regular basis.

A kinesiologist might say that calisthenics movements are more *authentic* than weight-lifting techniques. When the body has to lift itself, in a pullup or squat, for example, the skeleto-muscular structure naturally aligns to the most efficient and natural output ratio. When lifting weights, this natural shift does not occur—in fact the bodybuilder has to learn to move as *unnaturally* as possible to force maximum emphasis onto the muscles. Pullups are a good example of the "authentic" nature of calisthenics; humans evolved, like our primate relatives, pulling ourselves up into trees by the branches. This anatomical heritage still exists in the human body, which is why people adapt very quickly and safely to pullup training. A bodybuilding alternative to pullups is the *bent-over row*; humans did not evolve to execute this movement, and as a result many lifters quickly injure their spine, lower back and shoulders when performing this exercise.

The authentic movements offered by calisthenics apply the power of the joints naturally, as they evolved to be used. The result is that they develop *in proportion* to the muscular system, becoming more powerful over time rather than weaker and worn down. As the joint tissue rebuilds itself, former aches and pains are worked out of the system, and future injuries are avoided.

5. Bodyweight Training Quickly Develops the Physique to Perfection

Strength and health should be the major goals of your training. You need to be as powerful and functional as you possibly can be, for a long time into your old age. Calisthenics can give you that.

But let's be honest—we all want a little *muscle*, too. A lot, preferably. A big, beefy physique adds to the self-esteem and sends a message to other males saying "don't mess with me." This is an important part of prison culture. On the outside, it doesn't hurt with the ladies, either.

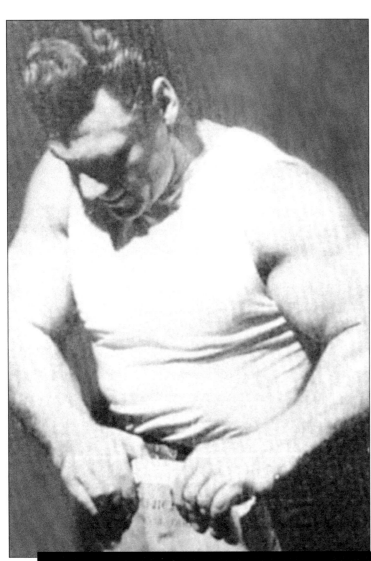

The practice of *modern* calisthenics mainly builds endurance and a little aerobic toning, but it does virtually nothing for the physique. Old school calisthenics on the other hand, will pack slabs of muscle onto any frame, and take the physique to its optimal development via the shortest route possible. What's more, the final result won't be the freaky, artificial "pumped up" gorilla costume worn by modern steroid-using bodybuilders. It will be natural, healthy and in perfect proportion, like the athletes of Greece who modeled for the statues of the Greek gods which—even today—are seen as being the archetype of the perfect human body.

In the pre-steroid era, the man widely thought of as possessing the most muscular—and most *aesthetic*—physique of all time was John Grimek. John Grimek won the 1939 "Perfect Man" title, and was the only man in history to win the Mr. America title more than once, in 1940 and 1941.

The legendary John Grimek prepares to tear a thick telephone book as easily as the average man would rip a piece of paper. Grimek's pumped arms stretched the measuring tape well over the eighteen-inch mark, at a height of 5'9. The man achieved his strength and mass in a pre-steroid era and did most of his training after twelve-hour shifts in a steel foundry. Traditional calisthenics played a major part in his success story.

His physique was awe inspiring, and is still widely regarded now. Rugged and masculine, Grimek was the ultimate specimen. Unlike today's muscle-bound bodybuilders, he was also a phenomenal athlete. To finish his posing routine, he flipped onto his hands and did a handstand pushup, before lowering his feet to the ground in a perfect bridge, and spreading his legs until he was sitting in the splits. Grimek was an avid weightlifter, but he also claimed that he got much of his upper body muscle from handstand exercises. He preached the value of calisthenics, but few, it seems, listened.

For indisputable proof that bodyweight training can develop a massive, muscular physique, take a look at the men's gymnastics next time it comes on TV. Those guys have massive biceps, shoulders like coconuts and lats that look like wings—all built simply by moving their own bodies against gravity. The way men *used* to train.

6. Bodyweight Training Normalizes and Regulates Your Body Fat Levels

Conventional bodybuilding is conducive to overeating. Forget the ripped pros you see in the magazines—no way do they look like that most of the time. They only do their photo shoots during the brief competition season, after months of strict and unhealthy dieting. In the off-season, these men are much heavier, carrying twenty, thirty or more pounds of superfluous body fat. And that's the top guys. The average bodybuilder is in a much worse situation; the magazines he reads religiously all tell him he needs way more protein than he actually does (in a cynical attempt to sell supplements) and as a result he chokes muscle-building foods down himself any chance he gets. Because the majority of amateur lifters are not on large doses of steroids, their metabolisms just aren't powerful enough to turn all those extra calories into muscle. The end result is that most guys become over-nourished and chubby when they begin lifting weights seriously.

Weight-training and the psychology of overeating go hand in hand. Before a hard session, an athlete convinces himself that if he eats more, he'll lift better and put on beef. After a hard session, an athlete is artificially depleted and his appetite increases accordingly.

The opposite dynamic occurs when an athlete begins training seriously in calisthenics. If obesity and bodybuilding are best friends, obesity and calisthenics are natural enemies. If your goal is to bent-over row 400 lbs., you could overeat as much as you like and probably still meet your goal despite carrying around a massive gut. But you couldn't set a goal of doing one-arm pullups without watching your bodyweight. Nobody ever became better at calisthenics by bulking up into a big fat pig.

The goal of calisthenics is to master lifting one's own body. The fatter you are, the more difficult this becomes. Once you begin training regularly in calisthenics, the subconscious mind makes the connection between a leaner bodyweight and easier training, and regulates the appetite and eating habits automatically. I know this is true—I've seen it myself on many occasions. Guys who take up bodyweight training naturally drop flab. Try it and see.

Lights Out

Many different types of people will read this book. Some will be beginners, looking to gain some strength and muscle on their journey through life. Many will be people who are already dedicated bodybuilders, weight-trainers and gym-goers, shopping around for some additional techniques and methods they can throw into their repertoire—maybe for when they're on holiday, on a weights layoff, or away from the gym altogether. Some readers will be convicts themselves, interested in the ideal cell routine to pass the time during their stretch inside. A few will be those devotees interested in exercise generally, who might want to know a little bit about how we do it in prison.

Whichever one of these you may be, I hope I've made you reflect on the values of bodyweight training. I'm passionate about spreading this message, because I know that *all* modern athletes can gain an *enormous* amount from the knowledge and methods that survive in prisons and penitentiaries. To me, this book is about more than just exercise techniques. It's a manifesto for revolutionizing modern strength training—a *convict manifesto*.

So far in this book I've been trying to sell you on the theory behind the kind of "old school" calisthenics that has survived in prisons. But before you can get to the most vital part—the *practice*—you need an overview of the system, as it's set out in this book. You'll find everything you need to know in the next chapter.

4: CONVICT CONDITIONING

ABOUT THIS BOOK

I first got the idea for this book when I was in Angola Penitentiary. I was in year six of an eight-year stretch, and I'd been training a lot of guys to reach their peak. As a result, I had a huge pile of loose notes, jotted ideas and scribbled training programs wrapped up in a big card file. The idea of writing a book actually wasn't my own—it wasn't even another convict who came up with it. It was a hack, named Ronnie.

Ronnie was a big, beefed up black guy who got a lot of respect from the inmates because he was a high-ranking local powerlifter who looked as big as a truck, and was about as strong, too. Although he was softly spoken, Ronnie didn't take any shit. And you certainly didn't want him to take you down, because he'd nearly tear your arm off in the process. But I always got along with Ronnie, partly because of our mutual interest in strength. Sometimes on his evening rounds he would stop at my cell and we'd chat about this or that exercise, or I'd tell him stories about the history of the iron game. One day I was talking to Ronnie about the finer points of handstand training, when he just blurted out "you know, you should write some of this down. Nobody knows any of this stuff on the outside anymore. It's all been lost." Having read exercise magazines and books in various prison libraries and on the outside for years, I had to agree with him.

Over the next couple of years I gradually transferred my techniques and methods into book form. It wasn't too hard in the sense that the system already existed. I had been teaching it for years. But condensing and distilling everything into a manual-sized book took a lot of effort. I was new to writing, but gradually made my way in the spare hours.

This book, *Convict Conditioning*, is the result of all those efforts. To make my teachings digestible, I thought it might be useful to the reader if I presented an overview of the structure of the book in this chapter, so you know what to expect and how best to use it. In doing this, I also want to introduce and outline some of the core concepts of *Convict Conditioning*, in particular the "Big Six" and the "ten steps."

Here's a summary of the book and its contents:

PART I: PRELIMINARIES

The first part, *Preliminaries*, will give you a great background to the system of *Convict Conditioning*. It contains an introduction, a chapter on old school calisthenics, a chapter on the benefits of bodyweight training relative to modern in-gym training, and the current chapter. These four chapters will teach you everything you need to know about the theory of the system, its nature, rewards and advantages. You'll also learn something about the long tradition of prison training, and the origin and history of *Convict Conditioning*. These chapters are all useful for learning about the system and clearing up any misconceptions you might have picked up about prison training or calisthenics from inauthentic sources.

PART II:
THE BIG SIX: POWER MOVES

The second part of the book is called *The Big Six: Power Moves*. This part contains the real meat of the system. As the title of Part Two implies, *Convict Conditioning* is based around *six* types of movements—the "Big Six."

As any competent weight-training coach will tell you, there are thousands of exercises you can do to train your muscles; but actually, a really good routine only requires a handful of big, basic exercises. This is because although the body contains well over five hundred muscles, these muscles have evolved to work in harmony; both with other muscles and with the body as a whole. Trying to work muscles individually neglects this fact, and de-trains the natural instincts of the body to function as a coordinated, unified whole. Therefore to work your muscles properly, the best approach is to select the fewest exercises you can to completely work the body, and continue to get stronger and stronger in those core exercises.

The Big Six

In our system there are *six* basic movements we use to work the entire body—everything from the muscles of the scalp down to the toes! The choice of six exercises is the result of centuries of tradition, and trial and error, as well as a basic knowledge of anatomy and kinesiology. The Big Six movements and the primary muscle groups they work are listed on *table one*. A quick glance at *table one* will confirm that the Big Six work all the major muscle groups as primary movers. They meld together perfectly; just as bridges work almost all of the back of the body, leg raises work the front; pushups work the pushing muscles of the upper body, pullups work the pulling muscles, and so on. Everything gets its ideal share of work. But there is also some overlap between these movements. For example, in addition to thoroughly working the main groups listed, pushups also work the abs, bridges also work the triceps, and so on. The Big Six chart is merely intended to indicate the *major* target groups of each movement. You can see from this brief list that six exercises are all that's required to work the body. Any more would be overkill; any less would leave gaps in your ability.

TABLE 1:
THE "BIG SIX" MOVEMENTS

Movement type:	Main muscle groups worked:
1. Pushups:	Pectorals (major and minor), anterior (front) deltoid, triceps
2. Squats:	Quadriceps, gluteal muscles (the butt), hamstrings and inner thighs, hips, calves and feet
3. Pullups:	latissimus dorsi (the "wings") teres, rhomboid and trapezius, biceps, forearms and hands
4. Leg raises:	Rectus abdominis ("six-pack"), obliques (waist muscles), serratus (outer rib muscles), intercostals (inner rib muscles), diaphragm and transversus, grip muscles, rectus femoris (quadriceps), sartorius (quadriceps), the entire frontal hip complex
5. Bridges:	All the spinal muscles, lower back, rear hips, biceps femoris, (leg biceps)
6. Handstand pushups:	Triceps, the entire shoulder girdle, trapezius muscles, hands, fingers, forearms

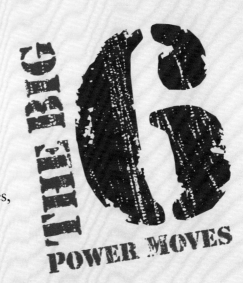

The Ten Steps

Learning to do high reps is fine. But as explained in chapter 2, just adding reps to your pushups or pullups will add stamina but very little strength and muscle. Strength and muscle are key areas in almost any prison training routine, and this principle is the backbone of the *Convict Conditioning* system. For this reason, *each of the big six movements is broken down into ten different exercises.*

These ten exercises are called the "ten steps." This is because they gradually allow the athlete to move onwards and upwards through the difficulty levels of the movement, from rank beginner through to master. You will be expected to slowly progress through the different exercises.

The ten steps are variations of the basic "Big Six" movements. There are ten steps for each of the movements of the Big Six; *pushups, pullups, squats, leg raises, bridges* and *handstand pushups*. In Part Two of this book, each of these movements is given its own chapter, which contains full details about the ten steps. For example, the chapter on *squats* contains information on ten different exercises. These exercises are all variations of the squat movement, and are graded by their difficulty; with exercise *one* being the easiest technique and exercise *ten* being the hardest:

Step 1, the *shoulderstand squat*, is the easiest version of the movement; Step 10, the full *one-leg squat*, is the hardest variation. Almost everybody will be able to do *shoulderstand squats* straight away, no matter how weak or infirm they are; hardly anybody will be able to do *one-leg squats* on the first time of asking, no matter how fit or strong they are. The purpose of this structure is to allow the individual trainee—training alone as his own coach, and with no special equipment—to work his way up gradually to be able to do *one-leg squats* for sets of twenty to fifty reps.

TABLE 2:
THE TEN STEPS FOR SQUATS

Step 1:	Shoulderstand squats
Step 2:	Jackknife squats
Step 3:	Supported squats
Step 4:	Half squats
Step 5:	Full squats
Step 6:	Close squats
Step 7:	Uneven squats
Step 8:	Half one-leg squats
Step 9:	Assisted one-leg squats
Step 10:	One-leg squats

The guy who can master Step 10 will have stronger, healthier and more functional legs than any muscle-bound gym rat who can squat 400 lbs. It's an *amazing* feat of athleticism. But—until now—very few people have had access to the old school knowledge of how to accomplish this feat. They try *controlled* single leg squatting once, and even one rep seems impossible. But if they knew how to pass through the ten steps, they'd actually master the exercise very quickly, earning a truckload of fitness and psychological satisfaction along the way. Somehow, in commercial gyms, this hard-earned traditional knowledge has gotten lost or been smothered in favor of gadgets, gimmicks, and new systems that aren't worth a dime unless you are all jacked up on steroids.

The inclusion of the ten steps is possibly the most important and revolutionary feature of *Convict Conditioning*. When properly applied, knowledge of these steps can take an individual from puny to powerful in a short span of time, and for this reason the system is jealously guarded by those I've taught it to on the inside. Knowledge is power. Information on the system only rarely goes beyond the prison walls, and nothing has previously been published. The book you are holding marks the first time the full details regarding the ten steps have ever been released for consumption by the public.

One thing's for sure. A lot of guys inside are gonna be pretty pissed at me that this system—given complete—is now "out there," in the public domain.

The Master Steps

The goal of your progress through the different exercises is to get you to a level where you can perform the hardest versions of each movement—the tenth step of each series. Because these tenth step exercises represent the zenith of the various movements, they are sometimes known as the *Master Steps*. Because there is one tenth step technique for each of the Big Six, there are *six* Master Step exercises that you should seek to conquer and perfect over time. These six "ultimate" bodyweight exercises are:

TABLE 3: THE MASTER STEPS

MOVEMENT-TYPE:	MASTER STEP:
Pushup:	One-arm pushup
Squat:	Full one-leg squat
Pullup:	Full one-arm pullup
Leg raise:	Hanging straight leg raise
Bridge:	Stand-to-stand bridge
Handstand pushup:	One-arm handstand pushup

Very few athletes will be able to perform all six of the Master Steps in perfect form and for multiple reps. You will find a few trainees who can do one, or perhaps two of these six. This is because a lot of guys tend to specialize on a strong point—very few train so that their entire body is all-over strong and powerful. This is a major mistake. It's also the reason why you'll be able to find several men who can do one-arm pushups but hardly any—anywhere outside of the toughest penitentiaries, or an elite gymnastics camp—who can perform all six movements properly. Only a handful of athletes in the world are able to correctly perform the Master Step techniques for all of the Big Six movements. You must resolve to become one of those few.

Progression Charts

In each exercise chapter, after the ten steps for the given movement are fully detailed, you'll find a clear but concise *Progression Chart* to help you move up through the ten steps. These six charts (one for each of the Big Six movements) detail each of the ten steps in order and, crucially, contain the information the trainee requires in order to know when he has met the *progression standard* for any given exercise—that is, when he can consider himself to have mastered that step and be ready to begin working on the next step in the series. It's important that athletes follow this advice because trying to move forwards too quickly can lead to disaster; poor technique, injury and ultimately de-motivation.

Variants

Every Big Six chapter rounds off with a short section called simply *Variants*. There are a great many different variations of the Big Six, and not all of these are included within the ten steps. This is partly because not all variations are suitable, and partly because to include every possible variation of the movement in a single program would be overkill.

To give a couple of examples, *dips* work similar muscles to *pushups*, and are therefore seen as a variant. *Tiger bends* are a famous old-time exercise related to *handstand pushups*, and are seen as a variant. *Jumping squats* and *box jumps* are explosive versions of *squats*, and are considered to be variants.

These variants are not *substitutes* for the ten steps. All the same, it's handy to know some of the variants in case you fancy adding some variety into your routine or if you're working around injuries.

PART THREE: SELF-COACHING

In prison I was known as *El Entrenador*—The Coach—because I was willing to teach strength training techniques and skills, for a price. But I was an exception—knowledge is power, and is jealously guarded inside prison, like all useful possessions. On the outside you can pick up a personal trainer at any gym. They are overpriced, and most of them know jack about genuine, productive training. You may get lucky and find a good one, but these are rare. In the final two chapters of the book, I want to give you the power to become your own coach.

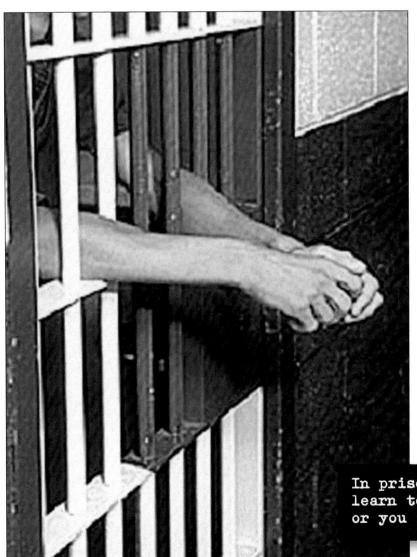

In chapter 11: *Body Wisdom*, I try to pass on some of the useful training philosophy I've garnered over the years. I'll give you tips on subjects ranging from proper warm up protocols to the best way to make real and permanent progress as a drug-free strength athlete. The approaches and strategies in this chapter could save you years of wasted efforts and yo-yo training.

Chapter 12: *Routines*, will teach you how to put the information in earlier chapters together, to construct your own training routine—no matter what your level of development.

In prison, you either learn to train yourself or you fail.

Lights Out!

Hopefully this chapter has given you a good overview of what the book is all about. This is important, because *Convict Conditioning* is not just another exercise book with lots of techniques and ideas. It's a complete system, a philosophy, a *way of life* that myself and others have lived for decades. It's kept us from going haywire, and in some cases it's been a slim line of hope that's meant the difference between life and death.

This book represents the condensed training knowledge of all my time inside. I've learned it there and I'm sharing it so that you don't have to go there. I wrote this book so that it would be used. Not just *read*—used! So get started. The best way to start would be to make sure you understand the benefits of the system, outlined in chapter 3, *The Convict Manifesto*. When you've got this, read all of chapters five to ten. Learn about the "Big Six"; proper exercise performance and mistakes to avoid.

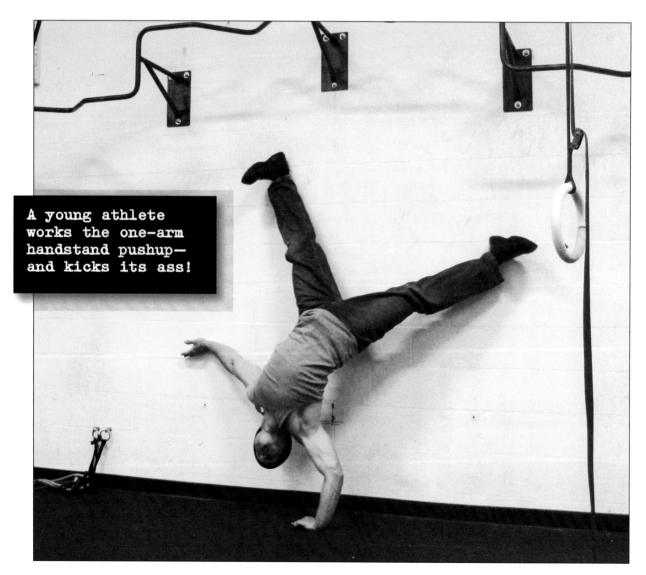

A young athlete works the one-arm handstand pushup— and kicks its ass!

Get started *now*. You don't need any special equipment. Begin by trying out the very first exercises in the ten steps for the *pushup, squat, pullup* and *leg raise* movements. Unless you are injured or disabled, these will be easy. Get to know the progress charts and over time read the entire book and develop your own routine with some help from chapter 12.

From the moment you begin *Convict Conditioning*—today!—your ultimate goal must be to finally perfect the Master Steps. Not just one or two of them, either—all of them! It's so important, I'm gonna say it again:

Your ultimate goal must be to perfect all six of the Master Step exercises.*

I don't care what kind of shape you are in, how old you are, or any of that crap. You might do it fast, or have to commit years to training to reach your personal peak. It doesn't matter. Nothing matters but effort and guts. You *do* have the power to get there. In this book I have given you all the tools you need to make it. The time for excuses is over. I'm not going to take them. In prison, we had no time for weakness. The kind of emotional and physical vulnerabilities people on the outside seem to wear as badges of honor would have been seen as invitations to attack and humiliation. None of this is acceptable for a student of my system.

The lights are out. You are alone in your cell with only your body and mind for company.

Let's train.

*The Master Steps are listed on page 33.

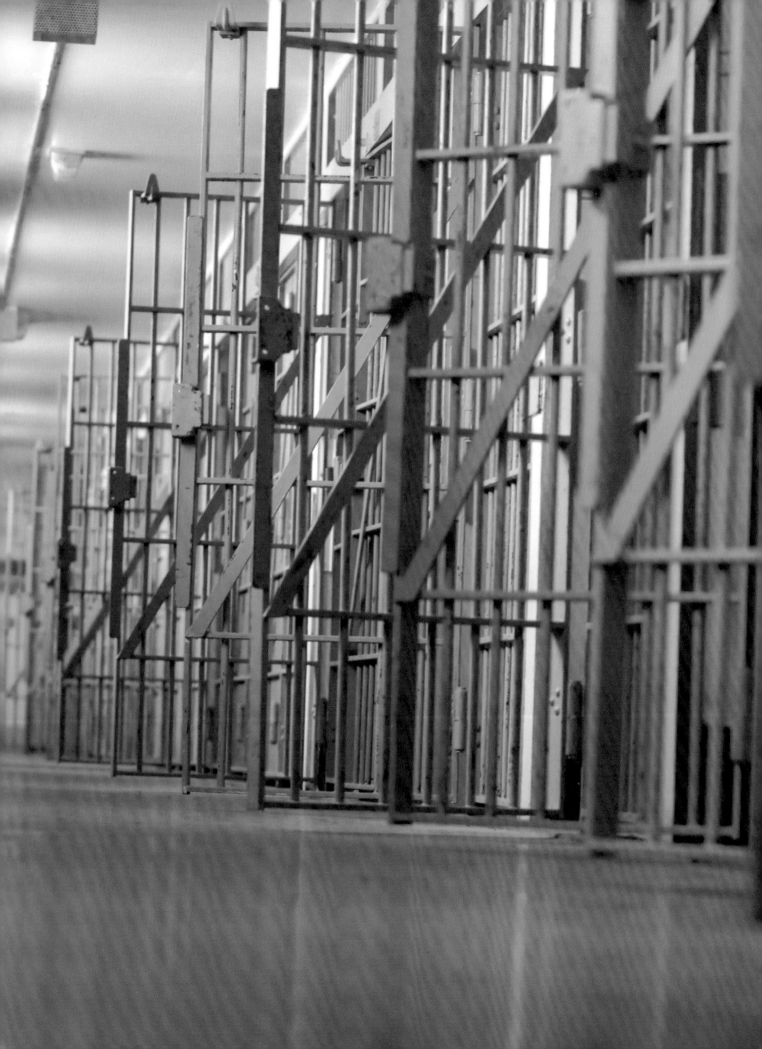

— PART II —

THE BIG SIX: POWER MOVES

This section of the manual sets out the Big Six exercises of *Convict Conditioning*. Over the following chapters, you will learn everything you need to know about these fine movements, including:

- Theories and benefits for each motion;
- The ten steps for each movement-type;
- Technical instruction;
- Tips and pointers on performance;
- Desired set and rep ranges;
- Alternative variant techniques.

After absorbing this section, you will know ten times more about calisthenics techniques than the average personal trainer. It's all here.

5: THE PUSHUP

ARMOR-PLATED PECS AND STEEL TRICEPS

The pushup is the *ultimate* upper body exercise. It generates strength, builds muscle, develops powerful tendons and trains the upper body pressing muscles to work in coordination with the midsection and the lower body. No other exercise in the world can achieve all these things. The bench press is often touted as a superior upper body exercise, but this is a fallacy. Not only does bench pressing isolate the upper body in an artificial way, it also destroys the rotator cuff muscles as well as irritating the elbow and wrist joints when performed over even short periods. The pushup *protects* the joints and builds functional strength, *real-world* strength—not just the kind of strength that can be used in a gym. This is why the pushup is the number one muscle-building exercise in military training camps and academies the world over. It always has been, since the first warriors trained for strength.

Unfortunately, because the bench press became the favorite kid on the block, pushups have been relegated to a high repetition endurance exercise. This is a shame—if you know how to *progressively* master the pushup movements, you can develop crushing upper body strength that will rival and surpass any bodybuilder or powerlifter. And your shoulders will thank you! This chapter will teach you everything you need to know to become an *ultimate master* of this movement.

Benefits of the Pushup

Different forms of pushup work the muscles to different degrees, but all the variations of the pushup provide great strength and muscle-building benefits. Pushups dynamically develop the network of pressing muscles around the torso, strongly working the *pec major*, *anterior deltoid* and *pec minor*. Pushups also build up all three heads of the *triceps*, the major muscle of the upper arm.

Pushups train these important muscles through their ideal range of motion, but in a correct pushup many additional muscles get a good *isometric* workout—meaning that they have to contract statically, to lock the body into place. Muscles trained isometrically during pushups include the *lats*, all the deep muscles of the chest and ribcage, the spinal muscles, the abdomen and waist, the hip muscles, the *glutes*, the *quadriceps* and the *anterior tibialis* (which is the shin muscle). Even the feet and toes gain some isometric benefit!

When performed progressively and with correct form, pushups also have a strengthening effect on the joints and tendons, adding to their overall power and health. The tiny yet vital deep muscles and tissues which support the fingers, wrist, forearm and elbow become much stronger over time when pushups are performed, reducing the chances of carpal tunnel syndrome, tennis elbow, Golfer's elbow and general aches and pains. Some pushup variants (such as *uneven pushups*—see pages 58—59) utilize unstable surfaces, and this effectively bulletproofs the vulnerable rotator cuff muscles of the shoulder, muscles which cause a great many strength athletes endless injury problems. The increased blood flow associated with pushups removes waste products built up in the joints, eliminates glue-like adhesions and relaxes old scar tissue. Weight-trainers who include progressive pushups in their routine suffer a lot less from joint injuries in these important areas than guys who only pump iron.

Perfect Technique = Perfect Results

In my time I must have read hundreds of pages on "correct" pushup technique, in everything from martial arts books to old military manuals. These descriptions are often dissimilar. In reality, everybody's "perfect" technique will be slightly different. This is purely due to different body types—variations in limb length, relative strength, body fat ratio and injury history all play subtle roles. For this reason, rather than write out an iron-clad description of the "perfect" pushup, I'd like to share a few general rules and ideas:

- Avoid bizarre angles and hand positions. Find an exercise groove that's comfortable for you.

- Keep the torso, hips and legs in alignment. Sticking the butt in the air during pushups only occurs because the waist is too weak to lock the body in place.

- Keep the legs together. Splaying the legs apart removes the need to stabilize the torso during motion and makes the exercises easier.

- The arms should be straight at the top of the movement, but don't hyperextend the elbows— keep a slight kink in your elbows to prevent the joint from pinching. (This is sometimes called keeping your arms "soft.")

- Breathing should be smooth. As a rule of thumb, breathe out on the way up, and in on the way down. If breathing becomes labored and you have trouble following this formula, take extra breaths.

Speed

A lot of guys recommend doing pushups fast—maybe as fast as possible. Some even favor "ply-ometric" pushups—which is just the modern flashy name for the old "clapping" pushups where you push yourself up explosively enough to be able to clap once, twice or even three times while in mid-air.

Being able to do pushups fast definitely has its benefits. Quick movements stimulate and train the nervous system by a mechanism called the "myotatic reflex." If you are competitive, many pushup events have a time limit, so the faster you can do the exercise the more likely you are to win. Besides, it's just good to know you can move your muscles fast. For these reasons, once in a while—when you are beyond beginner level and your joints and muscles are conditioned—you should do some work with higher speed pushups. However advanced you are, be sure to increase your speed gradually, over a few sessions, to allow your body to adapt.

A couple of fast sets every few workouts will be good for athleticism and variety. But despite this fact, the majority of your pushups should be done *relatively* slowly; for a count of *two seconds* down to the bottom position, a *one second* pause, and *two seconds* back up to the top position before immediately descending again.

There are two reasons why you should try to cultivate this kind of steady pace. Firstly, *smooth* technique develops higher levels of pure strength. When you move explosively, you inevitably rely on momentum during some portion of the movement. If momentum is doing the work, it means your muscles aren't. It's also far easier to cheat when you perform a motion quickly. We've all seen people "bouncing" out of the bottom position of exercises, because they lack the pure muscle power to move themselves.

Secondly, human joints adapt much better to regular movements than explosive ones. There's less risk of chronic or acute injury. Fast movements are pretty safe to use from time to time, but only once your joints have adapted to the regular, smoother-paced techniques. Explosive motions can be a useful adjunct to your training if you wish, but they shouldn't become the mainstay. People who exclusively train fast wind up with aches and pains and crackling joints sooner rather than later.

Basketballs, Baseballs, and Kissing-the-Baby

Some of the pushup movements I'll describe a little later on involve the use of objects to enhance your exercises. Utilizing objects to assist you with performing techniques and to monitor your depth of movement is not essential, but it's very useful—particularly if you are training alone. It's also a strategy that's widely used in prison.

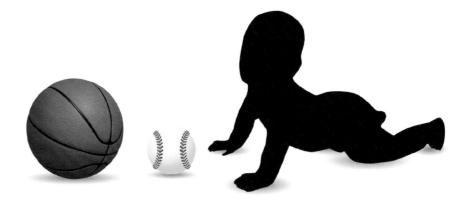

The only objects you'll need are a basketball and a baseball. These can be picked up cheaply at almost any big store. The old-timers used to use heavy medicine balls rather than basketballs, but basketballs are cheaper and just as good. If you don't wish to use basketballs or baseballs, you can substitute any other objects of an approximate size. Bricks are a handy alternative; a flat stack of three bricks is about the same size as a basketball, and one flat brick is nearly as thick as a baseball. Whatever you use, make sure it's something safe, that won't break and potentially injure you. Anything brittle or with jagged edges is out of the question.

When you use an object to determine your pushup depth, it's important not to *collide* with that object. Descend gently until you very lightly touch the basketball, baseball, or whatever your use. To determine how much pressure you should touch with, we had a saying in prison; *kiss the baby*. If your upper chest (for example) touches a baseball at the bottom of the pushup, it should only make contact with the amount of force you would use to kiss a baby on the forehead. No more, no less.

This technique of pausing briefly at the bottom of a pushup removes any momentum and builds excellent muscle strength and control. It's why I advocate a one second pause at the bottom of all movements. Incidentally, the kiss-the-baby technique can be applied to weight-training exercises, like the bench press or shoulder press. If you cannot very gently "kiss" your body with the bar in the bottom position—if you have to either bounce it or stop short—the weight you're using is too heavy. What do I mean by "too heavy"? Simply this—if you can't absolutely control a weight throughout a technique's range of motion, it's too heavy.

Palms, Knuckles, Wrists or Fingers?

I advise that you do the majority of your pushups with your palm or palms flat on the floor. A lot of trainees revel in their ability to perform pushups in exotic hand positions—they use their knuckles, their fingers, thumbs, and even the backs of their wrists. I want all my students to be doing pushups their whole lives—this means using hand positions that are easiest on the joints. For the majority of people, the most comfortable position will be the classic style of palm or palms flat on the floor. A rare exception might made be made for athletes with wrist injuries, who will find it easiest to do pushups on their knuckles with the wrists locked.

Fingertip pushups strengthen the hands and forearms and are a useful addition to your routine, particularly if you are also doing a lot of grip work. Build up to full fingertip pushups slowly, by using them with Step 1, *wall pushups* (pages 46—47), gradually working through the steps as your fingers adapt. For most people, a couple of sets of classic fingertip pushups using all the extended fingers performed every week or two will be enough to maintain hands which are vastly stronger and healthier than the those of the average man. It's all you really need.

For some of you, this will not be enough; you'll want more. If this is the case, rather than being tempted to use fewer fingers, it's safer to work through the ten steps using *all* your fingers until you can do one-arm pushups that way. Very few people ever get to such an advanced stage though. But trust me, by the time you can do fingertip pushups with four fingers and a thumb on one-arm pushups, your digits will be like steel rods.

Doing pushups on the backs of the hands or on the wrist joints is excruciating, and limits your muscular output—your wrists give out before your muscles do. Unless you are a classical karate expert and you need to toughen this area for strikes, I wouldn't even attempt it.

The Pushup Series

Most pushup routines contain very little variation. The only progression trainees are usually advised to make is to increase the number of reps, or maybe put their feet up on something as the exercise becomes easier. This is wrong, wrong, wrong! All this does once the athlete has adapted to the technique is increase endurance.

In *all* strength training, progression is the name of the game. In terms of muscle heft and power, *if you do what you've always done, you'll always get what you always got*—no matter how many reps you mindlessly add. The *Convict Conditioning* system contains ten distinctly different pushup movements. These movements are called the *ten steps*, and each individual movement is a little harder than the one before. The first three steps of *all* the Big Six movements will be relatively easy for most people, and can be thought of as a useful *therapy sequence* for athletes coming back from injury. They will also be helpful for rank beginners or the overweight to condition themselves gently. The remaining steps become increasingly difficult, until the final and hardest possible variation is reached—the tenth, or *Master Step*. The athlete is encouraged to progress from step to step, exercise to exercise, following the *Beginner, Intermediate* and *Progression standard* repetition ranges given with the descriptions.

Each of the exercises can be gradually refined over time by applying little nuances and tricks, and details on how to do this can be found in the *perfecting your technique* section of each description. By using these minor variations, each exercise actually becomes several exercises; and as a result, the pushup series contains not just ten, but over a hundred slightly different types of pushup movement. The illustrated descriptions of the ten steps of the pushup series conclude with a two-page *Progression Chart* which acts as an easy to reference summary. If you still want more, the chapter ends with *Variants* (pages 70—74). This section contains descriptions of more than a dozen other pushups or pushup alternatives.

You can find the *ten steps*, fully illustrated, on the following pages (46—65).

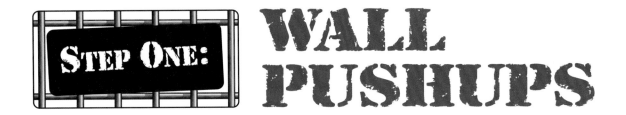

STEP ONE: WALL PUSHUPS

Performance

Face a wall. With your feet together, place your palms flat against the wall. This is the start position (fig. 1). Your arms should be straight and shoulder width apart, with the hands at chest level. Bend the shoulders and elbows until the forehead gently touches the wall. This is the finish position (fig. 2). Press back to the start position and repeat.

Exercise X-Ray

Wall pushups are the first step of the ten step series required for complete mastery of the pushup family of movements. As the first step, this technique represents the easiest version of the pushup. Every able-bodied person should be able to do this exercise without a problem. Wall pushups are also the first movement in the *therapy sequence* of the pushup series. This exercise will be of great benefit to somebody coming out of an injury or following an operation, who is looking to promote healing and rebuild their strength slowly. The elbows, wrists and shoulders—most notably the delicate rotator cuff muscles within the shoulders—are particularly prone to chronic and acute injury. This exercise gently activates these areas, stimulating them, developing blood flow and tone. Beginners new to calisthenics must start any training program very gently to develop their technique and ability. They should start with this exercise.

Training Goals

- Beginner standard: 1 set of 10
- Intermediate standard: 2 sets of 25
- Progression standard: 3 sets of 50

Perfecting Your Technique

Every person reading this book should be able to do this exercise, unless they are disabled, badly injured or ill. If coming back from an injury or operation, this movement is a good "tester," allowing the athlete to feel out any weak points during rehabilitation.

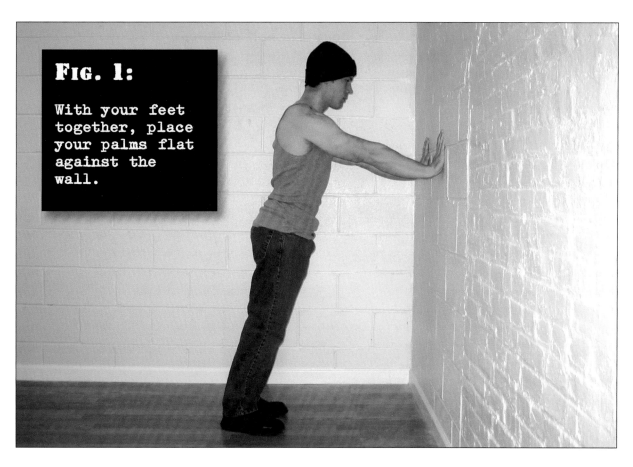

FIG. 1:

With your feet together, place your palms flat against the wall.

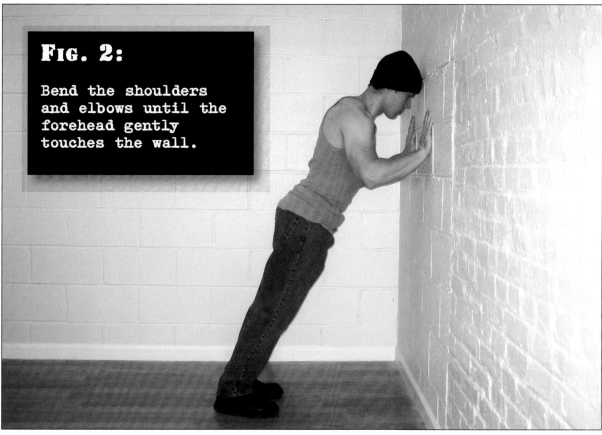

FIG. 2:

Bend the shoulders and elbows until the forehead gently touches the wall.

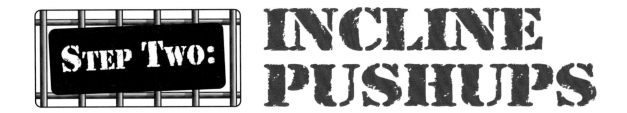

Performance

To do this exercise you will need to find a secure object or piece of furniture which is about half your height—it should reach the midpoint of your body (roughly around the level of the hips). Good options might be desks, tall chairs, work surfaces, kitchen tops, low walls or solid fences. In most prisons, I've found that the cell basin fits the bill nicely—but make sure it's strong enough to accommodate the demands of the exercise. With your feet together and your body aligned, lean over and grasp the object with the arms straight and shoulder width apart. This is the start position of the exercise and—if the object reaches your midpoint—should put you at about 45 degrees from the floor (see fig. 3). Bending at the elbows and shoulders, lower yourself until your torso gently touches the top of the object (fig. 4). Pause briefly before pressing back up to the start position, and repeat.

Exercise X-Ray

This exercise continues where Step 1 (the *wall pushup*) leaves off, with the lower pressing angle meaning that more bodyweight has to be moved by the muscles of the upper body. The *incline pushup* is easier than the classic *full pushup* (Step 5). For most athletes this exercise won't place very great demands on the muscles, but it will be useful for the beginner to continue their training gently, or for rehabilitation purposes.

Training Goals

- Beginner standard: 1 set of 10
- Intermediate standard: 2 sets of 20
- Progression standard: 3 sets of 40

Perfecting Your Technique

Incline pushups should be done at 45 degree angle. If the beginner standard can't be met at this angle, use a greater (more upright) angle—simply place the hands on an object higher than the body's midpoint. Once this is mastered, gradually use lesser angles until 45 degrees becomes easy. Harder angles can be attempted using progressively lower steps on a set of stairs.

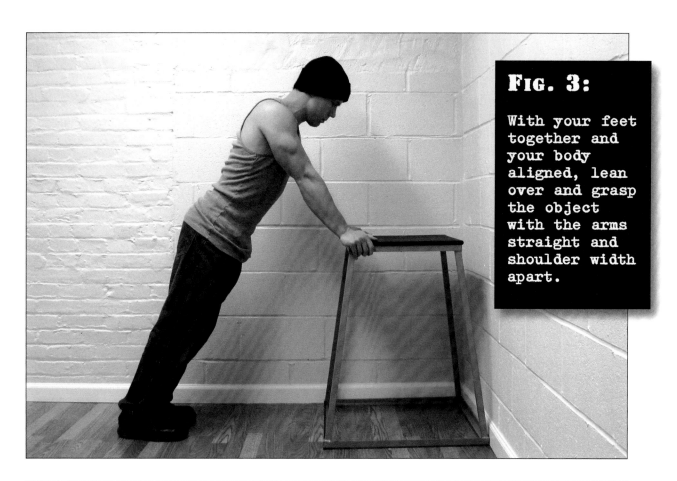

FIG. 3:

With your feet together and your body aligned, lean over and grasp the object with the arms straight and shoulder width apart.

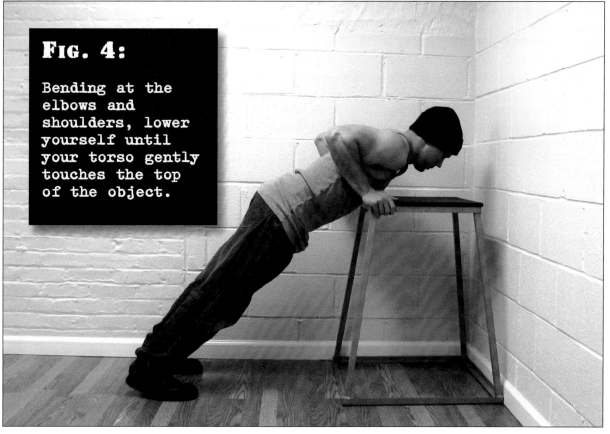

FIG. 4:

Bending at the elbows and shoulders, lower yourself until your torso gently touches the top of the object.

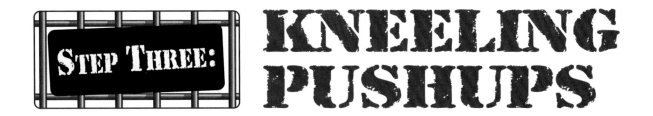

STEP THREE: KNEELING PUSHUPS

Performance

Kneel on the floor with your feet together, and your palms flat on the ground in front of you. The arms should be straight, shoulder width apart, and in line with your chest. Link one ankle around the other, and keep the hips straight and in alignment with the trunk and head. This is the start position (fig. 5). Using the knees as a pivot, bend at the shoulders and elbows until your chest is approximately one fist's width from the floor (fig. 6). Pause and press back to the start position, then repeat.

Exercise X-Ray

Kneeling pushups are Step 3 in the pushup series. They are an important movement for beginners to master, because they are the easiest type of pushup that can be performed *prone*, i.e., flat on the floor. Because of this, they form an important link between the first two steps, which are performed standing, and the harder prone techniques later in the series. Women often do kneeling pushups because they lack the relative upper body strength to perform the *full pushup*, but this exercise offers great benefits to guys as well. It's a good starting exercise for somebody who's maybe overweight or out of shape, and because you can pump up the upper body with relative ease in this position, kneeling pushups make an excellent warm up exercise you can do before attempting harder forms of pushup.

Training Goals

- Beginner standard: 1 set of 10
- Intermediate standard: 2 sets of 15
- Progression standard: 3 sets of 30

Perfecting Your Technique

If you find it impossible to perform full *kneeling pushups*, lessen your range of motion. Don't go all the way down to a fist width from the ground. Use a higher number of reps (about twenty) over a shorter range of motion you can perform comfortably, then workout by workout (keeping the reps high) gradually keep adding an inch of depth until the full movement is mastered.

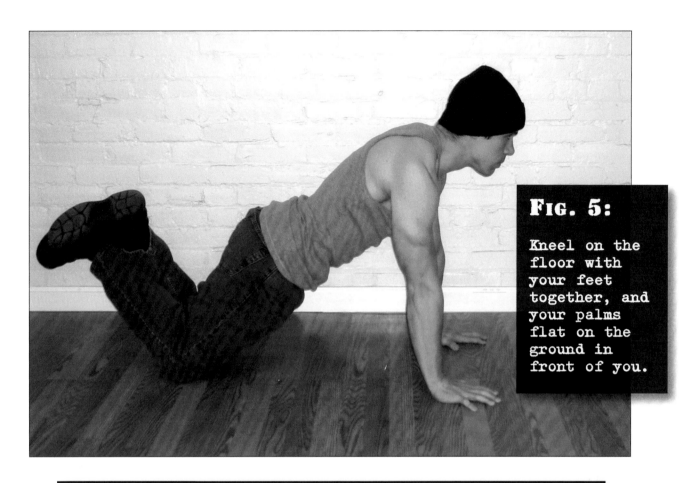

FIG. 5:

Kneel on the floor with your feet together, and your palms flat on the ground in front of you.

FIG. 6:

Using the knees as a pivot, bend at the shoulders and elbows until your chest is approximately one fist's width from the floor.

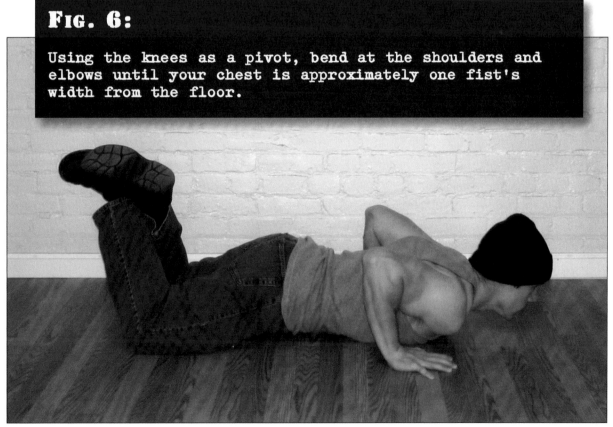

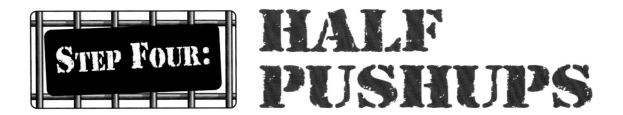

Performance

From the kneeling position, place your palms on the floor and stretch your legs out behind you. Your hands should be shoulder width apart, and directly below your upper chest. Your feet and legs should be kept together. Tighten your supporting muscles, so that your back, hips and legs stay locked in line. Starting with the arms straight, lower yourself approximately half the length of your extended arms, or until your elbows form a right angle. An excellent way to establish how far to descend is to use a standard basketball or soccer ball. Position yourself over the ball at the top of the movement, so that the ball is directly below your hips. This is the start position (fig. 7). Bend at the shoulders and elbows until your hips lightly make contact with the ball (fig. 8). On most people, this will be a good, objective indicator of the correct bottom position. Pause before pressing forcefully back to the start position.

Exercise X-Ray

The *half pushup* is an important exercise to master properly. You see a lot of guys doing pushups incorrectly, with their butt moving up as they bend at the hips. They do this because their waist and spinal muscles are weak. This exercise trains the waist and spine to keep the hips locked and aligned.

Training Goals

- Beginner standard: 1 set of 8
- Intermediate standard: 2 sets of 12
- Progression standard: 2 sets of 25

Perfecting Your Technique

If you can't do *half pushups*, shorten your range of motion until you are able to perform the technique as given above. If you are using a basketball to monitor your form, position yourself so that it's under your knees rather your hips. If you lower yourself from the arms extended position until your knees make contact with the ball, this will approximately equal a quarter pushup. Once you can do more than ten quarter pushups, position the ball a little higher up your thighs each time you practice until it is under your hips.

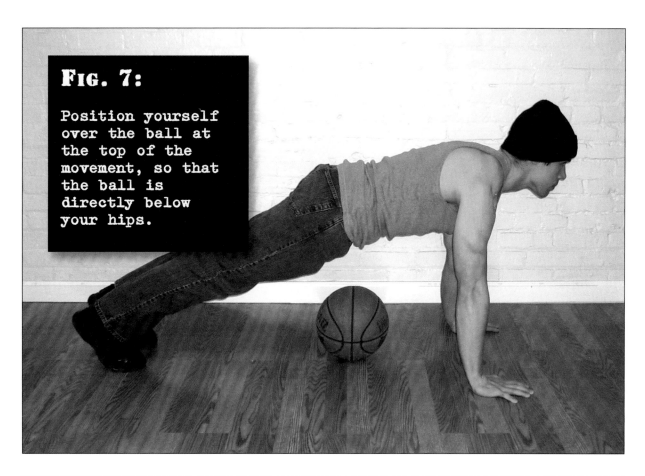

FIG. 7:

Position yourself over the ball at the top of the movement, so that the ball is directly below your hips.

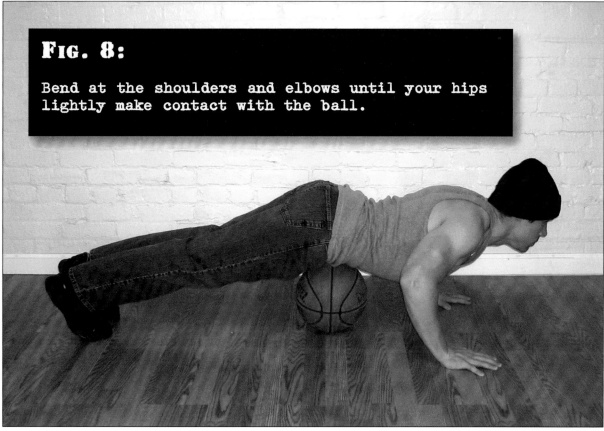

FIG. 8:

Bend at the shoulders and elbows until your hips lightly make contact with the ball.

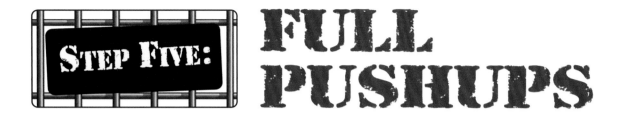

Performance

From the kneeling position, place your palms on the floor and stretch your legs out behind you. Keep your thighs and feet together, and ensure that the hands are below your upper chest and shoulder width apart. Straighten the arms. The hips and spine should be in line. This is the start position (fig 9). Bend at the elbows and shoulders until your breastbone comes to within a fist's width from the floor. In prison pushup competitions, a "counter" clenches his fist pinky side down on the floor, and counts out when the athlete's chest touches the knuckle of his thumb. If you're training alone and you wish to keep to the right depth, place a baseball or tennis ball directly below your chest (fig. 10). As your chest kisses the ball, pause and push up.

Exercise X-Ray

This technique is the "classic" pushup, the exercise most of us will remember from gym class. It's a fair guess that if you say the word "pushup" to most people, they will naturally picture the *full pushup*. The full pushup is an excellent upper body exercise, working the arms, chest and shoulder girdle in an efficient manner. It's by no means the hardest form of pushup, however; in terms of difficulty it only represents Step 5 in a series of ten.

Training Goals

- Beginner standard: 1 set of 5
- Intermediate standard: 2 sets of 10
- Progression standard: 2 sets of 20

Perfecting Your Technique

You might be surprised how many people—even big, strong guys—cannot do *full pushups* properly. If you are in this group, return to *half pushups* using a basketball. If you have graduated from Step 4, you will be able to perform twenty-five reps with the ball under your hips. Gradually move the ball a few inches forward every workout, or whenever you can—keeping the reps the same. When you can go from the arms straight position to a bottom position where your *jaw* touches the ball, attempt the full version again.

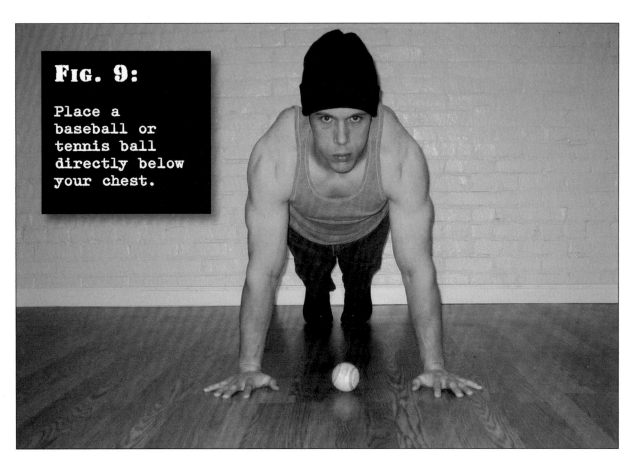

FIG. 9:

Place a baseball or tennis ball directly below your chest.

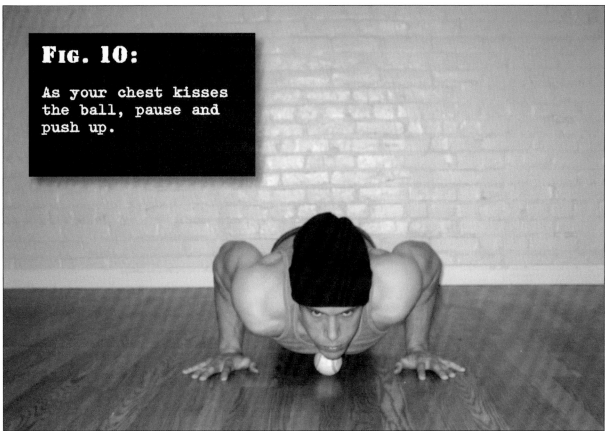

FIG. 10:

As your chest kisses the ball, pause and push up.

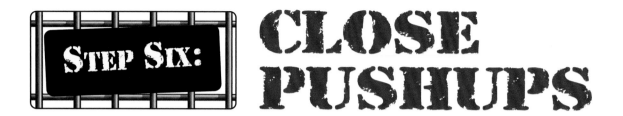

STEP SIX: CLOSE PUSHUPS

Performance

Begin this technique in the same top position as *full pushups* (Step 5), but with the hands touching. You don't need to overlap the hands or form a "diamond" between the thumbs and index fingers; it is sufficient for the tips of the index fingers to touch. From the straight arm start position (fig. 11), lower yourself until your chest gently touches the backs of your hands (fig. 12). Pause briefly before pressing back to the start position.

Exercise X-Ray

Close pushups are as old as the hills. They're a vitally important exercise in the pushup series, but are often overlooked in favor of flashier techniques like *plyometric* (clapping) *pushups* and *decline pushups*. This is a tragedy, because the close pushup is an essential tool to help you in your journey to mastering the *one-arm pushup*. Most athletes have trouble with the one-arm pushup because they find it difficult to press themselves up from the bottom position, when the arm is bent most acutely. This is because their elbows are weak when bent beyond a right angle. Because of the placement of the hands during close pushups, the athlete naturally bends his elbows to a greater degree to reach the bottom position than is the case with *full pushups*. This increased elbow flexion trains the triceps and strengthens the tendons of the elbow and wrist. As a result, athletes who have become comfortable with this movement will find one-arm pushups much more manageable when the time comes.

Training Goals

- Beginner standard: 1 set of 5
- Intermediate standard: 2 sets of 10
- Progression standard: 2 sets of 20

Perfecting Your Technique

If you cannot do *close pushups* with the hands touching (as described above), simply return to *full pushups*, and move the hands an inch or two closer every workout, keeping the reps quite high.

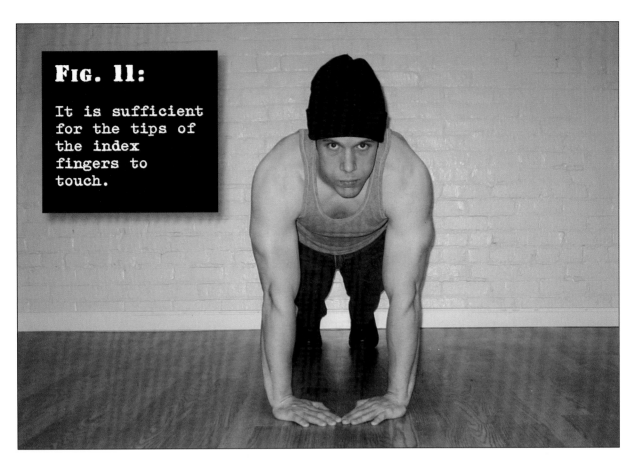

FIG. 11:

It is sufficient for the tips of the index fingers to touch.

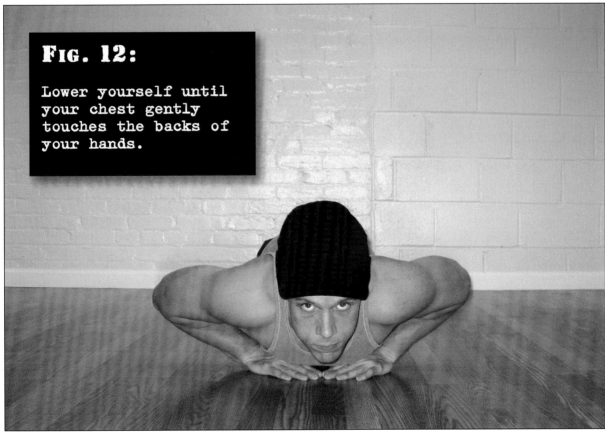

FIG. 12:

Lower yourself until your chest gently touches the backs of your hands.

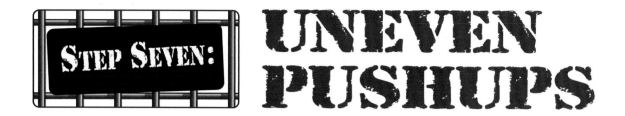

Performance

Get into the classic pushup position; feet together, legs, hips and back aligned, and arms straight with the palms on the floor beneath your upper chest. With one arm firmly supporting you, place the other hand on a basketball. Both your hands should be directly below your shoulders for stability. This is the start position (fig. 13). Once you have found your balance, do your best to evenly distribute your weight through both hands. At first this will not be easy, but persevere. Bend at the elbows and shoulders until your chest touches the top of whichever hand is on the ball (fig. 14). Pause briefly before pressing back up to the start position.

Exercise X-Ray

This is the first of the advanced pushup exercises that will take the athlete from double arm pushups to the single arm variety. You can use stable objects—like bricks or a cinderblock—instead of a basketball, but the basketball is best. The act of stabilizing the ball brings the seldom-used rotator cuff muscles into play, strengthening them for the more intense exercises to come. You can use a sturdy soccer ball rather than a basketball, but a classic basketball is king because its tacky surface helps the palm grip.

Training Goals

- Beginner standard: 1 set of 5   (both sides)
- Intermediate standard: 2 sets of 10   (both sides)
- Progression standard: 2 sets of 20   (both sides)

Perfecting Your Technique

Anybody who can do *close pushups* properly should be ready to attempt this exercise with confidence. If there are problems at first, they will be due to a lack of coordination rather than insufficient strength. If you have trouble, try using stable objects rather than an unstable basketball—a simple house brick is a good alternative. Once you can do twenty reps with one hand on a flat brick, try two flat bricks, one on top of the other. When you can do twenty reps with three stacked bricks, attempt the exercise with the basketball again.

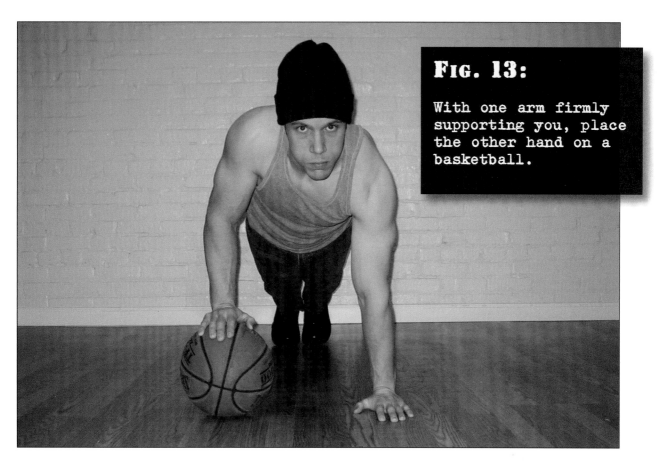

FIG. 13:

With one arm firmly supporting you, place the other hand on a basketball.

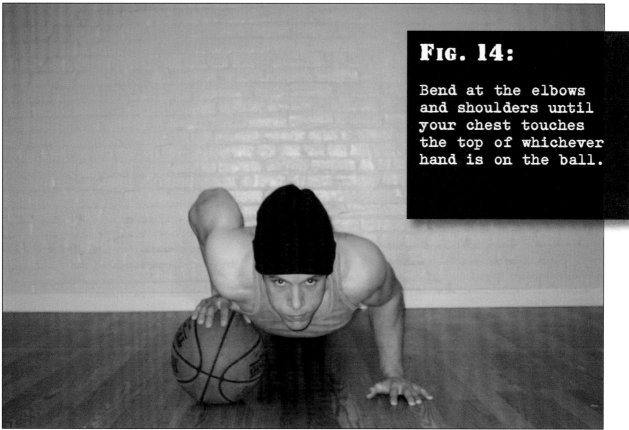

FIG. 14:

Bend at the elbows and shoulders until your chest touches the top of whichever hand is on the ball.

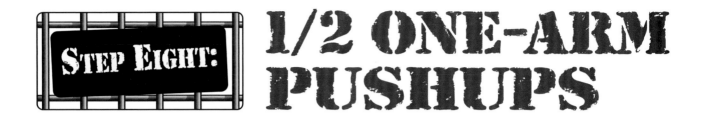

STEP EIGHT: 1/2 ONE-ARM PUSHUPS

Performance

Get into the *half pushup* top position, with a basketball located below your hips, as described in Step 4. Place one hand on the floor beneath your breastbone with your arm straight and your other hand in the small of your back. This is the start position (fig. 15). Bend at the shoulder and elbow until your hips reach the top of the basketball. This is the finish position (fig. 16). Pause and press back to the start position. If your triceps is weak, you'll have a tendency to twist your torso as you move. Don't—the whole body should be kept straight. This is true for all pushups.

Exercise X-Ray

Half one-arm pushups are Step 8 of the pushup series of movements. With this technique, the athlete finally moves from bilateral (two-sided) exercises to unilateral (one-sided) work. This is an important stage in the series. Working on half one-arm pushups will teach the athlete the balance and positioning necessary to master full *one-arm pushups*. Because only one limb transmits the moving forces, this exercise will also prepare the hand, wrist and shoulder joints for subsequent steps. Half one-arm pushups are an essential exercise in the series, and must be mastered for the reasons given above. However, the elbows are not required to bend very greatly in this exercise, so it must never be performed by itself as the sum total of any pushup program. It should always be followed with a movement where the elbows are bent *beyond* ninety degrees in the bottom position; either *close pushups* or *uneven pushups* should be added afterwards.

Training Goals

- Beginner standard: 1 set of 5   (both sides)
- Intermediate standard: 2 sets of 10   (both sides)
- Progression standard: 2 sets of 20   (both sides)

Perfecting Your Technique

If you can't do *half one-arm pushups*, start with quarter one-arm pushups with the ball under your knees. Gradually lengthen your range of motion by moving the basketball forwards over time, as with *half pushups* (see Step 4).

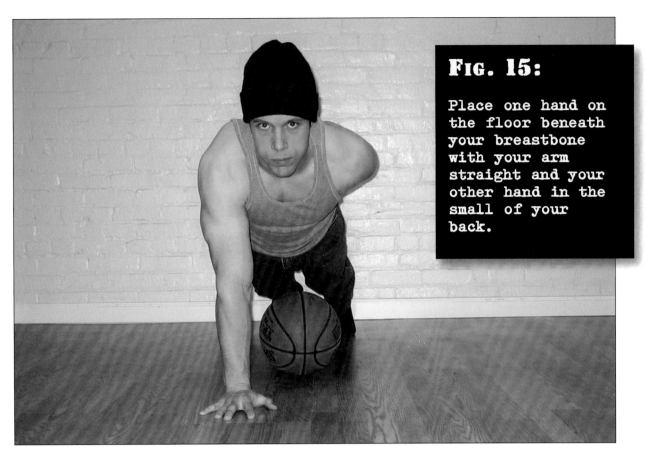

FIG. 15:

Place one hand on the floor beneath your breastbone with your arm straight and your other hand in the small of your back.

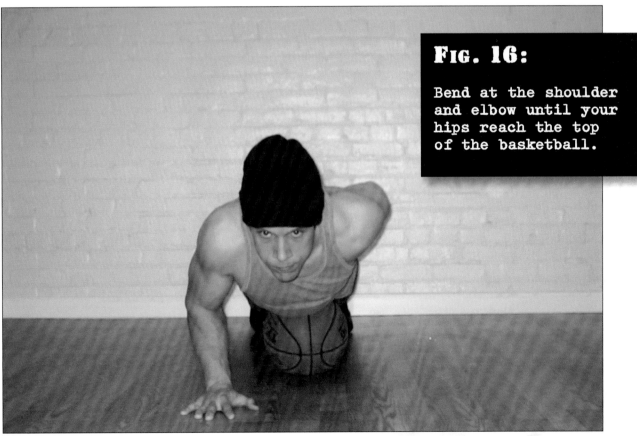

FIG. 16:

Bend at the shoulder and elbow until your hips reach the top of the basketball.

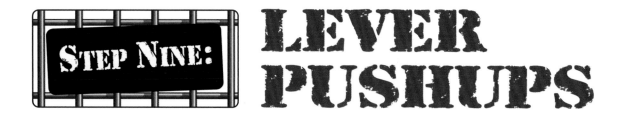

Performance

Get into a pushup position, with your body aligned and supported by the feet and one hand flat on the floor directly below your breastbone. Place your free hand on a basketball which is out to the side of the body. It should be as far away as you can reach while keeping your palm flat on the ball. Both your arms should be straight. This is the start position (fig. 17). Slowly, and under full control, lower yourself down until your chest is one fist's width away from the floor. As with *full pushups*, you can use a baseball or tennis ball to check your depth if you are training alone. The act of lowering yourself will cause the basketball to roll out further to your side (fig. 18). Pause briefly in the bottom position, then push yourself back up.

Exercise X-Ray

The *lever pushup*, when performed properly, is very nearly as difficult as the *one-arm pushup*. This is precisely why this exercise forms such a useful penultimate step in the series. You will find that the arm on the ball can contribute very little force, due to its position stabilizing the ball away from the body—this forces the non-ball arm to work very powerfully. If you are not yet strong enough to come out of the bottom position of the one-arm pushup, you can use this exercise to gently assist yourself until you get there.

Training Goals

- Beginner standard: 1 set of 5   (both sides)
- Intermediate standard: 2 sets of 10   (both sides)
- Progression standard: 2 sets of 20   (both sides)

Perfecting Your Technique

It's difficult to apply much force with the arm out straight, due to leverage. To make the exercise easier, bend the elbow of the arm on the basketball, bringing the ball closer to your body. Don't go too far—bringing it all the way under your body will transform this exercise into Step 7, *uneven pushups*. As you get stronger over time, gradually move the ball out away from your body until you can do the exercise with a straight arm.

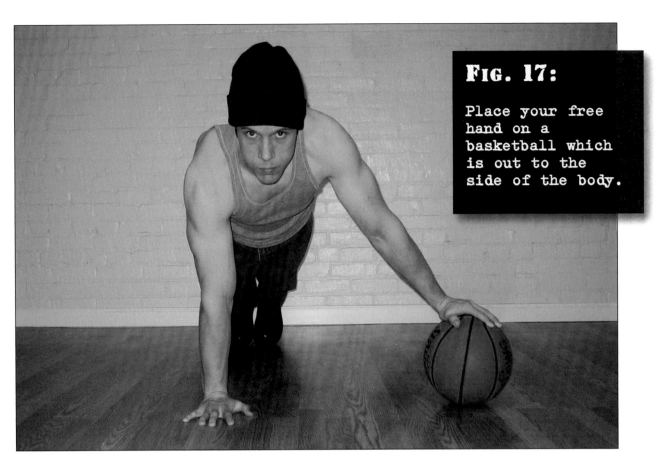

FIG. 17:

Place your free hand on a basketball which is out to the side of the body.

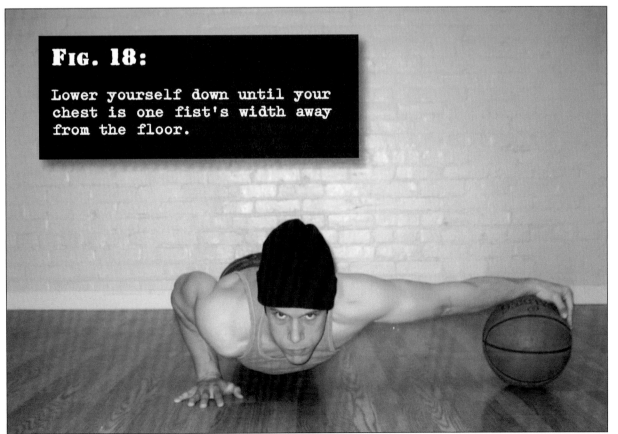

FIG. 18:

Lower yourself down until your chest is one fist's width away from the floor.

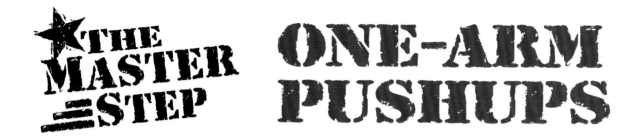

Performance

Kneel on the floor, with one palm out on the ground directly in front of you. Stretch your legs out behind you, until they are straight and supported by the toes. Keep the spine and hips aligned, and shift your bodyweight so that your supporting arm goes straight down below your chest—not out to the side or in front of you. Once you are stable, place your non-supporting hand in the small of your back. This is the start position (fig. 19). Bend at the shoulder and elbow, lowering yourself under full control until your jaw is approximately one fist width away from the floor (fig. 20). Pause momentarily, before pressing back up to the start position.

Exercise X-Ray

The *one-arm pushup* when performed with pure form, is the gold standard of chest and elbow power, and it's an impressive sight to see. Many athletes *claim* to be able to do this exercise without any problems, but don't be fooled. When you ask them to put their money where their mouth is, their pushups are a joke—they splay out their legs, twist their torsos into ugly shapes to make the exercise easier, and violently strain for shallow reps on wobbly, weak arms. Without doubt, the *true* master of the one-arm pushup is a rare beast. Make sure you become one of this endangered species.

Training Goals

- Beginner standard: 1 set of 5   (both sides)
- Intermediate standard: 2 sets of 10   (both sides)
- Elite standard: 1 set of 100   (both sides)

Perfecting Your Technique

If you have mastered the *lever pushup*, the *one-arm pushup* shouldn't be too intimidating. But if you have trouble doing five reps of the one-arm pushup in good form, go back to Step 9, and ensure that you are can use *perfect* form for twenty repetitions of the lever pushup. If you can do this but still have trouble with the one-arm pushup, keep working with lever pushups until you can do thirty repetitions, before trying again.

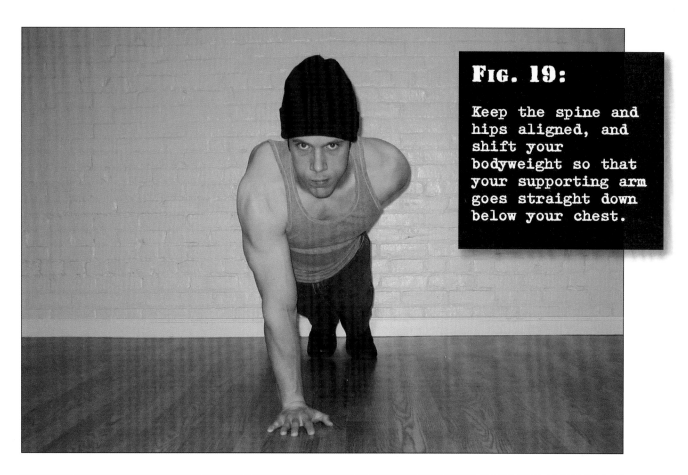

FIG. 19:

Keep the spine and hips aligned, and shift your bodyweight so that your supporting arm goes straight down below your chest.

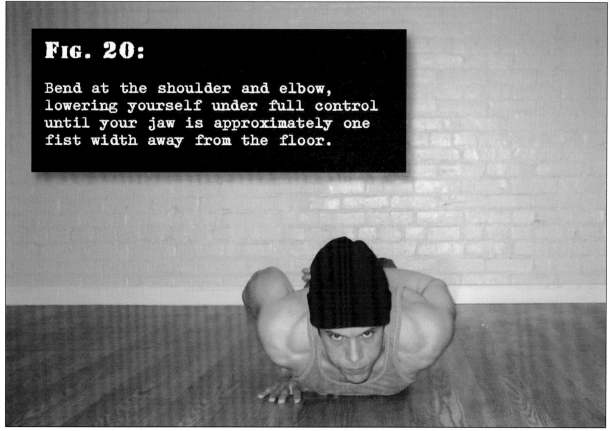

FIG. 20:

Bend at the shoulder and elbow, lowering yourself under full control until your jaw is approximately one fist width away from the floor.

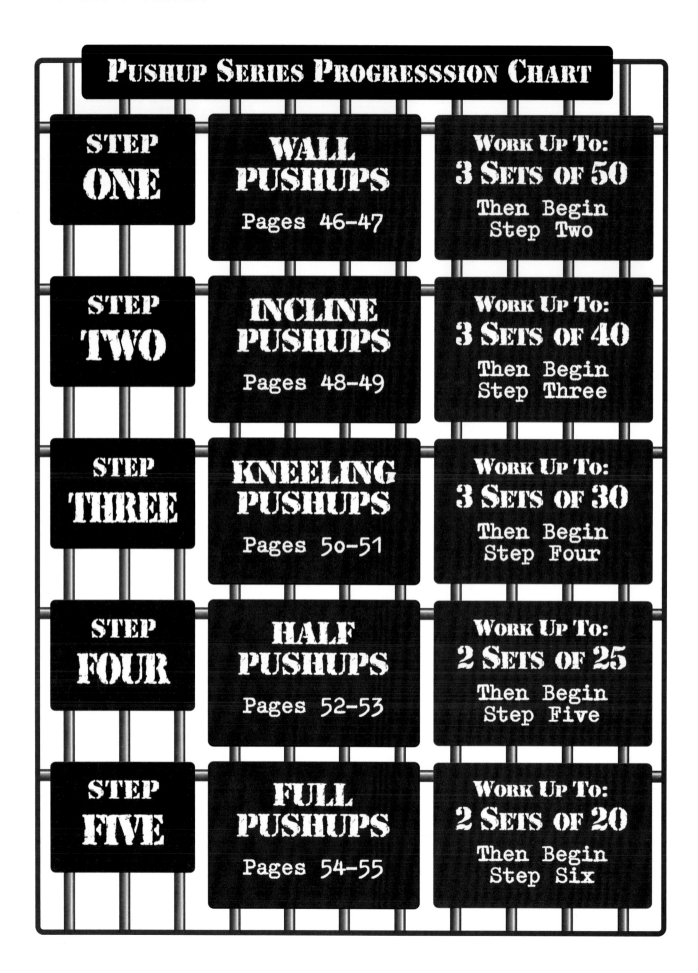

PUSHUP SERIES PROGRESSSION CHART

STEP ONE	WALL PUSHUPS Pages 46-47	WORK UP TO: 3 SETS OF 50 Then Begin Step Two
STEP TWO	INCLINE PUSHUPS Pages 48-49	WORK UP TO: 3 SETS OF 40 Then Begin Step Three
STEP THREE	KNEELING PUSHUPS Pages 5o-51	WORK UP TO: 3 SETS OF 30 Then Begin Step Four
STEP FOUR	HALF PUSHUPS Pages 52-53	WORK UP TO: 2 SETS OF 25 Then Begin Step Five
STEP FIVE	FULL PUSHUPS Pages 54-55	WORK UP TO: 2 SETS OF 20 Then Begin Step Six

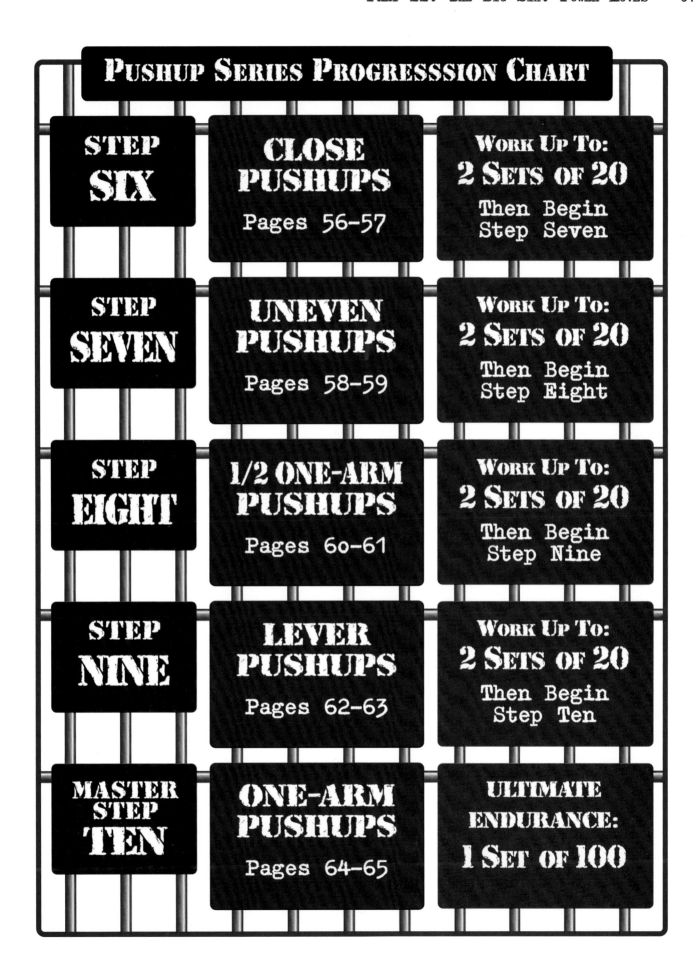

PUSHUP SERIES PROGRESSSION CHART

STEP SIX	CLOSE PUSHUPS Pages 56-57	WORK UP TO: 2 SETS OF 20 Then Begin Step Seven
STEP SEVEN	UNEVEN PUSHUPS Pages 58-59	WORK UP TO: 2 SETS OF 20 Then Begin Step Eight
STEP EIGHT	1/2 ONE-ARM PUSHUPS Pages 60-61	WORK UP TO: 2 SETS OF 20 Then Begin Step Nine
STEP NINE	LEVER PUSHUPS Pages 62-63	WORK UP TO: 2 SETS OF 20 Then Begin Step Ten
MASTER STEP TEN	ONE-ARM PUSHUPS Pages 64-65	ULTIMATE ENDURANCE: 1 SET OF 100

Going Beyond

Whoever you are, the ability to perform full *one-arm pushups* deeply, slowly and for reps—with picture perfect form—is an incredible achievement. Unless you are over seventy years of age or are carrying a permanent disability, you *will* be able to achieve this goal if you diligently work through the ten steps as outlined in the previous section.

How swiftly you achieve this goal is another matter. It will depend on your dedication, your body fat ratio, your arm length and natural strength, amongst other things. Only one thing's for sure—grit your teeth and put the work in, and you'll achieve where others fail. But perfection is a journey, not a destination. Where you chose to go when you become master of the one-arm pushup depends upon your goals.

One possibility could be to increase your reps. You'd be surprised how easy it is to do this once you've mastered a bodyweight technique—just a rep every workout or two, and before long your stamina will be through the roof. For determined trainees, two sets of fifty repetitions are an impressive but achievable medium-term goal.

Two sets of fifty is an amazing achievement. It should be considered an *elite level* of mastery. If you get to that level, you'll be able to challenge virtually any athlete in any gymnasium to the world and they'll be unable to match you. But for a dedicated athlete with good potential, the ultimate muscular endurance goal has to be *one hundred reps*. You read that right—one set of a hundred. Lifting the bulk of your bodyweight one hundred times *with only one arm* might sound like something only a super-hero could do, but it's achievable with training. At the time of writing, the Guinness World Record for most one-arm pushups over thirty minutes is held by Canadian athlete Doug Pruden. He cranked out a phenomenal 1382 repetitions! So there's really no excuse why a motivated trainee can't achieve a hundred reps with training.

Although the development of endurance is an interesting and satisfying sideline, I'm a big believer that bodyweight training should be first and foremost a *strength discipline*. Increasing your reps will improve endurance, but after you hit double figures it won't do very much for strength. If you want to increase your muscle and might, you'll have to find ways of making the one-arm pushup *harder*. At first you should do this by tightening up your technique to the max; slow down your movements to ensure that there is zero momentum taking the pressure from your muscles. Once your movements are hypnotically slow and smooth, try adding isometric tension from the antagonistic muscles. This basically means that as you are moving you tense your arms, shoulders and back as much as possible so that you have to fight for every inch of motion. This kind of training is murder and will really take your workouts up a notch.

If you are still finding that one-arm pushups are no problem, focus more of your attention and energy on developing your *one-arm handstand pushup* (pages 248—249). This exercise works the upper body pressing muscles in a comparable way to the one-arm pushup, but is much harder due to the angle and the fact that the entire bodyweight is lifted.

These tactics will allow you to continue gaining strength from your bodyweight training for years—until you reach your genetic limit. Weight-training is not necessary to perfect your body-power. But if you really *must* try weight-training, how about some hybrid techniques? If one-arm pushups become really easy, try them while holding a dumbbell in your free hand. This will really separate the iron men from the baby-weight pumpers!

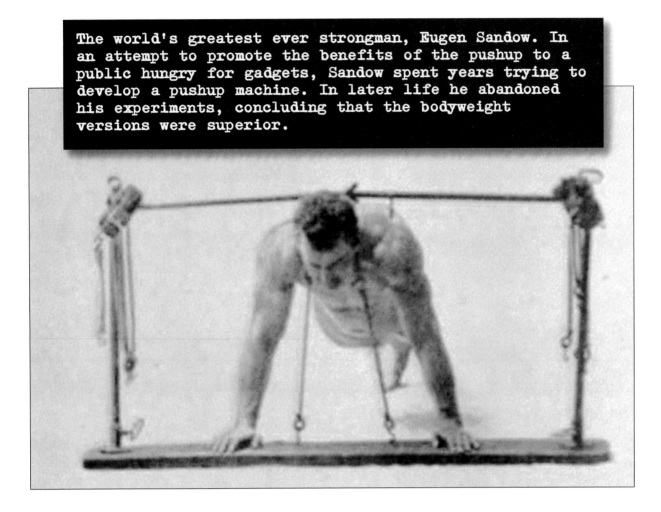

The world's greatest ever strongman, Eugen Sandow. In an attempt to promote the benefits of the pushup to a public hungry for gadgets, Sandow spent years trying to develop a pushup machine. In later life he abandoned his experiments, concluding that the bodyweight versions were superior.

Variants

There are numerous variants of the basic pushup movement. While you should endeavor to spend the majority of your training time working through the ten steps of the pushup series outlined earlier, you may, on occasion, want to experiment with these alternatives—perhaps as finishing exercises, when working around a light injury, or for the sake of variety. In this section you will find descriptions of some of the most useful alternative variations of the pushup.

Dips

This is a classic high school exercise. Take hold of parallel bars or two surfaces on either side of your body, lift your feet off the ground and bend at the elbows and shoulders to lower yourself down. Keep bending the elbows until the upper arms are parallel with the ground then press back up. Try to keep your torso erect as you go. This exercise can be made easier by raising the feet onto a surface level with the hips. In this version the hands can be placed behind the trainee, perhaps on a bed, table, bench, etc. As a result, this easier version is sometimes called *bench dips*. Dips and bench dips are not true pushup movements, but they strongly work many of the same pressing muscles. They also powerfully effect the lats, the large muscles on the side of the upper back, in a dynamic way.

Handstand Pushups

See *chapter 10*.

Decline Pushups

Confusingly, these are sometimes wrongly called *incline pushups*. They simply involve doing your pushups with the feet raised onto any surface higher than the hands. In prison a lot of guys use their bunk, but you can go higher with a desk or basin. Some men even wedge their feet high against the wall, but it requires a lot of body tension to retain this position. Raising the feet makes the exercise harder by transferring a greater proportion of the bodyweight through the hands. Because of the increased angle, this movement effects the shoulders and upper portions of the chest more intensely than the prone pushup. I don't advise my students to spend time on the decline pushup, because *handstand pushups* (see *chapter 10*) convey all the benefits of decline pushups in a more concentrated way. If you are doing handstand pushups, you are simply covering the same ground (but less efficiently) if you do decline pushups too. You are also risking overtraining.

Wide Pushups

These are the opposite of *close pushups*—instead of putting your hands together, you place them wider than usual, up to twice shoulder width. This variation takes much of the stress off the triceps and elbow joint and places more pressure on the pectorals at the point where they meet the front of the shoulder. In layman's terms, it works the chest more than the triceps. This type of pushup won't make you much stronger at doing pushups, because the chest/shoulder girdle is normally already proportionately much stronger than the elbow joint; doing this exercise consistently will only enhance that differential. That said, it's a useful exercise to master if you are specializing on your pectorals.

Superman Pushups

Full pushups are usually done with the hands at shoulder level or in line with the chest. In Superman pushups you do your reps with your hands flat on the floor way out in front of you, at nearly arm's length. In this position, you'll look a little like you're flying—hence the name. Due to the increased leverage of this technique, Superman pushups strongly work the upper pectorals and pec minor, as well as the lats and the tendons around the armpits. On the downside, due to the arm position, the range of motion of the exercise is decreased, and the important shoulders and triceps get significantly less work than in classic full pushups. For this reason, this exercise (like *wide pushups*) won't make you stronger at doing pushups, so unless you're trying to fix a relative weakness in your chest area, I'd avoid them.

Gecko Pushups

There are four levels of difficulty to the gecko pushup. In the easiest version the athlete does *full pushups*, but with one ankle hooked over the other so that only one foot is making contact with the floor. These are sometimes called *three-point pushups*. In the second version, the athlete raises one leg off the floor, but keeps it locked straight out behind him as he does his pushups. This nuance doubles the isometric involvement of the movement's stabilizers; the legs, hips, waist and spinal muscles. It also requires greater balance and focus than the normal pushup. In the third version the athlete keeps both legs on the floor, but stretches one arm out straight in front of him, level with his head. This is essentially a *one-arm pushup*, but with one limb pointing forward instead of being secured next to the lower back. In the fourth and hardest version of the gecko pushup, the athlete combines the second and third versions. He lifts one arm out straight in front, *as well as* stretching the opposite leg out behind him as he performs the movement. Doing pushups in this manner requires significant upper body strength and a lower back of steel in order to remain stable. In this position, the athlete resembles a lizard lifting alternate feet from the baking desert floor, hence the name "gecko" pushups. Gecko pushups are a fun finishing exercise to include in your routine when you have the strength. Be sure to do an equal number of reps on either side to keep development symmetrical.

Plyometric Pushups

Also known as *clapping pushups*. This is the standard pushup, but done explosively. Keeping the body ramrod stiff, descend quickly into the bottom position before driving up so hard that the hands leave the floor briefly. While in mid-air, clap the hands together in the split second before your palms meet the floor again and then repeat the exercise. The more powerfully you push, the further away you'll be able to get from the floor, and the more times you'll be able to quickly clap before coming back down. Many guys are able to do triple or even quadruple claps. An extremely difficult version is the *one-arm clapping* pushup, where you push up with just one arm before clapping. Clapping pushups add speed and are an excellent addition to your routine, once in a while. They can lead to injury however, so work into them slowly and don't even attempt them until you have at least mastered *uneven pushups*.

Stretch Pushups

This is the standard pushup, but performed with the hands on two raised objects on either side of the torso. You can buy specially made pushup handles for this, but placing the palms on two chairs will have the same effect. When you do pushups with your hands on a flat surface (like the floor), your range of motion is limited by that surface; but doing pushups with your hands on raised objects means you can lower your chest further than the point where it would normally be stopped by the floor. The feet can either be below the hands, or level (or higher) through being put on a bed, desk, another chair, etc. I'm not a big believer in stretch pushups. Stretching the muscles under resistance is painful, and does lead to increased soreness after the workout, but this is entirely due to microtrauma within the muscle tissue—it doesn't mean the muscles will get bigger or stronger. Stretching muscles won't increase your size or strength. If you want to make your pecs burn, do stretch pushups. If you want all-over upper body muscle and might, work through the ten steps and give stretch pushups a miss.

Jackknife Pushups

With your toes flat on the floor, place your palms on the ground at some point in front of you so that you are bent approximately ninety degrees at the hips. (This angle is called the *jackknife* position, because your body resembles an opening pocket knife.) Your hands should be about shoulder width apart, and despite the angle at the hips, your torso should be straight. Retain a gentle bend at the knee. Bending at the arms and shoulders, lower your chin until it kisses the floor at a point between your hands. Now continue moving your chin in an upwards arc, as your hips drop to brush the ground. You should finish the movement with your arms and legs straight, your shoulders high and your hips low. Keeping your arms straight, push your butt out and back until you are in the starting position again, and repeat. This exercise is easier on the upper body muscles than regular pushups, although the jackknife bending and straightening motion builds strong, flexible hips. For this reason, the exercise is popular with martial artists and wrestlers. Sometimes this exercise is known as a *cat pushup*, or by its Indian name, the *dand*.

Divebomber Pushups

These used to be popular in the Marine corps, back in the 70s. They are similar to *jackknife pushups*, except you bend your arms on the way back to the start position (in jackknife pushups, bend your arms as the hips move down, but you keep your arms straight when they go back up). Bending the arms a second time increases upper arm involvement, but lessens the effectiveness of the exercise as a flexibility movement.

Diagonal Pushups

Get into same the bent-over pushup position used to begin *jackknife pushups*. Your body should be bent well at the waist, with the hips high in the air, and your arms and legs almost straight. Keeping the legs together will make things harder. Now bend at the arms and shoulders, but instead of dropping your hips—as you would for jackknife or *divebomber pushups*—keep your body locked at a ninety-degree angle. Keep bending your arms until the top of your forehead gently touches the floor, and push back up. The body must stay at the same angle until you finish all your reps. It's easier to do this if your heels are jammed up against a wall. This exercise works the shoulders more than the conventional pushup. It's fun to do, but just like *decline pushups*, the *handstand pushup* is a far better alternative if you want to work your shoulders hard.

The Plank

The plank is not really a pushup. It's a static feat of strength that was a favorite amongst the strongmen of the second Golden Age, although it stretches back much further than that. The old-timers loved this exercise, and not without reason—the plank requires strength in almost every single muscle of the body, as well as balance and coordination. Besides which, it makes for a cool party trick. Place your palms on the floor shoulder width apart, bend your arms, tucking your elbows into your torso, and lean forwards until your feet are off the ground with the legs locked. To maintain this position, your back and legs have to be stiff as a board—hence the name "plank." This is an extremely difficult exercise to visualize without a picture, so I've included a photo below to help. The exercise is a tough one to pull off; the key is persistence along with the development of basic strength through practicing the ten steps. Keep it up and I guarantee you'll get there. The plank was popular amongst Canadian strongmen and for this reason it's still often known by its French name, *the planche*. In English-speaking countries it is sometimes known by its gymnastics name, *the elbow lever*.

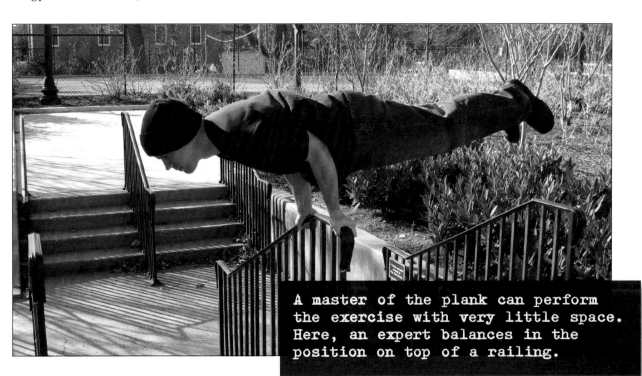

A master of the plank can perform the exercise with very little space. Here, an expert balances in the position on top of a railing.

Incline Tiger Bends

This is an exercise performed by a lot of bodybuilders who find themselves in prison and want to maintain their arm size. Although it's a bodyweight exercise, it's more like a *barbell triceps extension* than a true pushup, because it works the triceps but not the pectorals or shoulders. Lean forwards at a forty-five degree angle, grabbing a solid object in front of you. In prison, wash basins usually fit the bill, but if you are training at home you might want to use a kitchen counter or a work surface You can even do the exercise with your palms flat on a wall, opposite your chest. Keeping the elbows pointing down, bend at the elbows but *not at the shoulders*. Continue moving forwards as far as you can or until your upper arms meet your torso, then press yourself up. Plenty of strict reps will have your triceps screaming for mercy.

Maltese Pushups

These are an obscure variation of the pushup often used by gymnasts, because they partially mimic training on the rings. Maltese pushups look a little like *full pushups*, but the hands are placed in line with the hips, and quite far out from the body. If you were to draw a line up the athlete's torso and another from palm to palm in this position, the two lines would approximate a Maltese cross, hence the name of the exercise. The movement required by this type of pushup is difficult to appreciate unless you actually see an expert doing it. Maltese pushups work the biceps as well as the triceps, but the technique can be rough on the inner elbows. Unless you are a gymnast, I'd disregard them.

6: THE SQUAT

ELEVATOR CABLE THIGHS

The average person associates strength with the upper body. Broad shoulders, a deep chest, and thick arms are seen as the primary signs of a big, strong guy. Nobody really thinks about the legs. If you ask somebody—even a little kid—to make a muscle, he'll pull up his sleeve and show you a biceps shot. No one ever drops their pants and flexes a thigh at you!

This attitude is reflected in the training of the average gym-goer. Take a look at any gym in the world, and check out what's going on at the weights section. You'll see guys working shoulders, torsos and arms. You'll see teenagers queuing up to train on the bench press, and practically knocking each other over to get to the preacher curl unit or the cable pushdown station to pump up their triceps. Probably ninety percent of the strength exercises done in gyms the world over are for the upper body; and I'd estimate that nearly fifty percent of that amount is arm work. In an average gym, you'll see only a few individuals doing hard leg training.

Before his incarceration, a fellow inmate of mine in San Quentin was a regular trainee at one of the busiest gyms in the world—the Gold's Gym in Venice Beach (a.k.a. "Muscle Beach"), California. The Venice Beach Gold's Gym can probably count more serious bodybuilders and elite strength athletes as members than any other gym in the world. He told me once that the squat racks were right at the back of the gym. Despite visiting the place frequently over years, he said that he never, ever saw a queue for those squat racks. In fact, the majority of the day, they stood empty. If that's true of the world-famous Gold's Gym, how much more so for local gyms throughout the land?

The Source of Power

In fact, this attitude is totally backwards. The real strength of an athlete lies in his hips and legs, *not* his upper body and arms. Unless we are in mid-air, or seated with the legs raised off the ground, all movements of the upper limbs rely on forces transmitted through the legs. Upper body strength is important in many athletic motions, but if that strength isn't founded on a powerful lower body, it's totally useless.

True strength athletes understand this fact much better than weekend warriors, or "beach body" trainees. Big biceps and veiny pecs might look good, but they contribute little to maximum power. Take the classic Olympic lift, the *clean and jerk* as an example. This is probably the ultimate example of total body power. But despite the fact that the lifter holds the weight above his head, most of the force generated to achieve this lift comes from the *thighs*—the weight is *never* pressed up by the arms. It's far too heavy for that. Next time the event is televised, watch and you'll see. What actually happens is that the lifter powers the weight up to his shoulders, and then dips down before exploding the bar up a few inches with *leg* strength. He then bends his legs and drops his own body down, *under* the weight, in a full squat position with his arms locked out. From there, he powers out of the squat with his legs, to finish the movement. The upper body and arms are actually of secondary importance in the clean and jerk. Olympic lifters have massive thighs, because they spend much more time doing squats than any other exercise. They understand the value of leg power.

The heaviest exercise known to man is probably the *deadlift,* in which the athlete picks a heavy barbell off the floor and up to the hips. The world record is currently held by famous powerlifter Andy Bolton, who lifted 1003 lbs. under official conditions. That's over half a ton! Although this exercise works pretty much every muscle in the body, the lion's share of active lifting is done by the thighs and hips; in particular the glutes (which cross the hips), hamstrings (which cross the hips and knees at the rear) and the quads (which cross the hips and knees at the front). Even in direct upper body exercises like the bench press, the legs play a major role in generating strength. Wheelchair-bound Paralympian powerlifters may have hulking upper bodies, but their weights in the bench press are always drastically below their Olympian counterparts purely because they cannot transmit moving forces through their legs. Given these examples, it's easy to see that *true power* comes from the lower body—*not* the upper body.

The above illustrations relate to power sports, but the overemphasis on upper body strength seems to apply to most other sports too. Unfortunately, for many athletes, the importance of lower body strength and stability only becomes apparent when they suffer a leg injury. Following a knee impairment or hamstring tear, the trainee understands the vital importance of the lower body only too plainly. Try "upper body" motions like wrestling, punching, pushing, or pulling when you have a leg injury and you'll find them next to impossible. This is not to mention lower body movements, like running, hopping, jumping, kicking, etc. Most athletic movements are lower body based, and it goes without saying that these movements rely largely on leg strength. Upper body involvement is relatively minimal.

There is an old saying in field sports that a competitor is only as young as his legs. Traditionally, that "spring" in the legs is the first thing to go as an athlete begins to age. This loss of strength in the lower body can be postponed and even actively reversed, but no amount of upper body training will get the job done. You need to learn how to train your legs. This chapter will teach you everything you need to know.

Modern Methods Can De-Train the Legs

There are numerous exercises for the legs. Many of them isolate individual muscles within the thighs; leg extensions and sissy squats isolate the quadriceps, leg curls isolate the leg biceps, hyper-extensions focus on the glutes. In addition there are dozens of other leg machines and cable exercises which work on particular leg muscles or groups of leg muscles.

Far from being a bonus for the modern trainee, this excess of modern training techniques is actually a *negative* thing in most cases. This is precisely because many of these newer leg exercises have been designed to *isolate* different leg muscles. This practice might be useful for an advanced bodybuilder who wants to emphasize certain distinct portions on his lower body; but it does very little for overall muscle mass and functional strength because the leg muscles have evolved to worked as an *holistic system*, not as separate parts. In fact, the current practice of training the legs with multiple isolation exercises can even *reduce* functional strength and lower body athleticism because it de-trains the natural reflexes of the leg muscles to fire in a synergistic, coordinated way.

The best way to develop truly powerful, athletic legs is to use the *fewest* exercises—provided they work as many leg muscles as possible. The *ideal* would be to use only a single exercise—as long as you could find an exercise that dynamically works *all* the muscles of the lower body.

Such an exercise does exist, and it has been well known to athletes since ancient times. Because of its deep significance to physical culture the world over, this exercise goes by many names. In English-speaking countries it is called the *squat*, or *deep knee-bend*. In India—where physical culture is practically built on bodyweight squatting—it is called the *baithak*.

Muscles Worked by the Squat

Some will balk at the idea that a single exercise can work the entire lower body, but in the case of squatting the reputation is well deserved.

Precisely what constitutes a squatting motion? By *squatting* I basically mean lowing the torso by bending the three major pairs of joints in the lower body; the hips, knees and ankles. Writers usually focus on the bend in the knee when describing squats—in fact, squats are sometimes called *knee-bends*, or *deep knee-bends*. But in reality you need to bend all three types of joint in order to squat down unassisted. If you try to bend your knees without also moving the ankles and bending forward at the hips, you would topple backwards. It's *impossible* to squat without moving at all three axes. These major lower body joints have evolved to work in unison.

The bend at the hip primarily involves the powerful *gluteus maximus* (the buttock muscles), as well as the *gluteus minimus* higher up and the *gluteus medius* round the side. About a dozen smaller muscles like the *tensor faciae latae* and *piriformis* also play a role. A chain is only as strong

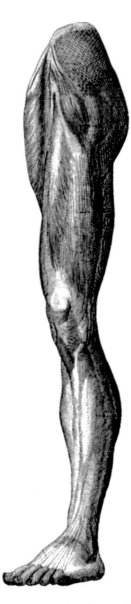

as its weakest link, and this is definitely true where the hip girdle is concerned. Despite the fact that these other hip muscles are relatively small, their strength is vital for healthy, powerful hips. Due to the forwards motion, the muscles along the spinal column and waist also receive their share of work during squatting, particularly the important lumbar muscles. Deep squatting puts pressure on the internal organs, and as a result, the *transversus* and abdominal muscles—which act as a muscular corset for these organs—also become more powerful.

The bend at the knee strongly works the *quadriceps* at the front of the thigh. As the name suggests, the quadriceps is made up of four heads; the *vastus lateralis*, which is the broad muscle up the outside of the thigh; the *vastus intermedius*, which is a deep muscle running up the center of the thigh; the *rectus femoris* which is the "detail" muscle at the front of the thigh; and the *vastus medialis*, the "teardrop" muscle next to the knee. These heads all have slightly different roles in extending the knee. Which head gets the majority of work depends on the depth of any given motion; lockout motions will mostly work the *vastus medialis*, and shallow motions mostly work the *vastus lateralis*. All four heads get a strong workout from *full* squatting motions, however. It's well known in bodybuilding circles that squats are the best motion for building the quads—bar none.

The squat also works the *semitendinosus*, *semimembranosus* and *biceps femoris* muscles—the complex at the rear of the thigh, most commonly known as the *hamstrings*. The fact that squats work the *back* of the thigh is not well known nowadays, and as a result most athletes train their hamstrings on specially constructed leg curl machines. This is a real shame, because leg curls put the hamstrings in the worst possible biomechanical position for strength, and as a result they don't do much to add muscle or power. The old-time strongmen and physical culturalists used to understand that squats worked the entire thigh—the hamstrings as well as the quads, and as a result most of them only focused on squatting motions for the legs. Their whole bodies got stronger as a result. If you don't believe that squatting works the hamstrings, test it for yourself. Firmly grab the back of your thigh as you do a deep squat, and you'll feel the muscles there all powerfully contract. In theory, the quadriceps and hamstrings shouldn't contract at the same time to move the body, because they are *antagonistic*—i.e., on opposite sides of the limb. But they do, and they do so strongly. Kinesiologists call this phenomenon *Lombard's Paradox*.

The *femur* (the thighbone) is the longest, strongest bone in the human body. Whilst an athlete descends into the squat, the bottom of the femur moves forwards. This causes the *tibia* and *fibia* (the shinbones) to correspondingly move forwards, where they are attached to the femur at the knee joint. This in turn forces the ankle to flex automatically, stretching the calves and Achilles' tendon and contracting and strengthening the shin muscles (*anterior tibialis*). When the athlete pushes back up, the ankle has to return to its original position. This seemingly small motion powerfully works every muscle in the lower leg; not only the calves (the flat *soleus* and diamond-shaped *gastrocnemius* muscles), but also the smaller muscles and tendons of the ankle. Even the muscles of the foot have to fire strongly to keep the body balanced and stable during squats. Many bodybuilders don't even train their calves directly—squatting keeps them thick and strong.

All these muscles—and more—are vigorously and dynamically worked by squatting motions. But even more important than the fact that the squat works all these muscles is the fact that it works them in synergy, in an *authentic* way—by which I mean, in a manner which is in perfect harmony with the way that muscles *naturally* work together. If you look at the basic kinesiology of fundamental athletic motions like:

- Running
- Jumping
- Bracing yourself
- Sitting down
- Standing up
- Stamping
- Heavy pushing (e.g., pushing a vehicle)
- Heavy pulling, (e.g., tug-of-war type pulls)

You'll see that they all require a bend at the leg and hips, just the same as squats. It's precisely because *all* the muscles of the lower leg are able to work together synergistically that the lower body—in fact, the entire human body—has such a capacity for enormous strength.

Lose the Barbell

That last section sounded a little like an anatomy lesson. Sorry about that. But my goal was to provide you with as much evidence as possible to prove that the squat really *is* the greatest lower body exercise, and that it works practically every lower body muscle. Whether you agree with what I've said or not, I hope I've gone at least some of the way towards establishing the fact that squatting is one hell of an exercise.

What I haven't established yet—at all—is why bodyweight squats are superior to squatting motions with a barbell. Surely they are the same motion, after all? In fact—on the face of it—barbell squats may even appear to be the superior exercise, because the trainee can progressively add weight to the barbell as they get stronger.

Well, if you've been reading up until this point, you'll pretty much be able to anticipate what my philosophy on this matter is going to be. Bodyweight squats blow barbell squats away!

There are several problems with barbell squats, and exercises on machines designed to mimic barbell squats. The major problem is that the legs contain the biggest and strongest muscles in the human body. This means that in order to work them, heavy weights are required. Because the lower body muscles are conditioned just by carrying the body around all day, they adapt quickly to training. As a result, heavier and heavier weights have to be used over time. Eventually, long-term squatters need to use *enormous* weights just to continue improving. Barbells loaded to in excess of five hundred pounds are not uncommon amongst master squatters—and this is for genetically average guys who are drug-free! When you squat with weights, this big heavy bar has to be placed on the upper back. (Some guys squat holding the bar on their upper chests, but the movement is awkward, can cause upper body injuries, and requires a drop in weight.) Placing this heavy weight on the upper back vertically loads the spine with significant force. This in turn compresses the vertebrae, the discs in the spine, which can cause problems ranging from lumbago and muscle strains to sciatica and bulging or fully herniated discs. Placing the full load at a point near the top of the spine also promotes an exaggerated forward lean during squatting, which can strain lower back muscles. It can also cause the knees to track inwards, which increases shear force to the knee joint. All these problems are compounded for taller athletes, because long leg bones place the lifter at a significant biomechanical disadvantage. The taller you are, the more the above problems will apply to you. It's not by coincidence that all the truly great barbell squatters are short.

Bodyweight squatting relies upon *no* external loads; so no heavy weights dig into the back or shoulders, forcing the body into unnatural positions which irritate the spine or joints. In *Convict Conditioning*, the athlete progresses by mastering a series of harder bodyweight movements which culminate in the ultimate leg movement—the full *one-leg squat*.

The benefits of mastering the one-leg squat are enormous. The first obvious benefit is *strength*. If a 200 lbs. man learns to squat on one leg, it's essentially the equivalent of performing a two-leg squat with 200 lbs. on his back. Barbell squats only develop the muscles at the back of the hips, but one-leg squats simultaneously work the muscles at the front and side of the hips, due to the raised position of the non-squatting leg (see *figure 40* for an example.) This ensures harmonious development and prevents the recurrent hip problems that tend to plague barbell squatters. *Balance* is another major benefit. Hardly anybody has to stand on one leg during the course of a day, and as a result, very few people realize how much equilibrium it requires. Training the muscles hard while moving up and down—and huffing and puffing—is an incredibly intense coordination workout. Squatting on one leg is also much more *functional* than the two-leg barbell variety, because in nature, most movements involve favoring one limb at a time. Think of kicking, hopping up onto something, climbing, etc. The fact that bodyweight squatting is a more natural type of movement than squatting with an external load also means that the body recovers quicker between sessions. Surprising, but true. One-leg squats even encourage improved mind-body connection and mental focus, because the legs are performing radically different tasks throughout the exercise. Without doubt, single-leg squatting beats barbell squatting—hands down.

Thoughts on Squatting

Entire books have been written on how to squat. I'm a big believer that you need to squat throughout your entire athletic career—it's one of the few really *invaluable* exercises. For this reason, athletes need to get to know their own squatting abilities and structure over a long period of time (you *are* going to stay strong your whole life, right?). As a result, your individual technique will develop spontaneously. I give some technical pointers on the following pages, under the *exercise x-rays* sections, but rather than giving a formal list of specifications on the exercise I'll just throw some ideas out there to try and help you along the way. In some cases, owning a compass is better than being given a set of directions. Squats are one of those cases. Read, experiment, cultivate, practice. It doesn't matter if you agree or disagree with the following ideas. Just use them as a starting point. And get squatting!

- Different depths of motion in squatting develop different muscles. A *full* range of motion develops all the muscles equally. For this reason, you should aim to master full squats. Some of the steps are half-movements, but they exist only as stages in the process towards full squats. Half-movements must always be performed in conjunction with full movements.

- What is a full range of motion for the squat? It means squatting down until your hamstrings are pressing on your calves and you cannot descend any further, before pushing up with thigh and knee power until your legs are fully straight. Anything less is not a full squat.

- Some people believe that going all the way down is bad for the knees. This is not true. It's only bad for the knees if you have a pre-existing knee problem—and even then, it may help alleviate that problem. Knee tendons can be strained if they are not ready for the low position, but if you carefully follow the steps through, your knees will easily be strong enough to take on the full squat. No worries!

- Similarly, a lot of bodybuilders dislike the idea of totally straightening the legs at the top of the squat. They think that this allows the thigh muscles to rest, robbing them of work. It's true that straightening the legs fully takes pressure off the muscles momentarily, but provided that brief rest translates into greater levels of strength to pour into the next rep, it can only be a good thing. Straighten your legs fully during squatting.

- Control the negative portion of the movement as much as the positive. Don't just drop down. Lower yourself using muscular control.

- Bend forwards, but don't bend *too* far forwards when descending. This will overemphasize the hips, and underemphasize the thighs. A frontal tilt is necessary, but don't get into the habit of *bowing* forwards.

- In the bottom position, you will be virtually "sitting" into the squat. Thinking in terms of *sitting* rather than *squatting* can sometimes help athletes descend more naturally, because it facilitates correct hip positioning—which is a fancy way of saying the butt should stick out.

- The bottom position of the squat is the hardest portion of the motion to control. This is true for almost all exercises, but is particularly true for the squat. Despite the difficulty—particularly on one-leg squats—you must never *bounce* out of the squat, by dropping quickly and springing straight up. This can severely damage the cartilage in your knees, *for good*. Instead, slowly build up the tendon strength that's required by mastering the early steps carefully.

- As with all The Big Six: movements, I advocate a one second pause at the bottom. This is an excellent way to eliminate dangerous bouncing.

- A pause at the bottom is a good habit, but it's not a panacea. You can still cheat, even with a pause. To get out of the sitting position, some athletes tend to rock forwards. This provides momentum and makes the first few inches easier, but it places undesirable pressure on the knees. Stay sitting, and push up using leg power only. If you can't do this, you are too weak for the exercise you are attempting. Go back to easier steps and keep working at them.

• Some people find that they have to lift their heels off the ground when they squat, so they put a board or block under the heels to help them. This is a bad habit. Needing to elevate the heels has nothing to do with balance or body structure, and everything to do with lack of ankle mobility and inflexibility of the Achilles' tendon. If your ligaments and tendons are stiff, the ankle won't be able to bend sufficiently during the exercise, and your heels will rise. Don't use boards. Stretch your calves out until you can squat without assistance.

• As mentioned above, squatting works a lot of muscles—including the largest muscles in the body. This is a big benefit, but the down side is that the exercise requires a lot of effort. That's one of the reasons the squat has gradually become less popular, and numerous alternatives have been developed. Grit your teeth, and tough them out. Over the months, the body and mind will adapt to the pain, and the exercise becomes more tolerable. Heck, you'll even learn to love it. (Maybe.)

• I like to keep my arms straight out in front of me during squats. This tends to help balance in the bottom position—it throws some weight forwards, and can offset the tendency to fall back, especially for taller guys. Some bodyweight squatters like to put their hands on their hips, shoulders, or cross their arms on their chest. See what feels easiest for you, depending upon the given exercise.

• Many guys are afraid of the squat, because they think it will aggravate old knee injuries. In fact, the opposite is usually true. The increased blood flow and range of motion in full squats removes waste build-up and stretches old scar tissue, alleviating pain. The knees and surrounding muscles and tendons become stronger and more flexible, and the likelihood of future injuries is lessened.

• The most common knee injury is the tear of the ACL (the *anterior cruciate ligament*). The ACL is a ligament running through the knee that holds it together, and is often fully or partially torn when the foot is flat on the floor and the knee is forcibly twisted. ACL injuries are common in football, soccer, wrestling, martial arts, in fact *all* combat and contact sports. Knees are intricate, and sometimes a chunk of cartilage (called the *meniscus*) is ripped at the same time the ACL tears. If the ligament hasn't been surgically reconstructed—even if it has—the injured knee can be very unstable, sometimes popping right out of place. Far from worsening ACL injuries, squats will definitely *help* the athlete. The knee is very strong in squatting movements, and it's virtually impossible for the joint to become unstable and dislocate when the foot positioning is correct. Squats strengthen the quadriceps, which acts as a substitute ACL and holds the knee tight during other activities. If squatting does cause you pain following an injury—or if the knee locks—this is usually due to a torn piece of cartilage. Exercise can't help here—a surgeon will have to remove that torn piece. But it's keyhole surgery and you will be out of hospital the same day. If this is you, quit suffering and get it done.

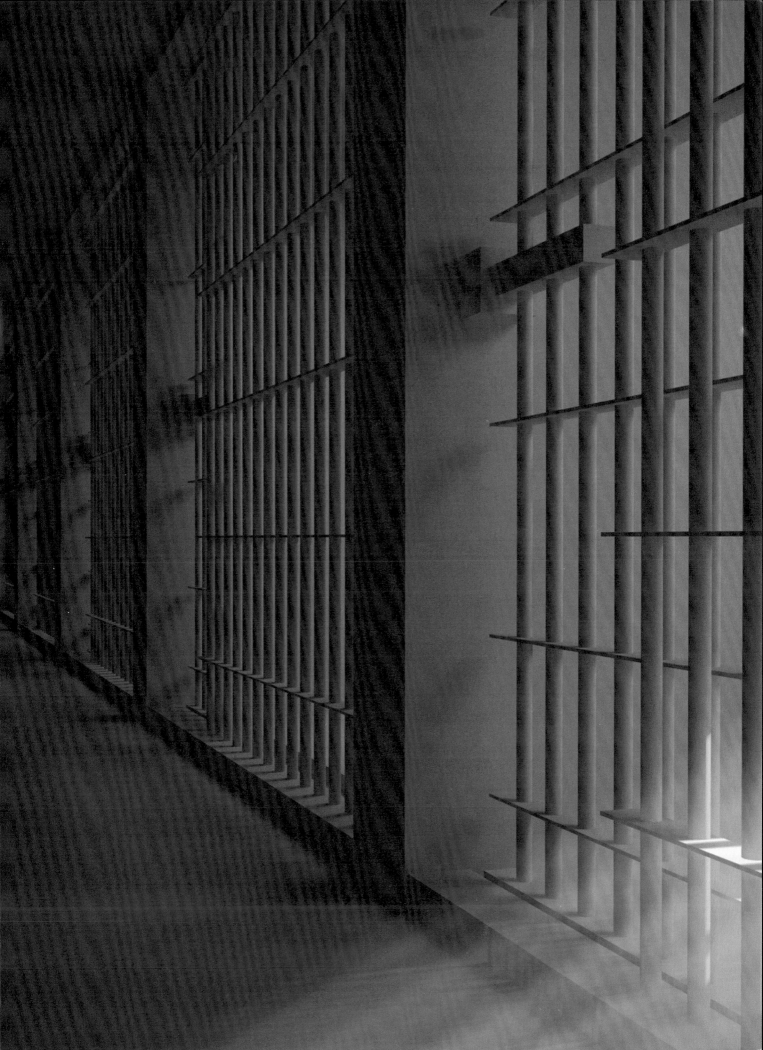

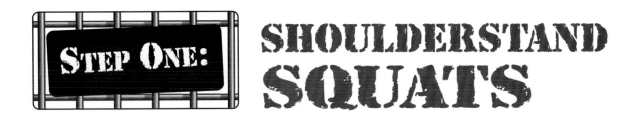

STEP ONE: SHOULDERSTAND SQUATS

Performance

Lie on your back, with your knees well bent. Kick against the floor while pushing with your hands until your feet are up in the air. As you reach this position, place your hands on your lower back for support, whilst keeping your upper arms firmly on the floor. You will now be in a shoulderstand position, supported by your shoulders and upper back, as well as the backs of your upper arms. Remember to constantly support your weight through these areas and keep any pressure off the neck. Your body should be locked straight, not bent at the hips. This is the start position (fig. 21). Keeping your torso as upright as possible, bend at the hips and knees until your knees touch your forehead. This is the finish position (fig. 22). Extend your legs directly back up, until your body is back in the start position. Repeat.

Exercise X-Ray

Shoulderstand squats are the perfect preliminary exercise for anybody who wants to start squatting. Due to the inverse position of the body, there is virtually no weight going through the knees and lower back. This makes them an ideal rehabilitation exercise to help those with back or knee injuries—perhaps coming out of surgery—to get back into sports where leg motion is crucial. In strength terms, shoulderstand squats are in fact harder on the upper body than the lower body. But they do free up tight joints, increase range of motion and set beginners on the road to *perfect* form.

Training Goals

- Beginner standard: 1 set of 10
- Intermediate standard: 2 sets of 25
- Progression standard: 3 sets of 50

Perfecting Your Technique

At the first attempt, not everybody will be able to touch the knees to the forehead. Try to increase the depth of your knees every workout and your joints will soon loosen. The technique will be virtually impossible for people with very fat stomachs, because the paunch gets in the way. Practicing on an empty stomach will help, until you shed those excess pounds.

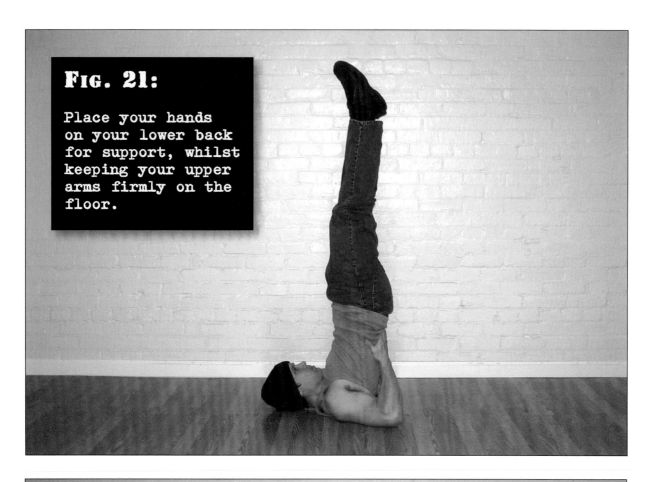

FIG. 21:

Place your hands on your lower back for support, whilst keeping your upper arms firmly on the floor.

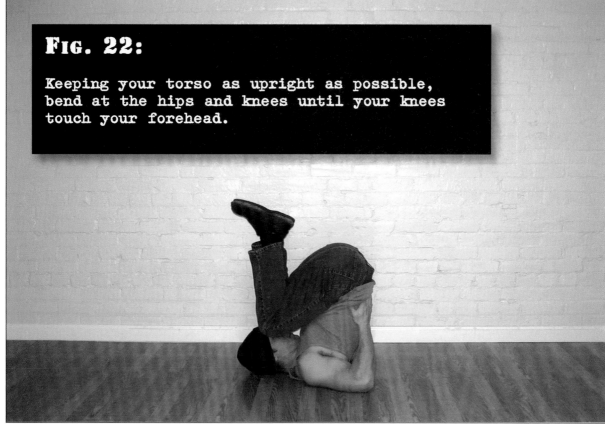

FIG. 22:

Keeping your torso as upright as possible, bend at the hips and knees until your knees touch your forehead.

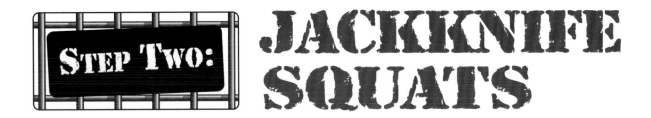

Performance

Stand in front of a sturdy object which comes up to your knees, or at least the tops of your shins. A small coffee table, chair or a bunk are good choices. Your legs should be shoulder width apart, or a little wider. Keeping your legs fairly straight, bend at your hips until your palms are in contact with the object. Tilt forwards slightly so that you can take some of your body's weight through your hands. This is the start position (fig. 23). Now, with your torso remaining as parallel to the floor as possible, bend at the knees and hips until your hamstrings reach your calves and you cannot go any further. This will require that you bend your arms, also. This is the finish position (fig. 24). Using combined leg and arm power, push yourself up to the start position. Do not raise the heels at any point during the exercise.

Exercise X-Ray

For *jackknife squats*, the torso is angled forwards so that it's not directly above the legs; as a result, part of the weight is transmitted through the arms. This exercise is about half as difficult as the standard bodyweight *full squat* (Step 5), and is a great way to prepare the lower body muscles and tendons for later steps. Performed correctly, it will also give beginners the balance and Achilles' tendon flexibility required to master the bottom position of a full squat.

Training Goals

- Beginner standard: 1 set of 10
- Intermediate standard: 2 sets of 20
- Progression standard: 3 sets of 40

Perfecting Your Technique

This exercise is hardest at the very bottom position, where the lower limbs take the majority of the body's weight. If this is difficult, gradually work to the bottom position by increasing your squatting depth by an inch or so each workout. An alternative method would be to use more arm power to share the load taken by your legs, and help you get out of the bottom position. Try to use less arm strength and rely on the legs more as they become stronger.

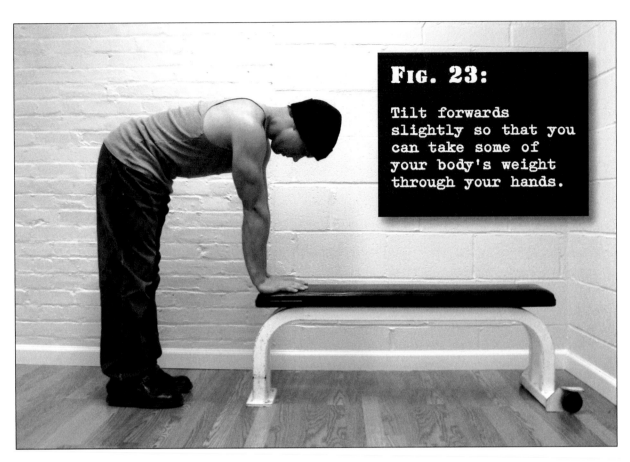

FIG. 23:

Tilt forwards slightly so that you can take some of your body's weight through your hands.

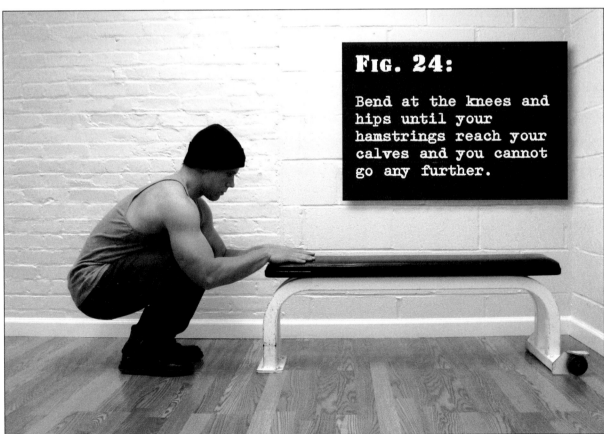

FIG. 24:

Bend at the knees and hips until your hamstrings reach your calves and you cannot go any further.

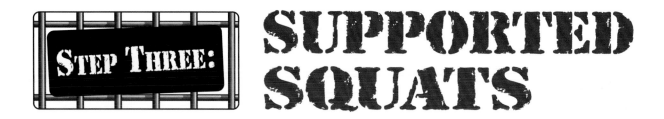

Performance

Stand up straight with the feet shoulder width apart, or slightly wider. Your arms should be out straight and angled down, holding onto a sturdy object higher than your thighs. A desk, robust basin or the back of a chair will do. This is the start position (fig. 25). Slowly lower yourself down by bending at the hips and the knees, keeping your back as straight as possible, until your hamstrings meet your calves and you cannot descend any further. This is the finish position (fig. 26). Pause for a moment, before pushing yourself up using mostly leg power. To take some of the pressure off your legs—particularly in the bottom position—pull yourself up slightly with your arms, by exerting downward force on the object you are holding. Try to keep the arms fairly straight. Your heels should remain flat on the floor throughout the exercise.

Exercise X-Ray

Supported squats are the last exercise before the athlete progresses onto *half squats*. This exercise forms an ideal link between the *jackknife squat* (where the legs move the majority of the body's weight) and the half squat (where the legs move virtually all the weight of the body). Supported squats continue adding flexibility and strength to the athlete's lower limbs. They condition the tendons, ligaments and soft tissues of the knees. They are a good way to continue perfecting form, most importantly the ability to push up from the bottom position using strength alone rather than momentum.

Training Goals

- Beginner standard: 1 set of 10
- Intermediate standard: 2 sets of 15
- Progression standard: 3 sets of 30

Perfecting Your Technique

Fine-tuning the amount of leg strength required on this exercise couldn't be simpler; to make the exercise easier on the lower body, simply use more upper body strength. As you become more comfortable in the bottom position, gradually use less arm strength to assist you in getting back up.

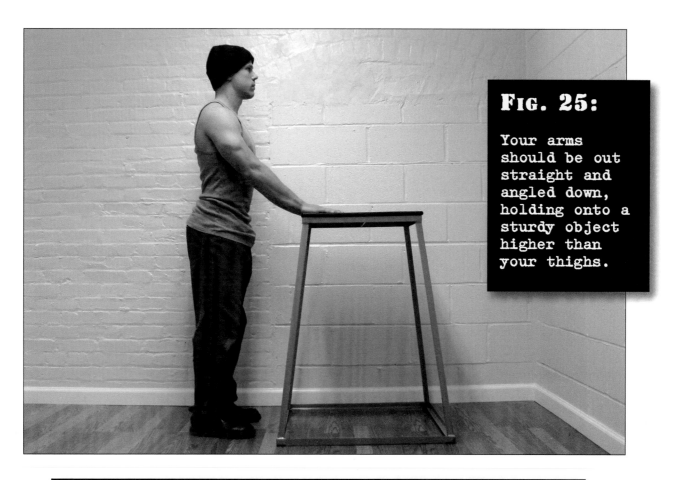

FIG. 25:

Your arms should be out straight and angled down, holding onto a sturdy object higher than your thighs.

FIG. 26:

Slowly lower yourself down by bending at the hips and the knees, keeping your back as straight as possible.

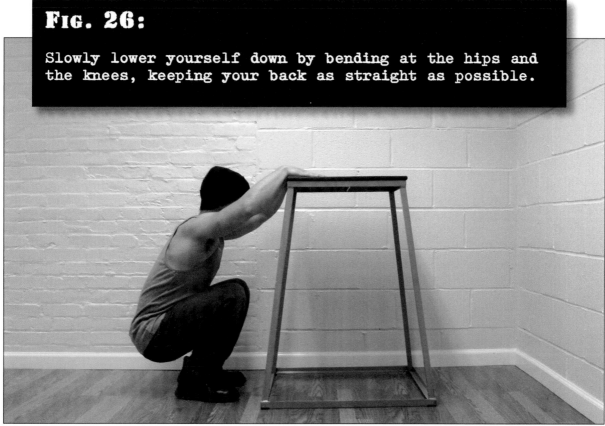

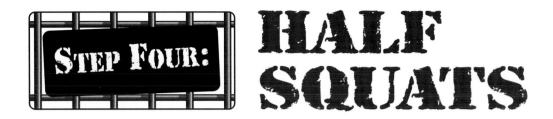

Performance

Stand with the feet shoulder width apart, or slightly wider. Don't keep your feet perfectly in line with one another; allow your toes to point very slightly outwards. Place your hands in a comfortable position—on your hips, chest or shoulders is fine. This is the start position (fig. 27). Now bend at the hips and knees until your knees are angled at ninety degrees, or (in other words) your thighs are parallel to the floor. This is the finish position (fig. 28). You can use a mirror or ask a friend the first few times until your body learns the right depth. Don't rush the technique, and never bounce; pause in mid-air at the bottom position for a one count before returning to the start position under full muscular control. Keep the back straight throughout the motion, and keep your heels flat on the floor. Your knees should always point in the same direction as your feet; don't ever allow the knees to "track" inwards as you squat. The outwards angle of your toes will assist you with this.

Exercise X-Ray

Half squats are the first step in the squatting series where you are handling your full bodyweight without any assistance. As such, they deserve respect. This exercise will teach you the balance and basic body positioning under gravity that you need to excel at harder forms of squatting. You will also begin to learn the optimum knee and foot positioning for your unique build. The thighs are very powerful in this top position, and for this reason the rep ranges given below are higher than normal. The muscles of your hips and inner thighs in particular will grow stronger as a result of mastering this movement.

Training Goals

- Beginner standard: 1 set of 8
- Intermediate standard: 2 sets of 35
- Progression standard: 2 sets of 50

Perfecting Your Technique

If you can't perform *half squats* in the style described above, start with quarter squats instead and add an inch of depth every time you can are able.

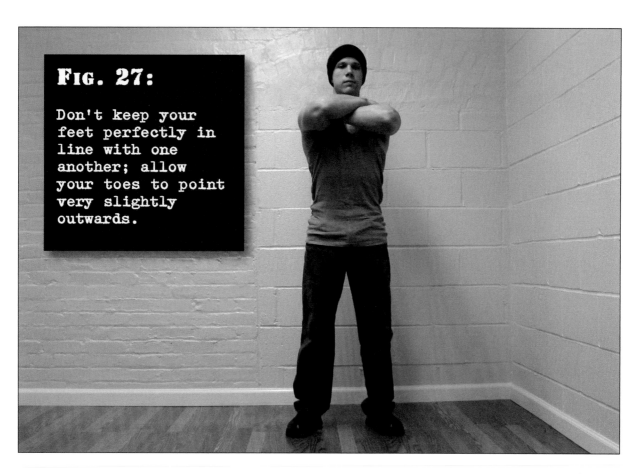

FIG. 27:

Don't keep your feet perfectly in line with one another; allow your toes to point very slightly outwards.

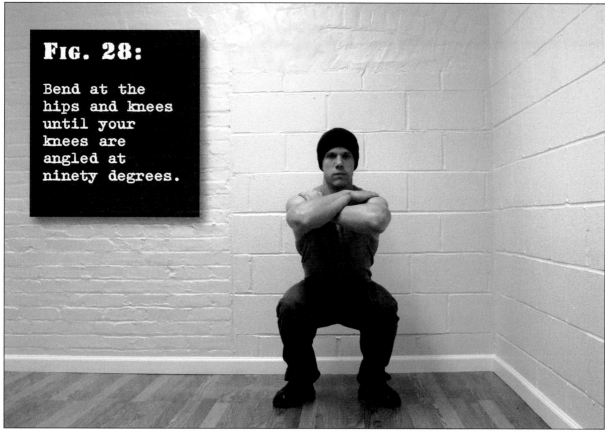

FIG. 28:

Bend at the hips and knees until your knees are angled at ninety degrees.

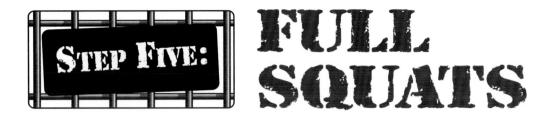

Performance

Stand tall, with the feet shoulder width apart or a little wider, depending upon your preference. Turn the toes slightly out, and place the arms in a comfortable position. This is the start of the movement (fig. 29). Bend at the hips and knees, keeping the back straight. When your thighs reach approximately parallel to the floor, shift your weight backwards as if you were about to sit down. Continue descending at a controlled speed until the backs of your thighs are resting against your calves. This is the finish position (fig. 30). Pause for a moment before pressing yourself back up with leg strength alone. Your upward motion should be the reverse of your downward motion. Don't raise the heels, or allow the knees to track inwards.

Exercise X-Ray

Full squats are the classic bodyweight leg exercise, used productively the world over for many thousands of years. And not without reason; full squats strengthen the knees, and add power and athleticism to every muscle in the thighs, as well as the glutes, spinal muscles and hips. The entire lower leg is conditioned, including the calves, *anterior tibialis* (shin muscles), ankles and even the soles of the feet. Full squats help legs retain their youthful vigor.

Training Goals

- Beginner standard: 1 set of 5
- Intermediate standard: 2 sets of 10
- Progression standard: 2 sets of 30

Perfecting Your Technique

If you have met the progression standard for *half squats, full squats* won't prove much of a problem. Due to leverage, the exercise will be hardest in the bottom position. This will be particularly true for tall people with long femurs (i.e., thighbones). If you cannot meet the beginner standard, return to doing half squats and slowly add an inch of depth to your technique whenever you get stronger. Don't rush, and resist the urge to bounce or rock forwards onto your toes. Use pure muscular power, or don't bother!

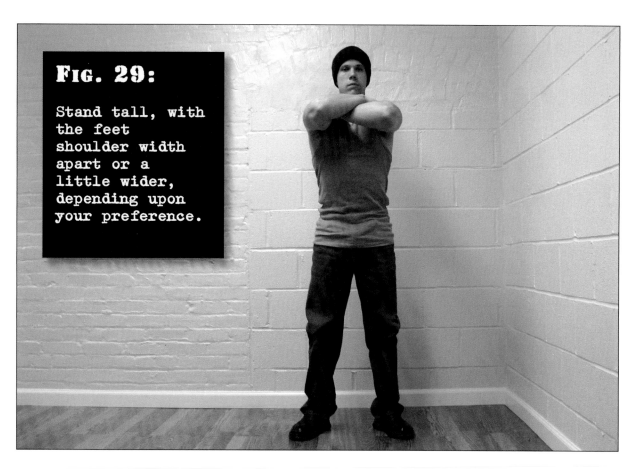

FIG. 29:

Stand tall, with the feet shoulder width apart or a little wider, depending upon your preference.

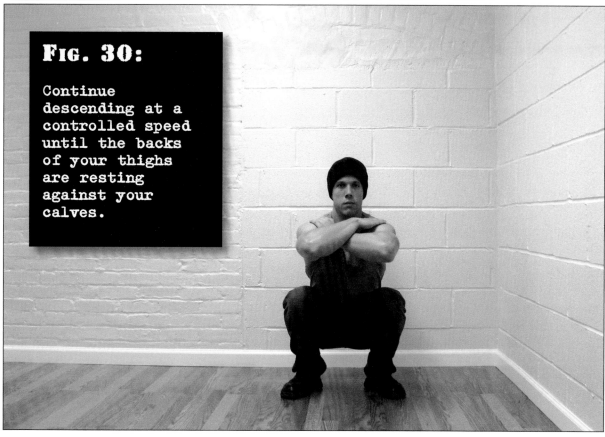

FIG. 30:

Continue descending at a controlled speed until the backs of your thighs are resting against your calves.

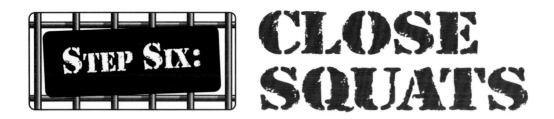

STEP SIX: CLOSE SQUATS

Performance

Stand up straight with your heels together, toes angled out very slightly. Your arms should be straight out in front of your chest. This is the start position (fig. 31). Bend at the knees and hips until your hamstrings are resting on your calves and you can go no further. Your chest will be pressed into your thighs (fig. 32). Do not raise the heels. To prevent yourself from tipping backwards, you may have to flex your shins to pull your toes up so that you ease forwards. Return to the start position using leg power only.

Exercise X-Ray

Close squats have all the benefits of *full squats*, but with an amplified effect on the quadriceps. Over time, this exercise really strengthens the knees, shins, and gluteal muscles, tightening up the butt better than any machine.

Training Goals

- Beginner standard: 1 set of 5
- Intermediate standard: 2 sets of 10
- Progression standard: 2 sets of 20

Perfecting Your Technique

Many trainees who have rushed through the earlier steps often experience problems with the *close squat*. The biggest problem is the tendency to overbalance and fall back in or near the bottom position. This tendency will be amplified for tall athletes with long thighs. The problem is caused by a lack of strength in the frontal shin muscles, combined with a lack of the correct equilibrium. If you have rushed the series so far, go back to Step 3 and follow the program properly. If you still have problems, go back to the *full squat*, and bring your feet an inch closer together every time you work out. Keeping your arms straight out in front will help throw your weight forwards. Holding a weight such as a light dumbbell, book or bottle of water in the outstretched hands will also help, but try to avoid this if you can. Some athletes really struggle with this exercise due to their structure. If this is you, completing this step with the heels one hand span apart is acceptable.

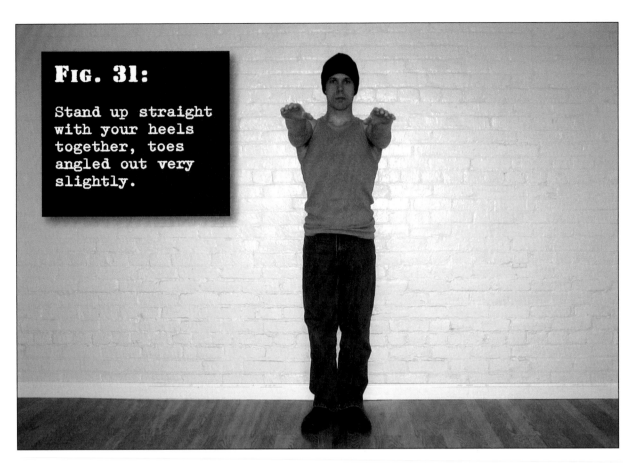

FIG. 31:

Stand up straight with your heels together, toes angled out very slightly.

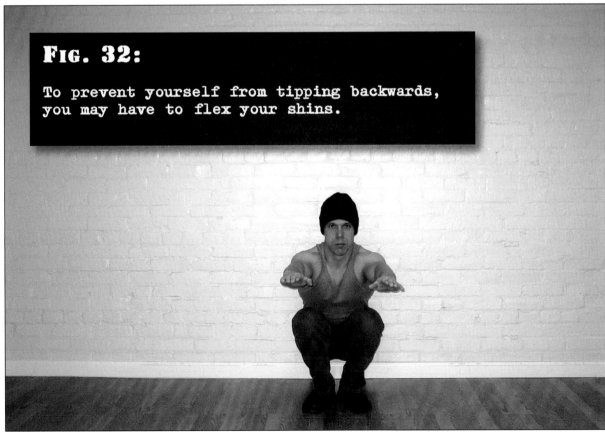

FIG. 32:

To prevent yourself from tipping backwards, you may have to flex your shins.

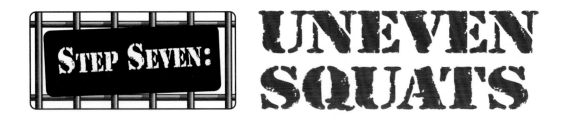

Performance

Stand up straight with one foot flat on the floor, and another resting firmly on a basketball located approximately one foot length in front of the other foot. The feet should be shoulder width apart or a little wider. Your arms should be out in front of you, directly opposite your chest. This is the start position (fig. 33). Bend at the knees and hips until the back of the thigh of your non-ball leg touches the corresponding calf. You will not be able to descend any further, despite the fact that your ball leg is not compressed as much. This is the finish position (fig. 34). While learning this position, you may tip backwards, so ensure that you have enough clear space behind you just in case. This applies to all deep squatting. Pause briefly, before pushing yourself back up to the start position with both legs. At no point during the exercise should you raise your heel, rock forwards or bounce, despite the fact that you may instinctively want to do these things at first. Use strength.

Exercise X-Ray

Uneven squats are the first big step towards mastering unilateral squats. Up until now, the effect of the steps in the squat series has been symmetrical; they have developed both legs equally. In this exercise, the leg on the ball cannot supply much power due to its raised position and the fact that it has to control the ball. The non-ball leg does most of the work, and acquires superior strength while still having enough help to push the athlete out of the difficult bottom position. The balance and coordination are also greatly improved as a result of this exercise.

Training Goals

- Beginner standard: 1 set of 5   (both sides)
- Intermediate standard: 2 sets of 10   (both sides)
- Progression standard: 2 sets of 20   (both sides)

Perfecting Your Technique

This exercise requires more skill *and* more strength than the earlier steps. If balancing on the basketball is a problem, use a stable alternative (e.g., three flat bricks) instead. If you still have trouble, use a lower object than the ball (e.g., one brick), and build up the height as you gain confidence and balance.

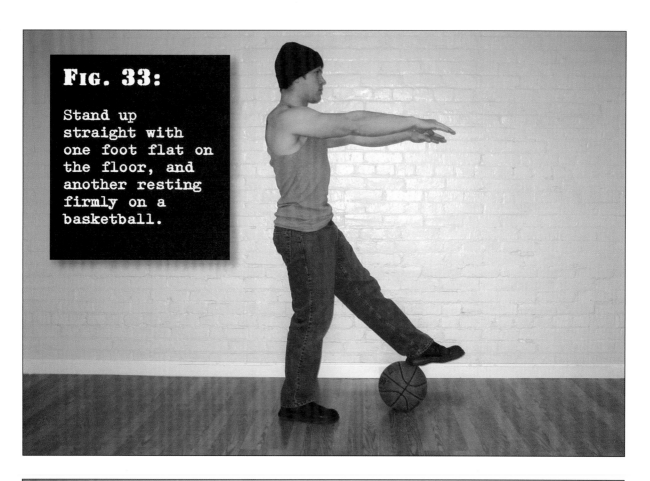

FIG. 33:

Stand up straight with one foot flat on the floor, and another resting firmly on a basketball.

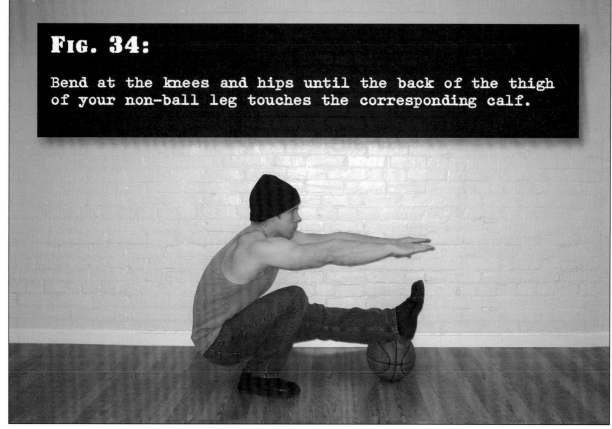

FIG. 34:

Bend at the knees and hips until the back of the thigh of your non-ball leg touches the corresponding calf.

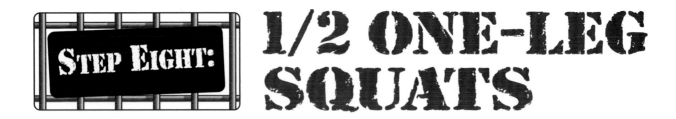

STEP EIGHT: 1/2 ONE-LEG SQUATS

Performance

Stand straight, with one foot flat on the floor, and the other foot up in the air in front of you. Your elevated foot should be at about the level of your opposite thigh, and the leg should be straight, or nearly so. Place your hands out in front of your chest. This is the start position (fig. 35). Bend the hip and knee of the leg which is supporting your bodyweight, until the knee is bent about ninety degrees. This will put your thigh approximately parallel with the floor. At this point, your raised foot should still be some way off the ground. This is the finish position (fig. 36). Pause for a moment under tension, before driving yourself up using the power of your single leg. Keep the back flat and the heel of your supporting leg on the floor at all times.

Exercise X-Ray

This exercise is the first full unilateral (one-limbed) movement in the series. It's an important stage to master, because it teaches the athlete the balance required before full *one-leg squats* can be attempted. It's during this exercise that the athlete also begins to learn the skill of holding the non-working leg above the ground for extended periods. This is not easy, and requires very strong hip flexors, muscles that are weak in most men. Because only one leg is moving the weight of the body, increased leg strength is developed—but only in the top range. For this reason, when the athlete is practicing this exercise, they should always follow it up with an exercise where a full range of motion is required; preferably *close squats* or *uneven squats*.

Training Goals

- Beginner standard: 1 set of 5   (both sides)
- Intermediate standard: 2 sets of 10   (both sides)
- Progression standard: 2 sets of 20   (both sides)

Perfecting Your Technique

This exercise should prove no problem to an athlete who has met the progression standard of *uneven squats*. If you still find it a challenge, just begin with a shorter range of motion, and gradually add depth over time.

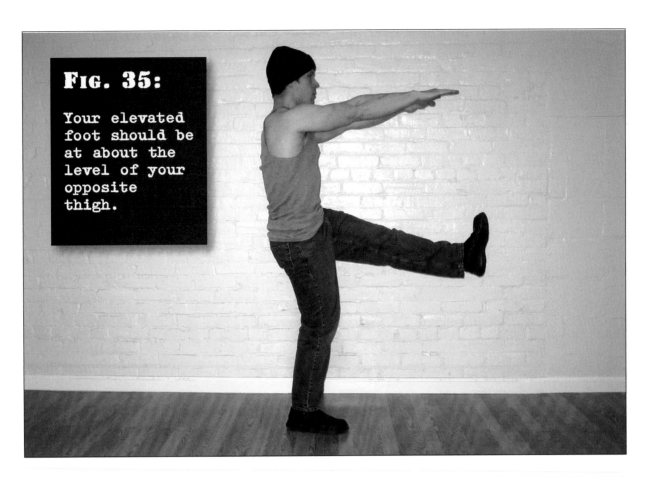

FIG. 35:

Your elevated foot should be at about the level of your opposite thigh.

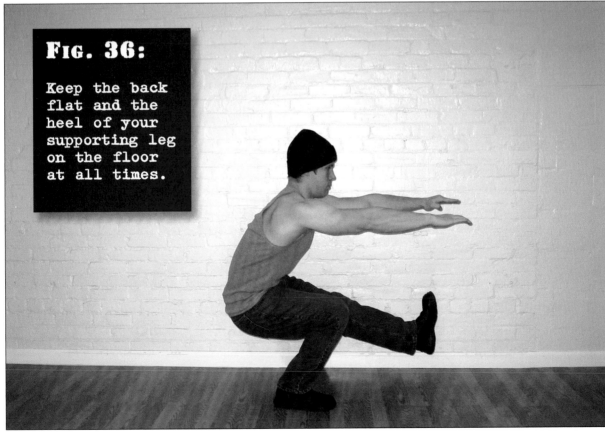

FIG. 36:

Keep the back flat and the heel of your supporting leg on the floor at all times.

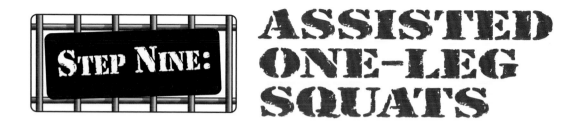

STEP NINE: ASSISTED ONE-LEG SQUATS

Performance

Place a basketball to the side of the foot of the leg you are planning to work. Stand up straight with one foot flat on the floor, and the other foot up in the air in front of you, as for *half one-leg squats* (Step 8). Place the arm corresponding to your raised leg out in front of you, and let your other arm hang by your side (fig. 37). Bend at the hip and knee of your supporting leg until your hamstrings meet your calf, and you cannot go any further. Place your hand firmly on the basketball. This is the finish position (fig. 38). Return to the standing position using mostly leg strength, but press down on the basketball to help you over the first few inches. Keep the heels flat.

Exercise X-Ray

The bottom position of any squatting movement is the hardest part, and this is true most of all for *one-leg squats*. This exercise will help you tackle the lowest position safely, by allowing your arms to help you through the crucial first few inches. This exercise will strengthen the knee ligaments and tendons, and allow the athlete to approach the Master Step—one-leg squats—with confidence. It will also force the hip flexors to work harder to keep the elevated leg higher than in *half-one leg squats*, and this may take some getting used to. Invest some training time in this important step.

Training Goals

- Beginner standard: 1 set of 5   (both sides)
- Intermediate standard: 2 sets of 10   (both sides)
- Progression standard: 2 sets of 20   (both sides)

Perfecting Your Technique

If you can't reach the beginner standard of this exercise, continue your unilateral training but try pressing off an object higher than the basketball. A chair seat or a low coffee table could be good choices. This will free your arms to provide more support over a longer range of motion than is possible when you use a basketball. Once you master the exercise with a higher object, work with progressively smaller objects until you are ready to try the basketball again.

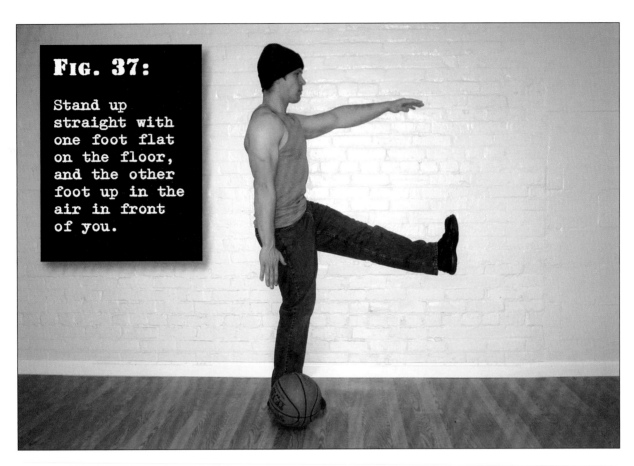

FIG. 37:

Stand up straight with one foot flat on the floor, and the other foot up in the air in front of you.

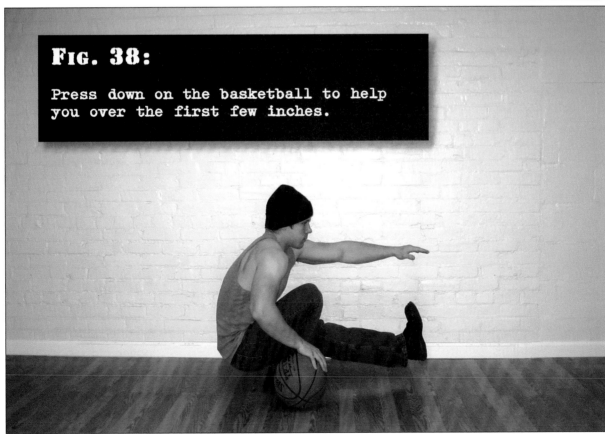

FIG. 38:

Press down on the basketball to help you over the first few inches.

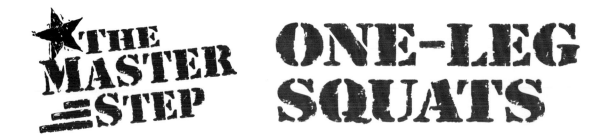

Performance

Stand tall. Raise one foot in the air, until it is approximately level with your hips. Keep your elevated leg as straight as possible. This will not be too difficult provided you have spent time mastering the previous steps. Place the arms directly out in front of your chest. This is the start position (fig. 39). Bend at the knee and hip of the supporting leg. Control your descent; do not allow yourself to just drop. Descend smoothly, until the back of the thigh of your supporting leg compresses against the calf and you cannot go any further. Your torso will also be tight against your working thigh. This is the finish position (fig. 40). Pause for a count of one, under tension. Push yourself back up to the start position using leg strength alone. There should be no momentum at all. Retain a straight back, hold the elevated foot off the ground, and keep the heels firmly on the floor. Pause at the top, and repeat.

Exercise X-Ray

The *one-leg squat* is the king of all squatting movements—in fact, it is the ultimate *lower body* exercise, *period*. It increases strength in the spine, hips, thighs, lower legs and feet, maximizes stamina and vastly improves athleticism. Over time, this exercise will transform skinny legs into pillars of power, complete with steel cord quads, rock-hard glutes and thick, shapely calves. The master of this movement will never lose the "spring" in his legs, and will be protected from all kinds of hip ailments and knee injuries.

Training Goals

- Beginner standard: 1 set of 5   (both sides)
- Intermediate standard: 2 sets of 10   (both sides)
- Elite standard: 2 sets of 50   (both sides)

Perfecting Your Technique

If you can't meet the beginner standard of *one-leg squats*, return to Step 9 (*assisted one-leg squats*) and use an object slightly *smaller* than a basketball—three stacked bricks, for example. Keep using progressively smaller objects to push against until you require no support at all.

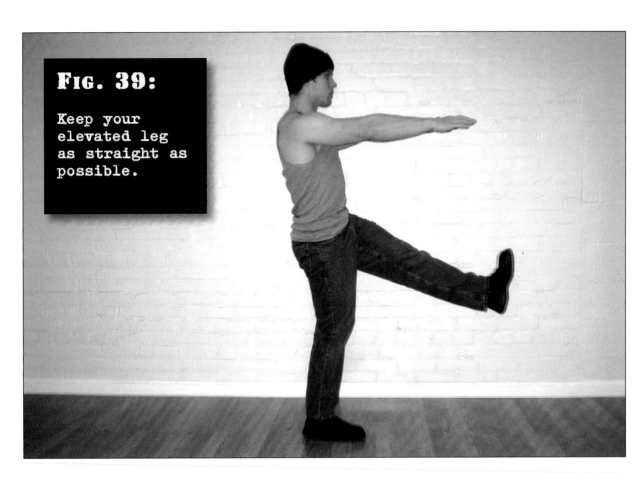

FIG. 39:

Keep your elevated leg as straight as possible.

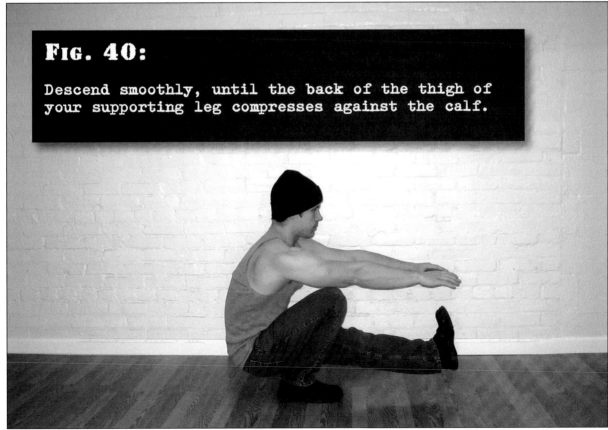

FIG. 40:

Descend smoothly, until the back of the thigh of your supporting leg compresses against the calf.

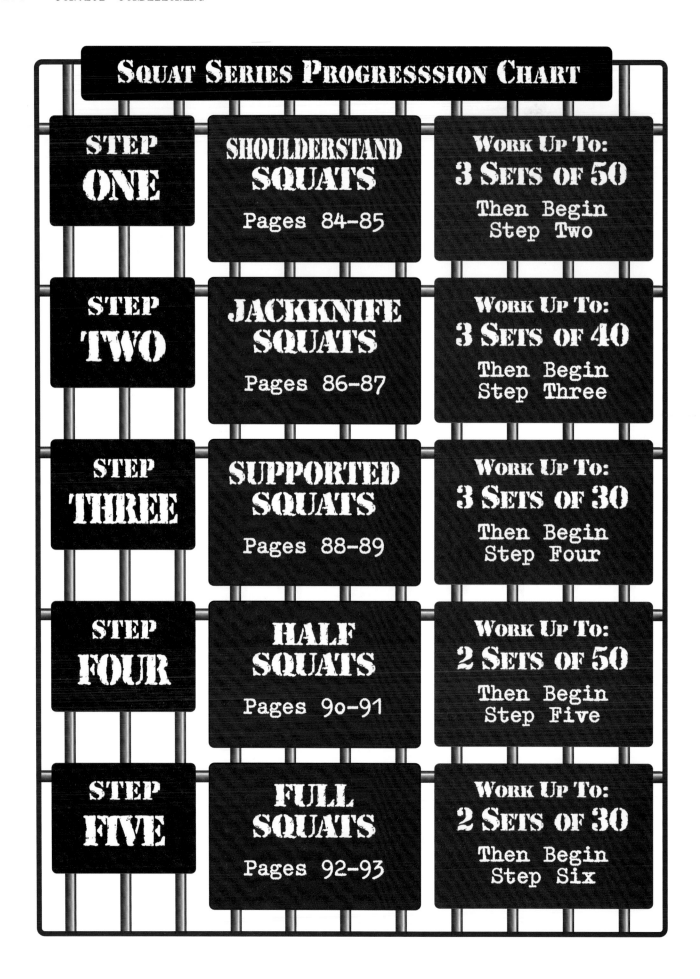

SQUAT SERIES PROGRESSSION CHART

STEP ONE	SHOULDERSTAND SQUATS Pages 84–85	WORK UP TO: 3 SETS OF 50 Then Begin Step Two
STEP TWO	JACKKNIFE SQUATS Pages 86–87	WORK UP TO: 3 SETS OF 40 Then Begin Step Three
STEP THREE	SUPPORTED SQUATS Pages 88–89	WORK UP TO: 3 SETS OF 30 Then Begin Step Four
STEP FOUR	HALF SQUATS Pages 9o–91	WORK UP TO: 2 SETS OF 50 Then Begin Step Five
STEP FIVE	FULL SQUATS Pages 92–93	WORK UP TO: 2 SETS OF 30 Then Begin Step Six

SQUAT SERIES PROGRESSSION CHART

STEP SIX	CLOSE SQUATS Pages 94–95	WORK UP TO: 2 SETS OF 20 Then Begin Step Seven
STEP SEVEN	UNEVEN SQUATS Pages 96–97	WORK UP TO: 2 SETS OF 20 Then Begin Step Eight
STEP EIGHT	1/2 ONE-LEG SQUATS Pages 98–99	WORK UP TO: 2 SETS OF 20 Then Begin Step Nine
STEP NINE	ASSISTED ONE-LEG SQUATS Pages 1oo–1o1	WORK UP TO: 2 SETS OF 20 Then Begin Step Ten
MASTER STEP TEN	ONE-LEG SQUATS Pages 1o2–1o3	ULTIMATE ENDURANCE: 2 SETS OF 50

Going Beyond

Once you master the *one-leg squat*, take a little time to build up your reps. This is good advice that should be followed for all the Master Steps. The ability to perform multiple strict reps guarantees muscular fitness and control. How far you choose to go is up to you. I've met convicts who could crank out more than a hundred reps of this exercise—several times throughout the day! I've also broken the triple-digit mark in my time, and could have kept going but I found very high rep squats boring. Provided you are committed, relatively young (under sixty) and not obese, fifty reps per leg is an impressive and achievable long-term goal. It's certainly fifty more reps than the average bloated bodybuilder could ever achieve.

Okay. Let's say you get to the stage where you can do fifty one-leg squats with perfect form. Well done! Were do you go from there?

The knee-jerk ('scuze the pun) reaction is to look for ways to get stronger and stronger. This is certainly how bodybuilders and powerlifters think; those guys are constantly working out ways to add another wheel to each side of the bar, or increase their hack squat and leg press weight. In some cases this quest can go on for a very long time—the legs have a natural capacity to get very strong. The tendons of the legs are naturally powerful, and the thighs and hips contain muscle cells in abundance, a factor that can be easily exploited in the drive for greater strength. Man-mountain powerlifter-turned-wrestler Mark Henry can squat *nearly a thousand pounds* without a lick of support gear. Not to be outdone, the ladies also have the capacity to build extremely powerful gams. Women can rarely match men in terms of upper body strength, but they can be capable of huge leg strength because their hips and thighs are naturally well developed for childbirth. American girl Becca Swanson—the strongest woman on the planet—has squatted well over eight-hundred pounds—despite weighing a hundred and forty pounds less than Henry. Strong legs on women is nothing new. Before the Middle Ages when oxen were scarce during furrowing season, the farmer would handle the plough—controlling it with his strong upper body and arms—while his wife literally pulled it through the soil, using her strong legs and butt.

So—assuming you've already reached the expert level in your one-leg squatting—I'm about to tell you how to get stronger and stronger, right? Spill lots of secret prison-guarded tips and tricks for building more and more power in the legs? Wrong. I'm all about strength, but in the case of the lower body I think the instinct of endlessly adding resistance is a mistake. Of course, it's easy to add weight to the one-leg squat if you want. The old school strongmen did it all the time. Just grab a dumbbell and hold it to your chest, or slap a barbell on your back (see the photo below). Training this way, Bert Assirati could do one-leg squats with two-hundred pounds. American female shot-putting champ Connie Price-Smith has used two hundred and forty-five pounds in the exercise.

Big figures look impressive, but in reality they are often associated with injury. *All* serious powerlifters are constantly plagued by knee and back problems. Most have to go under the knife sooner rather than later, and the majority are crippled into old age because they have whittled away their knee joints and vertebrae in the quest for ponderous poundages.

Don't be misled by the idea that strength is everything. For a prison athlete, *function* is everything. Where the legs are concerned, *mobility* is more important than strength. Once you have developed the strength to perform unilateral squats, you'll have piston-like legs and your joints will be incredibly powerful. Further resistance work will give you chunkier thighs, but you won't necessarily gain in athleticism. The next stage—if you haven't started already—is to learn to *use* your lower body strength. Explore stair sprints, jumping, car pushing, etc. (see the *Variants* section). These will add conditioning, speed, agility and endurance to legs that are already awesome. Don't get blinded by big numbers in your leg training journey

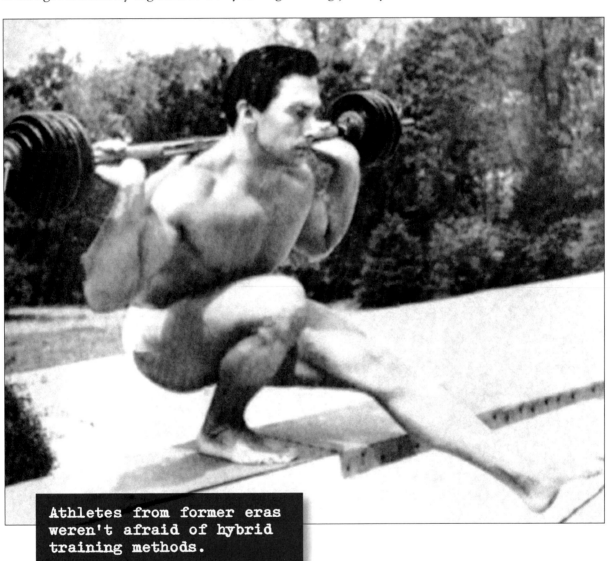

Athletes from former eras weren't afraid of hybrid training methods.

Variants

In bodybuilding, a great deal of emphasis is placed on different leg and foot positions during squatting or leg pressing, in the belief that different postures develop different parts of the quads. It's thought that a wide stance develops the inner quad, whereas a close stance works the outer quad; toes out works the teardrop by the knee, heels raised works the *rectus femoris*, and so on. In reality the four heads of the quadriceps tend to work as a group—the difference made by distinct stances or foot positions are relatively minor. Weird stances and angles place the knees and hips in unnatural positions and will hurt your body sooner rather than later. When doing squats, find a posture that is strong and comfortable for you, and stick with it. If you are looking for variety, don't mess about with your squatting formula; try a distinctly different movement like the ones given below.

Lunges

Lunges are a classic squat substitute. Stand with your feet together, and take a long step out in front of you. Bend at both knees, keeping the spine straight, until your front knee is bent at a right angle and your rear knee nearly touches the floor. Now rise back up, pushing through your feet until your knees are straight. At this point you can either continue the motion into a step backwards to the starting position and repeat, or step forwards and through with your rear leg so that you can lunge ahead, switching legs. Obviously confined to a cell we didn't have much space, so we stepped back to the start position and alternated our legs, lunging forwards with the right, stepping back, lunging forwards with the left, and so on. But if you have a long stretch of space ahead of you, you don't need to keep going back to the start position. You can just keep on stepping forwards with your opposite leg. If your legs are in good shape, you can cover long distances this way. I once met a kickboxer who swore by this method. He didn't even count reps—he judged his workout by lengths of his local football field!

Leg Press Lunges

This is a nice variation of the lunge which focuses on one leg at a time. Place one leg up on something at about knee height. For me, a bunk is about right, but using stairs can help you find the best level for you. Experiment with different steps. Your raised leg should be out in front of you, with a minor bend in the knee. Now—keeping your back straight—bend at the knee and hip of the raised leg, until your hamstring presses against your calf. At this point, your thigh should be close to your chest. You can bend the knee of the rear leg a bit to ensure that you are secure, but the main motion should come from the front leg. Pause for a moment before pushing back up again with your front leg until it's back to where you started. This motion looks like a kick, but obviously a lot slower and smoother. Complete your target reps, and then switch legs. A few hundred reps will sear delicious pain into your quads the next morning.

Sissy Squats

Grab something sturdy with one hand, for support. Stand up straight with your feet together or nearly so, and bend at the knees, keeping the hips locked straight. This will require rising onto your toes, and applying a mild backwards lean of the torso. At first this exercise is tricky, because you want to bend forwards at the waist, but eventually you'll get the hang of it. Most of the force is transmitted through the knees, so never bend them more than ninety degrees. At first, even this depth may seem impossible, so work up to it. Pause at the bottom, before pushing back to the start position and repeating. This is an unusual technique, and beyond simply adding reps, it's hard to make the exercise progressive. But it's a useful exercise to have in your training arsenal—sissy squats don't involve any significant bend at the hips, so it's a good way to keep the quadriceps conditioned while recovering from a lower back injury. There seems to be some dispute as to how this exercise got its name. Most sources seem to think it's because the leverage works against the muscles, making even a strong man feel like a sissy, but my mentor Joe Hartigen swore that the exercise was named after the Greek king, Sisyphus. According to mythology, Sisyphus was condemned to roll a huge boulder up a hill every day for eternity, only to be doomed to watch it roll back down as dusk arrived. Unfortunate. Bet he had great thighs though.

Hindu Squats

This is an exercise used by Indian wrestlers for centuries. With your feet shoulder width apart or a little wider, drop down onto your haunches, raising your heels as you do so. Immediately—with no pause—push yourself back up using leg power, rocking back on your heels as you go. This rocking movement back and forwards on the heels generates a kind of see-saw type rhythm as your center of gravity shifts forwards and back, up and down. This rhythm in turn encourages greater speed, greater explosiveness than in usual squats. Unlike regular squats, this ballistic performance is actually a core element of Hindu squats. Finding a way to gently swing your arms in tune with the movement will help cultivate and maintain the rhythm. Don't pause at the bottom or the top—to get the motion right, you need constant movement. There are good and bad pints about Hindu squats. On the down side, Hindu squats are no replacement for the regular squat series, because the only way you can make them progressive is by adding reps. This develops stamina, but not strength. In addition, the momentum used during the natural rhythm may irritate the knees of some athletes. On the plus side, the rhythmic nature of Hindu squats make them an excellent choice for a high rep alternative to running for those who wish to develop lower body endurance but with little floor space. They also provide great cardio benefits. If you chose to use them, work them into your program gradually, to allow your knee tendons to get used to the exercise.

Plyometric Jumping

Squatting develops muscular size and strength. But to be able to unleash this strength quickly, it's helpful to incorporate some plyometric work into your leg training once in a while. Fortunately, explosive leg training is easy—the legs are instinctively explosive during sprinting, hopping, kicking, etc. Perhaps the most focused form of plyometric training is *jumping*. Jumping is natural, safe, and can be done virtually anywhere. Plyometric trainees in gyms often use sturdy platforms for *box jumps*, which involve hopping up onto a box from a fixed stance. You really don't require any equipment to do plyometric jumping though. In San Quentin my first cellmate taught me a technique he learned in the military called *dead leaps*. Just place your feet together and dip quickly, before jumping forward as far as you can. Keep your feet together as you land, and try not to topple forwards or the jump doesn't count. This is actually harder than it looks, as people normally take a run-up—at least a step or two—before they jump anywhere. When jumping for explosiveness, emphasize *power* rather than high reps. Warm up, and repeat the jumps for two or three sets of four to six reps—that's all you need. As you progress, you'll naturally jump further. We marked the cell floor with a piece of chalk, and tried to beat our own records every week. If you run out of space (this is easy to do in a cell), begin doing your dead leaps with just a single leg. Stand on one leg and dip down, before jumping as far as you can. You need to land on the same foot you pushed from and land without falling otherwise the jump isn't valid. If you enjoy unilateral work, you can also experiment with box jumping using one leg. This advanced exercise involves jumping out of a one-leg squat onto a box (see the photos below), but don't even attempt this unless you have super-healthy knees. Traditional *high jumping* and *long jumping* are also good athletic training, but to me, dead leaps are the best jumping technique because they also teach balance and control—and without these, explosive power isn't as useful.

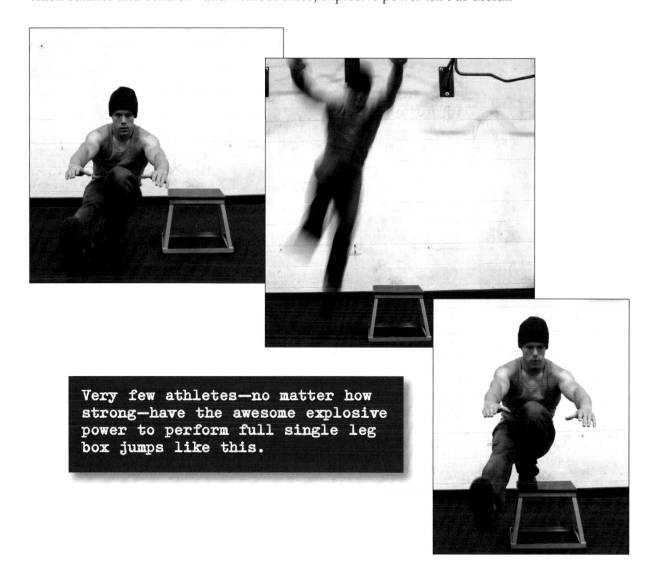

Very few athletes—no matter how strong—have the awesome explosive power to perform full single leg box jumps like this.

Stair/Hill Sprints

This was never an exercise I was able to get into in prison, but I have spoken to guys who swear by incline sprinting. Find yourself a big, ugly flight of stairs. One storey in a house isn't enough—try the stairs in a big apartment building, or preferably the stairs in a sports arena between events. The more intimidating the better. If you live in the country and can't find arena stairs, a nice steep hill will get the job done just as well. Starting at the bottom, just run up the incline. How easy is that? The answer is—*not easy at all*. Whether on stairs or a hill, carrying your bodyweight quickly upwards is incredibly demanding on your energy systems. After just a few seconds you are gasping to get your breath, and before your know it your legs are full of lactic acid. By the time you get to the top of the stairs (if you make it), your legs will be like jelly and you'll feel lucky to be alive. Whatever you do, *don't* run back down—your exhaustion will diminish your coordination and control, making a nasty tumble a possibility. Walk down instead. Over time, you can improve your performance by bettering your time or doing more laps of the stairs. Stair sprints are popular with combat athletes; it was the previous generation of UFC fighters—champs like Maurice Smith—who brought this old technique back to the attention of the training public. Many athletes practice this method instead of barbell squats, because it generates maximum lower body endurance with little risk to joints if done properly. It seems to have a lot of promise, and I regret not having access to big stairs when I was at my peak. Give it a try, but be warned—it's very intense and may well make you puke if you go too hard too soon.

Car Pushing

When I was a kid I saw a Dick Butkus interview where he talked about developing his awesome power for football by pushing a two-ton vehicle around when he was in high school. As a result, I became obsessed with the idea of pushing cars. It seemed like something only Superman could do. Whenever I got the chance, I would push my mom's scratched up Ford Maverick a short way along the block. My arms were like spaghetti when I was a kid and it took forever to get a few yards, but man was it a satisfying feeling! I don't follow the Chicago Bears much any more, but as soon as I got out of prison I quickly rediscovered my love of car pushing. Find a clear stretch of road or track, turn off your engine and stick your whip into neutral (you might experience a little trouble if you keep it in gear). Get round the back of your car and put your palms on the metal of the trunk—you don't want to be putting a load of force through a glass rear windshield just in case. Keep your arms nearly straight and lean into the movement as much as you can. Push away with your legs. Once you get over the vehicle's inertia, pushing gets a little easier. But not much. You'll have to push off your toes as you go, and this is fantastic for the calves. The legs get a massive workout, but so does the back, midsection, chest, shoulders and arms. Build up to pushing the car one hundred yards, if you can find a free strip that long. Measure the distance using strides— a hundred long steps will be about right. When you can do this, time yourself. Do the stretch two or three times once or twice a week, and try to beat your best time whenever you can. This builds *dangerous* levels of strength-athleticism! Car pushing is a phenomenally functional leg exercise, because it teaches you to transmit all the power you developed though squatting right through the body. Pushing this way helps your muscles understand how to express large forces, and this is useful in wrestling, martial arts, football and pretty much all truly athletic sports. It'll help if you get cornered by a couple of enemies in the yard, too.

Fireman Sprints

This is an intense method of sprinting that requires a training partner. Bend down and press your shoulder into your buddy's waist. As he doubles over you, stand up straight, hoisting him clean off the ground. This will have his head down around your back, with his feet dangling around your thighs. Hook your nearest arm around his legs for stability. This is the classic *fireman's lift*. From this position, run as fast as you safely can to a fixed goal about a hundred yards away. Then place your partner back on his feet, and have him carry you back. Repeat this torture on alternating sides for as many cycles as you can stomach. Like stair sprints and car pushing, this exercise is great for heart and lung capacity, cardiovascular stamina, leg metabolism and total body energy generation. It's an interesting and demanding technique, but—like any exercise involving external loads—there are inherent risks. Warm up well, wear solid boots to protect your ankles and retain mental focus throughout the exercise. This method isn't only popular with fire-fighters; it's also used extensively by bodyguards and close protection specialists, who might have to carry a client out of a dangerous area quickly.

7: THE PULLUP

BARN DOOR BACK
AND MAJOR GUNS

No matter what your opinion of bodyweight training, there's no denying it—*pullups are cool.* Who wasn't inspired watching Sylvester Stallone, jaw clenched, performing *uneven pullups* from that climbing frame in *Rocky II*? Perhaps my personal favorite example from the movies was the sight of a very lean and mean Linda Hamilton cranking out pullups from the legs of her upturned metal bunk in *Terminator 2*. I can remember, years back when I was new to prison, seeing a grey-haired black veteran inmate doing one-arm pullups from the door of his cell, and vowing that one day I would learn how perform such a seemingly impossible technique.

Human beings have *always* been attracted to pullups as a feat of strength. It's nothing new. In fact, the pullup is the oldest muscle-building exercise in existence. Evidence of pullups in ancient history are easy to find; several classical writers described the technique, which was popular with warriors, athletes, and even civilians who wanted to retain excellent levels of strength. Despite this, it's impossible to date the origin of the exercise, because in a sense it undoubtedly predates the human species. Evolutionary scientists tell us that prior to evolving into *Homo sapiens*, our distant ancestors were almost definitely tree-dwellers, just as chimpanzees and many other great apes still are. For the forerunners of humanity, pulling yourself up into the branches of a tree would have been as natural an event as taking a step is for us today.

Given this amazing anatomical heritage, it's surprising that the average trainee gives so little thought and attention to his back muscles. Go to any gym in the world, and you'll see guys (even intermediate athletes, who should know better) endlessly working their torsos with bench presses and other chest exercises, with only a few easy sets of rows or machine work thrown in for back, almost as an afterthought. Perhaps this is partly because it's so difficult to see the back muscles in a mirror—we tend to forget them. But I think culture also plays a part. Men are taught from a young age that being masculine involves *pushing*; we push against objects to show our dominance over them; we push and punch during combat, to defend ourselves; when times are tough, we *push forwards*, we *press on*; we even *psychologically* push other people away, to retain our personal space. It's women who are taught to *pull* things towards them—children, other people, their friends. Men are supposed to be more independent—strength means pushing things away!

Benefits of the Pullup

Maybe that last idea is a perceptive insight into the cultural anthropology of exercise techniques. Or maybe I'm just a guy who's spent way too much time alone in his cell thinking about pushups and pullups. Maybe a little of both. Who knows? But whether you buy my theory or not, there's no denying that the upper body pulling muscles are totally underrated by most athletes. When we think of torso muscles, we might think initially of a big chest, or broad, round shoulders. Although these pushing muscles are certainly important, they are positively puny in comparison with the musculature of the upper back—the *pulling* muscles. The largest muscles of the human torso are the *latissimus dorsi* (often known as the "lats") which run from the armpits down beyond the ribs, and which span out around the back like opening fans. Most of the other back muscles are worked by pullups, such as the *trapezius, rear deltoids* and the *teres* and *rhomboids* around the shoulder blades, but the lats definitely get the lion's share of the work. Not only are these muscles big, they are also astonishingly responsive—it's as though the muscle cells of the lats are genetically preprogrammed to get big and strong when stimulated. Take a look at a modern bodybuilder posing, and the most impressive muscles are not the arms or legs but the lats; a lot of these guys have lats that practically look like wings. Even hard-gaining bodybuilders who find it incredibly difficult to add beef to their chests discover that as soon as they start training their lats properly, they become bigger almost overnight. It's as if these muscles are major tools utilized by our forefathers, lying dormant yet faithfully waiting to explode into growth when called upon.

Sadly when trainees do actually devote time to training their backs, the exercises used are often unsuitable. They bend over with heavy weights to do barbell and dumbbells rows, exercises that place enormous pressures on the lower vertebrae of the spine. These techniques inevitably lead to injury and stiffness. Perhaps this is why machine exercises have recently become the number one choice for back training. Options here include cable rows and pulldowns, as well as more obscure and elaborate seated units. Why has machine work become so popular? Because it's easy! The back can be pumped up in relative comfort and with lighter weights. Unfortunately, because it's easy, machine work seldom delivers much by way of results unless the bodybuilder is already jacked up on large doses of steroids. These guys can get away with doing powder puff exercises and still get pumped up like balloons. Not *strong*—just pumped up.

Forget all these alternative exercises other people are doing in the gym. You really don't need them. The best—and *safest*—exercise to build a powerful upper back is the humble *pullup*. It really *is* the king of back exercises for the reasons given earlier—the human body has *evolved* to pull its own weight upwards vertically. We don't often have to do this in the modern world, but the genetics we are born with don't realize that. Master the pullup, and your lats will expand like crazy; the muscles around your shoulder blades will take on the appearance of coiled snakes, and your traps will get thicker and harder than iron girders. Every pulling muscle in the torso gets its share of work from pullups, and they get bigger and stronger as a result—fast.

Without doubt, pullups will give you bigger muscles quicker than any other torso exercise in existence. But this is really only a pleasant side benefit of the real gift of pullups, which is *functional strength*. A good friend of mine was a former Marine Drill Instructor. He once told me that every season, at least a few of his new recruits were big, heavy bodybuilders who usually thought that they were tougher than they really were. A lot of these men could do pushups all day, but when you asked them to pull their bodyweight up—maybe over a wall on the assault course, or during rope climbing—these guys often struggled and totally choked compared with smaller men. This is purely because modern bodybuilders tend to rely on weights to build their backs up. They neglect bodyweight work and as a result they lack the functional qualities so necessary for agility.

That vital attribute of true strength, the grip, also gets a hell of a whipping from pullups—holding onto that bar as you move your bodyweight up and down will give you fingers and palms much stronger than the average guy, even if you do no specific grip training. The flexor muscles on the forearm also benefit and become more powerful. Believe it or not, pullups even give the abs and hips—which, in daily life, are not used to holding both legs off the ground—a great isometric workout. Beginners who attempt the exercise often have stomachs that are sorer than their lats the next day.

Big Biceps

Even bodybuilders will concede the back-building benefits of the pullup, but few people these days seem to know that pullups are also the best *biceps* exercise known to man. Most modern trainees stick to exercises like curls to work the biceps, but in reality—no matter how much weight you use—curls are *isolation* exercises, because they only work the muscles through a single joint, the elbow joint. Pullups are a *compound* exercise. They work the biceps through *two* joints, the elbow *and* the shoulder. This is how the biceps has naturally evolved to work, and as a result this small arm muscle is very powerful when worked in this way. Think about it—if a 200 lbs. man does pullups, his biceps are working with 200 lbs. through a full range of motion. How many people do you know who can do strict 200 lbs. barbell curls? If the same man goes on to master the one-arm pullup, he is lifting 200 lbs. with *one biceps muscle*—the equivalent of curling a 200 lbs. dumbbell in the gym! It's no wonder gymnasts have gargantuan, melon-sized biceps! If you really want to unleash your full biceps strength and size potential, forget the curls. Get doing pullups.

The Safest Upper Back Exercise

The fact that humans were practically born to do this exercise also means that it's the *safest* back exercise in existence, because the movement works *with* your natural biomechanics, not *against* them. This is an important point, because (due to dangerous exercises) back training causes more injuries than any other type of training in the gym. Most of these injuries are suffered by the lower back, but lower back injuries caused by *pullups* are unheard of. The reason why is simple—because the legs are hanging during pullups, there is no external pressure on the spinal column. The lower and upper back retain their natural curves, locked into place by the spinal erector muscles which run up either side of the spine.

When performed consistently and correctly, pullups *protect* the body against injuries. On most lifters, the *anterior deltoid* at the front of the shoulder is artificially strong due to an over-attention to pressing movements in the routine. This results in an imbalance within the shoulder girdle, leading to injuries and the stiff, unnatural movements so common to bodybuilders. The pullup is the best exercise known for the *posterior deltoid* at the rear of the shoulder; adding progressive pullups to a routine will quickly iron out any imbalance and render shoulder function smooth and harmonious again, preventing future shoulder injuries. If they are worked correctly, pullups generate healthy joints and result in hardly any injuries—a claim that cannot be made for other forms of back training!

Pullups vs Chinups

A lot of new trainees get confused about the difference between a *chinup* and a *pullup*. For example, some coaches claim that a pullup must be done so that the chest is lifted all the way to the bar, whereas in a chinup only the chin goes over the bar. In Europe, the term chinup is used *instead* of pullup, although they mean exactly the same thing. In some places in the US both terms are used interchangeably. I've met ex-football players who swear that a pullup is done with an overhand grip, whereas a chinup is done with an underhand grip. There seems to be no universal agreement. No wonder people get confused.

In *Convict Conditioning* a pullup is *any* exercise where you pull the torso towards the hands against gravity, so the term casts a pretty wide net. But don't get too hung up on terminology. The names you use aren't as important as correct execution of the exercises.

The Ideal Range of Motion

The ideal range of motion for strength when you lift your bodyweight up to the bar goes from a point where your arms are nearly straight (but slightly kinked) to a point where your chin passes over the bar. Pulling up beyond this point—until the chest or even the sternum touches the bar—takes the lats out of the movement and emphasizes the weaker muscles between the shoulder blades. It limits strength potential and puts the upper body in a vulnerable position. Doing pullups until your chin passes the bar is best.

The slightly kinked elbow position at the start position serves two major functions. Firstly, it takes the pressure off the elbows, preventing them from becoming hyperextended. Secondly, it helps you brace your upper body for the powerful movement required. Despite what some bodybuilding pundits tell you about the motion, you should *never* relax into a full stretch in the bottom position of the pullup. Doing so will take the stress off your muscles and place them on the ligaments which hold your joints together. This is *not* what you want. Not only should you keep your elbows bent by about ten degrees in the bottom position, bracing your upper body also requires that you keep your shoulders "tight."

"Tight" Shoulders

To keep your shoulders safe in *all* hanging exercises, it's of vital importance that the athlete understands the importance of keeping the shoulders tight.

The shoulders are ball-and-socket joints. This kind of joint is incredibly versatile in terms of motion, but that versatility comes at a price—increased vulnerability. If you relax your shoulders while you are hanging from an overhead bar, the ball joint becomes stretched in the socket, and is only held in place by inflexible ligaments. This practice not only causes the ligaments irritation under great force, it can also result in partial or complete shoulder dislocation in some cases. This is rare, but it does happen, particularly where there is pre-existing injury. Keeping tight shoulders cradles the joint in a dense network of muscles, protecting the internal ligaments and making dislocation virtually impossible.

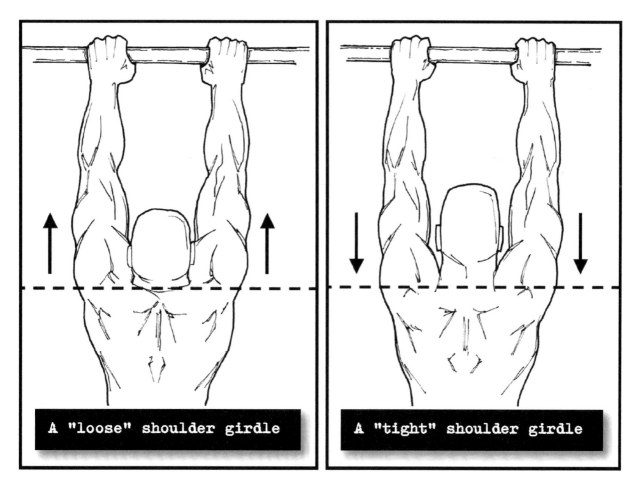

A "loose" shoulder girdle   A "tight" shoulder girdle

Hanging techniques—particularly pullups and leg raises—are fantastic exercises you should be enjoying throughout your career, so start practicing good form right from the beginning. Tightening your shoulders isn't a dramatic movement; from the outside, it's barely noticeable. All it involves is a downwards pull of your shoulder socket by an inch or two. (Check out the drawing above for an illustration.) This is easily done by firmly flexing the lat muscles. Keep your entire upper body braced as your proceed, and you'll soon get the knack.

Hanging Tough

Another point of contention on pullup form is *grip position*. You have *overhand* grip (knuckles facing you) *underhand* grip (i.e., curl grip), *hammer* grip (thumbs facing you)…Which is best?

It depends. The most important factor to consider is something kinesiologists call *pronation*. Pronation basically means *turning back*. In the context of the pullup it describes the phenomenon where your hands automatically try to turn inwards—palms turning down—the closer you pull them towards your body. This is a very small natural movement we all have. It might seem quite minor, and it usually doesn't interfere much with standard pullups, but it becomes more of a factor the further you progress through the pullup series.

The take home message is that during early steps you can use any kind of grip you find easiest. The exercise descriptions usually illustrate an overhand grip, as this is strongest for most people, but an underhand or hammer grip is also acceptable. As you progress beyond the *full pullup* however, the natural tendency to pronate may make a fixed position uncomfortable. If this is the case, experiment. Often a hammer grip feels stronger and more natural as the exercises become harder. Those with strong biceps who don't feel much of a pronation effect will prefer an underhand grip. Some athletes feel happier with an overhand grip throughout their careers and experience no problems. Use whatever seems to help you.

The best possible kind of grip for more advanced pullup techniques involves a hanging ring— the kind you see gymnasts use. They are ideal because the flexible rope they are attached to naturally allows your hands to pronate as much or as little as they want to during the movement. Solid bars lock your hands in place, limiting this kind of fluid motion. If you experience nagging wrist, elbow or shoulder problems during pullups, learning to use hanging rings can eliminate these problems by helping the arms find their natural groove during the exercise.

"Kipping"

Pullup movements should be performed using muscle strength rather than momentum. But if you lack the strength, you'll tend to kick upwards with your knees to give you the momentum to complete a rep. There's a special name for this kind of cheating technique—*kipping*.

Kipping puts unnecessary stress on the joints, gives a false sense of strength and encourages sloppy form. For that reason, it should never be used by beginners, who should stick with perfect form—two seconds up, a one second pause then two seconds down, followed by another one second pause. No momentum should be used. If you need momentum to do your reps, drop back down to easier exercises where you can complete your reps without cheating.

Once you become stronger at pullups—when you can do Step 5 without cheating—then you can begin to productively use kipping in your workouts. Do as many reps as you can strictly—at least three or four—then use kipping to generate the power to do another one, two or even three reps. This will allow you to push past your normal barriers and develop more muscular stamina than you otherwise could. But *don't* overexploit this technique, and *don't* use kipping as a substitute for muscular power. Only ever use kipping at the end of a set. Never the beginning.

Remember, when you are looking to progress to the next step in the series, the only reps you should count towards your progression standard should be reps where you don't use kipping.

Hanging Out

Prior to the nineteenth century, a lot of cells—especially local Sheriff's jails—were basically cages. As a result, they had roof bars. The convicts in the eighteenth century had no problem doing pullups off these. Gradually the bars fell out of favor due to increased suicide risk, and now convicts are mostly forced to do their pullups on the welded pullup/dip station out in the yard. You'll need to find somewhere, too. The human body is remarkably adaptive, and if you pay attention you'll find you can do pullups almost anywhere—from a rafter, a tree branch, a rugged heating pipe, even the edge of a roof or balcony (see page 145). If you want to be able to work out at home, I'd advise investing in a pullup bar to fit between doorframes. These are cheap and can be found in many stores. Something a bit higher—like a pipe strung from a roof—is even better, because you don't have to worry about pulling your feet up high. Another handy custom pullup station can be made simply by laying a metal bar or cylinder across the top of a loft hatch. This can also be an excellent place to savor some sneaky leg raises.

Given the opportunity, the best pullup tools are parallel hanging rings, as mentioned above. You can buy these, but provided you can find solid rings that'll fit your fist, you can make your own. Just loop a rope through each ring, and find somewhere robust to hang them.

Bodyweight and Pullups

Unlike most of The Big Six: exercises—pushups, for example—pullups require that an athlete moves the *total* weight of the body. This means that every extra pound you are carrying has to be lifted through every inch of motion during the exercise. The reality of the situation is that the more overweight you are, the harder it will be to progress through pullups. Pure *muscular* weight is no barrier to mastering the ten steps, but if you are more than thirty pounds overweight due to useless *fat*, your chances of getting beyond Step 5 or 6 are vanishingly small unless you possess freakish strength, or are cheating on the movements. If this applies to you, don't worry. Follow the ten steps of the pullup as far as you can, then remain working on the exercise you get up to. Put as much effort into that exercise—as well as the other Big Six movements—as possible, while you diet off the extra weight. You'll get there.

Serve Your Time

The pullup series is more challenging than most of the other movements of The Big Six:, largely because the entire bodyweight is moved by the upper body. As a result, it will inevitably take the athlete longer to progress through this series than, say, the pushup series (where only a proportion of the bodyweight is used) or the squatting series (where the powerful lower body muscles do the lifting).

Moving more slowly through the pullup series is normal. Once you are really working hard, it may sometimes take months to move from one step to the next. This mustn't be seen as a negative thing. Remember that you only *appear* to be moving slowly because the forces required are very impressive; this means that every little advancement you make translates into a very significant increase in ability. Focus on that, rather than the passage of time.

Don't ever feel the urge to rush from exercise to exercise, step to step. This is advice that applies to *all* your bodyweight work. Never forget that moving up to bodyweight exercises which are placed higher in a series simply *demonstrates* your strength increases. But those strength increases are only actually *built* through dedicated, repetitive work on the lower exercises in the series. Rushing won't build strength faster.

The most successful calisthenics athletes understand this fact. They don't hurry to move from exercise to exercise before they are ready. This path ultimately leads to failure and disappointment. Instead, they learn to love whatever movement they are occupied with at the time. They study it, become absorbed by it, master its nuances. They really dedicate time and energy to that exercise—as if it's the last one they'll ever do. They are patient, giving their bodies the time required to build real strength. When the time comes, you can bet they'll be ready to move to more advanced work. If you can cultivate this attitude, you'll get a lot further a lot *faster* in the long run.

The Pullup Series

Many people—particularly the overweight—approach pullups with enormous dread, as a supremely difficult exercise. If you are one of this group, don't worry. Once you begin training in the correct technique, your body adapts and actually gets good at the early exercises quite quickly; it's as if your muscles "remember" their heritage, and rapidly figure out what they are supposed to do.

Part of the fear of pullups these days is due to a misunderstanding—or *incomplete* understanding—as to their nature. When people talk about pullups, they generally only think of one exercise—*full pullups* (i.e., the full, two-handed pullup). When beginners try this exercise, it seems impossible, unless they are either abnormally strong or extremely skinny and light. Because of these early experiences, a lot of trainees steer clear of the pullup, and stick to lifting weights when training their backs so as not to embarrass themselves. This is a big mistake. In reality, there are numerous pullup movements—not just the one everybody knows. To be sure, some of these exercises are *harder* than the full pullup, but some are also much *easier*.

The *Convict Conditioning* system contains ten types of pullup movement. The classic full pullup is Step 5 in the series. Rather than jumping in at the deep end with the classic full pullup, the student of this system slowly works his way through the four steps which go before it. Each of these steps gradually increases the pulling strength of the athlete, and by the time he is ready for the full pullup, it won't seem nearly as intimidating as it otherwise would have. For many it will seem easy. When the student has mastered the full pullup, the journey is not over, however—there are a further five steps, culminating with one of the most coveted and admired strength feats of all time—the *one-arm pullup*.

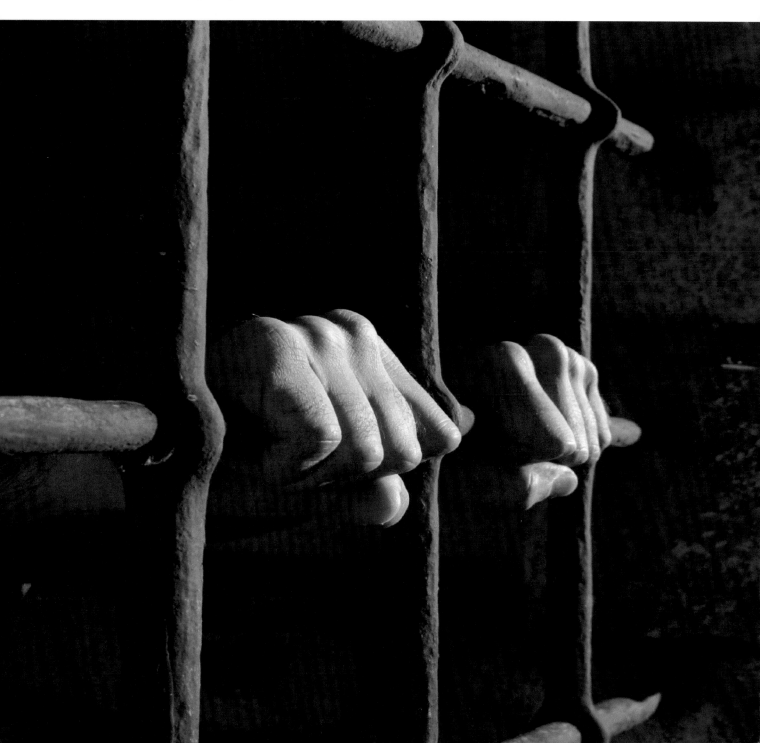

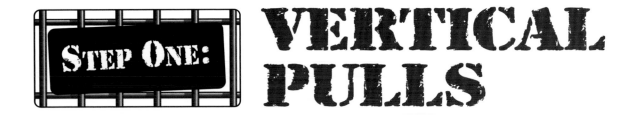

Performance

Find a vertical base you can hold on to. This base should be secure and allow you to grip it safely; a doorframe or high railings are excellent potential candidates. Stand close to the base—the tips of your toes should be between three and six inches out. Take hold of the object in a comfortable grip. Ideally your hands should be shoulder width but any symmetrical position will suffice. This is the start position (fig. 41). Because of your proximity to the base, your arms will be well bent. Now allow your bodyweight to shift back by leaning slightly. Extend your arms as you go, until they are very nearly straight, and your body is angled diagonally backwards. This is the finish position (fig. 42). At this point you will feel a gentle stretch in your upper back, and possibly your arms. Pause momentarily before pulling yourself back to the start position, by contracting the shoulder blades and bending the arms simultaneously. Pause and repeat.

Exercise X-Ray

Vertical pulls are a very gentle exercise. They are ideal for athletes rebuilding their back and arm strength, particularly following on from a shoulder, biceps or elbow injury. They increase blood flow and re-train the pulling "groove." This is also an excellent exercise for any beginner. Its low intensity allows athletes new to pulling to really feel the muscles at work in the shoulders and upper back, before things get too heavy.

Training Goals

- Beginner standard: 1 set of 10
- Intermediate standard: 2 sets of 20
- Progression standard: 3 sets of 40

Perfecting Your Technique

This should be an easy exercise that virtually everybody should be able to do. If you are in rehabilitation from an injury and you find the motion too severe on an involved area (perhaps you have stitches), simply reduce the range of motion, tighten the shoulders, and don't extend your arms as far.

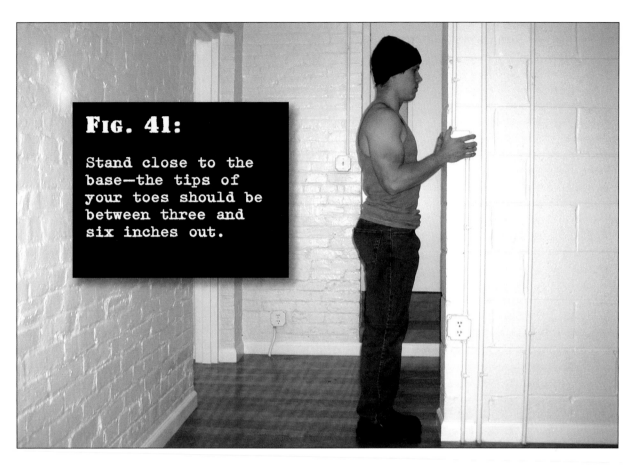

FIG. 41:

Stand close to the base—the tips of your toes should be between three and six inches out.

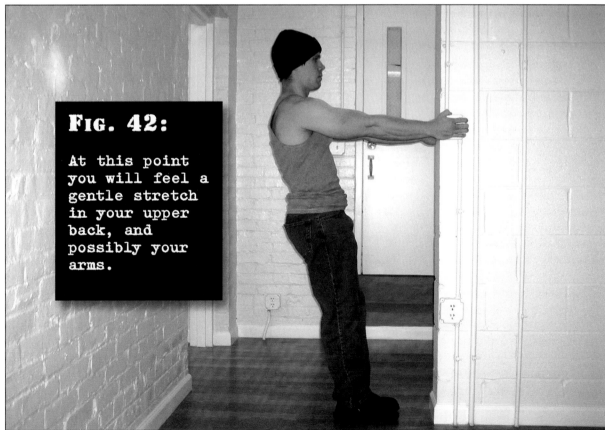

FIG. 42:

At this point you will feel a gentle stretch in your upper back, and possibly your arms.

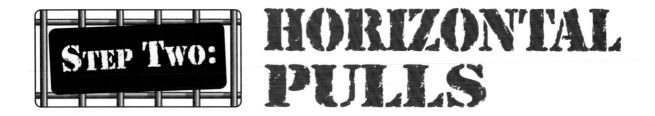

Performance

Find a horizontal base you can hold onto which will safely carry your bodyweight. It needs to be at least as high as your hips. The top of a big, sturdy, table or desk is usually the best option. Get down so that your chest and lower body are underneath the table and reach up so that you can hold the lip, using an overhand grip. Ideally your hands should be shoulder width but this will not always be possible depending upon what kind of table or desk you have access to. Now pull yourself up so that your back is off the floor. Depending upon the height of the table, your arms will probably have to be slightly bent for this. Keep your body tensed and locked straight, so that its weight goes only thorough your hands and heels. This is the start position (fig. 43). Now smoothly pull yourself up, keeping the body (especially the knees) aligned, until your chest touches the lip of the table at the point where your hands are gripping. This is the finish position (fig. 44). Pause for a count of one, before lowering back to the start position. Repeat.

Exercise X-Ray

Horizontal pulls are similar in theme to *vertical pulls*, but they place the body at a much more severe angle. As a result, the strength is tested more intensely. This is an excellent intermediate exercise to master before the athlete begins the hanging work on the horizontal bar which follows. This movement conditions the joints, significantly the vulnerable elbows and shoulders.

Training Goals

- Beginner standard: 1 set of 10
- Intermediate standard: 2 sets of 20
- Progression standard: 3 sets of 30

Perfecting Your Technique

The higher the object you are pulling up to, the less extreme the angle of the body, and the easier the exercise. If horizontal pulls are just too hard for you at first, try to find something higher than hip height to pull yourself up to. Once you can do thirty reps, try pulling from the hip height base again.

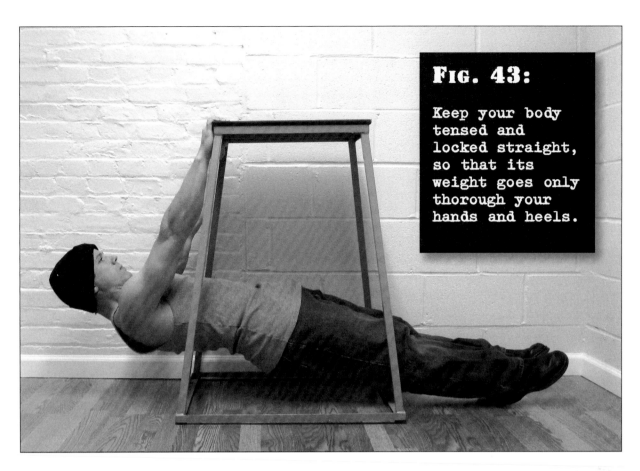

FIG. 43:

Keep your body tensed and locked straight, so that its weight goes only thorough your hands and heels.

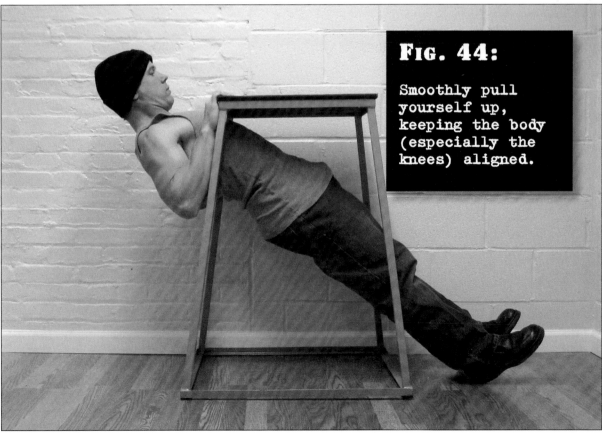

FIG. 44:

Smoothly pull yourself up, keeping the body (especially the knees) aligned.

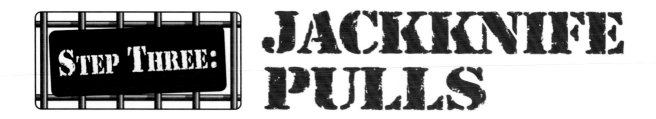

STEP THREE: JACKKNIFE PULLS

Performance

To perform this preliminary pullup exercise, you will require a high horizontal bar and a high-backed chair or similar object situated just in front of the bar. Jump up and grab hold of the bar. Your arms should be approximately shoulder width apart, in an overhand grip. When working with the bar, always keep your shoulders good and "tight" (see page 117). Don't fully relax your arms, either; keep them flexed and with a slight kink in the elbows. Now swing your legs up and rest your calves near the ankles on the back of the object you've placed in front of the bar. Arrange this object beforehand so that you'll be able to straighten your legs out. Ideally, the object should be high enough that the feet of your straight legs end up opposite your pelvis—the classic jack-knife angle. This is the start position (fig. 45). Now smoothly pull yourself up, using your straightened legs to assist you by pushing down with them. When your chin passes the bar, you are in the finish position (fig. 46). Pause before lowering yourself to the start position under full muscular control. Take care getting down when you've finished your set, and don't work to "failure." If your grip releases before your feet are directly below you, you risk falling and hurting yourself.

Exercise X-Ray

Jackknife pullups train the athlete in the basic full-range pullup motion, although this exercise is easier than *full pullups* because the legs take some of the weight and can provide assistance in the bottom position.

Training Goals

- Beginner standard: 1 set of 10
- Intermediate standard: 2 sets of 15
- Progression standard: 3 sets of 20

Perfecting Your Technique

The bottom position is the hardest portion of any pullup exercise. If you can't do full-range *jackknife pullups*, focus on the top position with the arms bent, and gradually add depth to your movement as you gain strength.

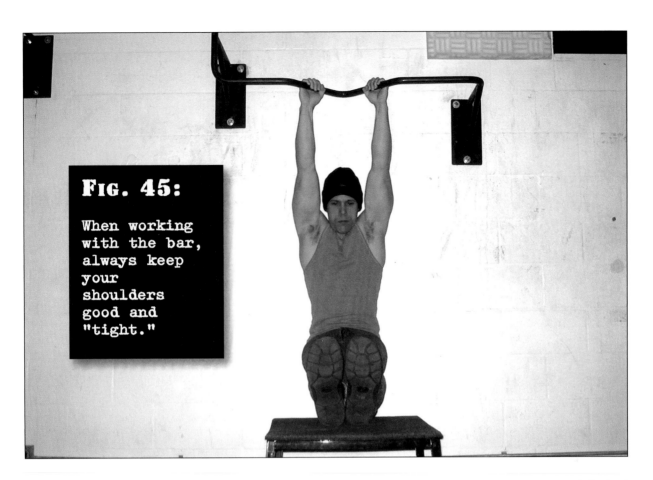

FIG. 45:

When working with the bar, always keep your shoulders good and "tight."

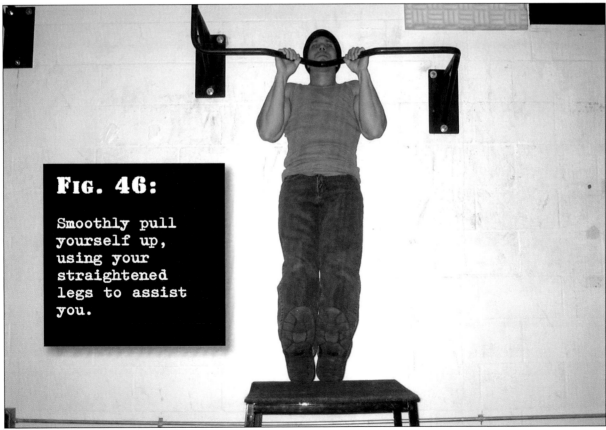

FIG. 46:

Smoothly pull yourself up, using your straightened legs to assist you.

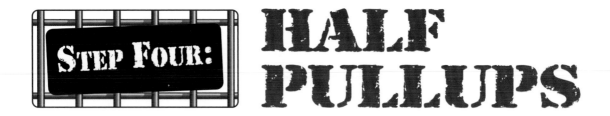

STEP FOUR: HALF PULLUPS

Performance

Take hold of a horizontal bar. The bar should be high enough that your feet are clear of the floor—even if only by an inch—when your body hangs down straight. Use an overhand grip which is shoulder width or a little wider. Jump up so that you are supporting your weight on arms that are bent approximately at right angles (your upper arms should be parallel to the floor). Keep your shoulders tight. Bend at the knees, looping one ankle over the other to take the legs out of the movement. This is the start position (fig. 47). Smoothly pull yourself up by bending at the shoulders and elbows until your chin clears the height of the bar. This is the finish position (fig. 48). Allow your elbows to travel forwards if it seems "right" for you. Pause at the top for a moment, before lowering to the start position under control. Repeat as needed. After you get set, keep the legs still throughout the entire motion.

Exercise X-Ray

Things are getting serious now. During *half pullups*, the upper body muscles exclusively move the entire weight of the body—certainly more than the average man can comfortably row or use on pulldowns. As a result the grip is strengthened and the back, biceps and forearms are developed.

Training Goals

- Beginner standard: 1 set of 8
- Intermediate standard: 2 sets of 11
- Progression standard: 2 sets of 15

Perfecting Your Technique

This is the first movement in the pullup series where the athlete is expected to move his full bodyweight through space without assistance. Consequently, it proves a sticking point for many trainees, particularly heavier or overweight guys. It's at this point when you need to start losing excess fat, if you have any—and most people do. You can still work on this exercise as you drop weight. If you find it difficult just reduce the range of motion, staying nearer the bar. As your weight decreases, your range of motion will increase.

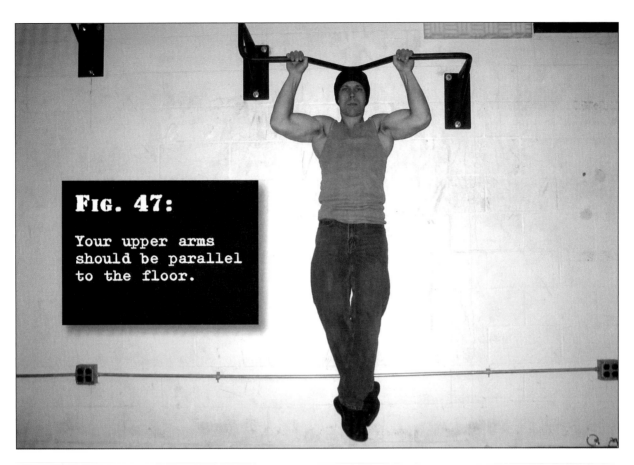

FIG. 47:

Your upper arms should be parallel to the floor.

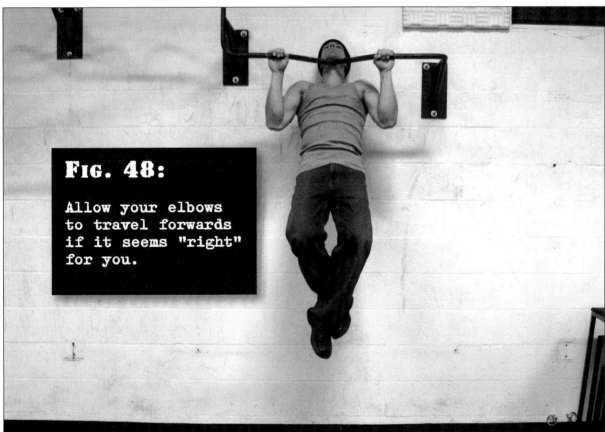

FIG. 48:

Allow your elbows to travel forwards if it seems "right" for you.

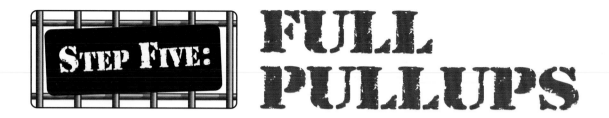

STEP FIVE: FULL PULLUPS

Performance

Grab hold of a horizontal bar with a shoulder width overhand grip. A slightly wider grip is acceptable—experiment to find out which width feels strongest for you. Bend at the knee and loop the ankles behind your body. Your feet should be clear of the ground. Tense the body, keep the shoulders down tight and retain a very slight (almost unnoticeable) bend in the elbows to take the stress off the arm joints and place it on the muscles instead. This is the start position (fig. 49). Bend at the elbows and shoulders until your chin passes over the bar. This is the finish position (fig. 50). Enjoy the view! Pause for a moment, before reversing the motion under full control. Don't be explosive—this means depending on momentum during the exercise. The perfect muscle-building technique is *smooth*. Try to take two seconds up and two seconds down, pausing for a second at the top and bottom.

Exercise X-Ray

The *full pullup* is the classic muscle and power exercise for the upper back and biceps. The master of this exercise will possess superior functional mobility and athletic strength. The human body evolved to pull itself up well—a man who cannot do pullups cannot be considered to be truly *strong*.

Training Goals

- Beginner standard: 1 set of 5
- Intermediate standard: 2 sets of 8
- Progression standard: 2 sets of 10

Perfecting Your Technique

Full pullups are a heavy calisthenics exercise. If you find them difficult, you are not alone. The key is perseverance. Resist the early urge to "kip" the body up (see page 118)—this will only ingrain the habit. Instead, help yourself out of the difficult bottom (extended arms) position by placing one foot on a chair and gently pressing down. Use less foot pressure every time you train, until eventually you are only using your foot through the first three or four inches. Eventually you'll be able to do full pullups unassisted.

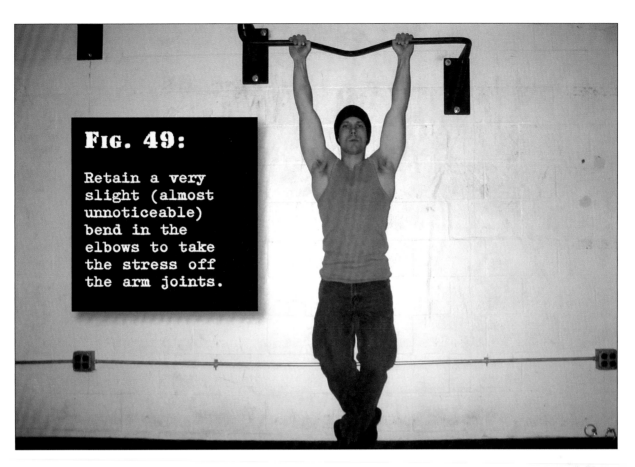

FIG. 49:

Retain a very slight (almost unnoticeable) bend in the elbows to take the stress off the arm joints.

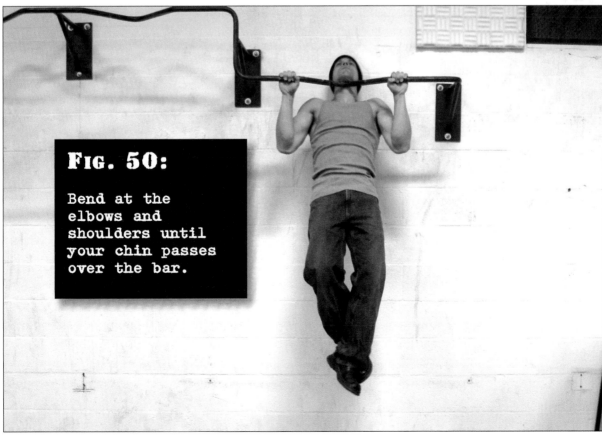

FIG. 50:

Bend at the elbows and shoulders until your chin passes over the bar.

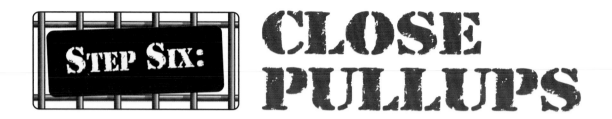

STEP SIX: CLOSE PULLUPS

Performance

Jump up and grab a bar with an overhand grip. Your hands should be next to each other—four inches apart at the maximum, if a very close grip irritates your joints. Bend at the knees with your ankles looped behind your vertical plane to keep them out of the motion. Kink the elbows very slightly and keep your shoulders tight. This is the start position (fig. 51). Bend at the elbows and shoulders to raise your body, slowly levering yourself up until your chin passes the bar. This is the finish position (fig. 52). Pause for a count of one, before slowly lowering yourself back down to the start position. Pause and repeat. Try to minimize leg movement during the set.

Exercise X-Ray

The weakest link in all pullup movements are the arm flexors—the biceps and related upper arm/forearm muscles. If an athlete has mastered two-arm pullups and wishes to progress to the single arm version, he will have to spend time radically strengthening his biceps. This is what *close pullups* do—bringing the hands nearer together puts the bigger, stronger back muscles at a disadvantage and forces more of the load on the arm flexors. Close pullups will force your biceps to grow larger and more powerful.

Training Goals

- Beginner standard: 1 set of 5
- Intermediate standard: 2 sets of 8
- Progression standard: 2 sets of 10

Perfecting Your Technique

Some athletes trained in the *full pullup* find this exercise difficult, because during *close pullups* the arms try to *pronate* (turn inwards) as you pull. Sometimes an overhand grip limits this natural twisting motion. This is a good time to experiment with your grip; try a side on, or underhand grip. Experiment with ring work if you can (see page 118). See what works for you. If strength is a problem, continue with full pullups, bringing your arms an inch closer every workout or so. Over time, you'll master the close grip.

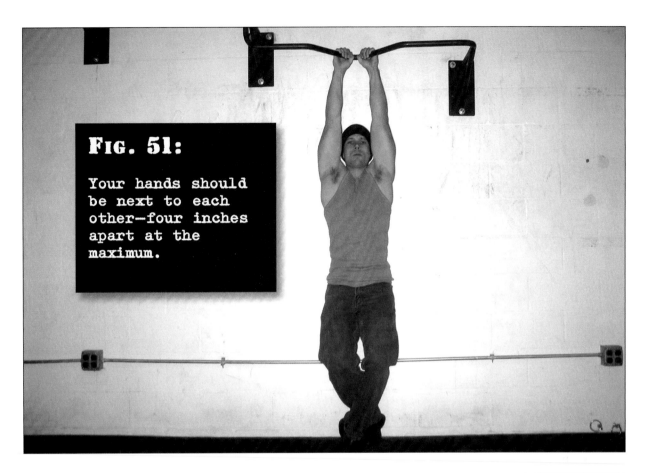

FIG. 51:

Your hands should be next to each other—four inches apart at the maximum.

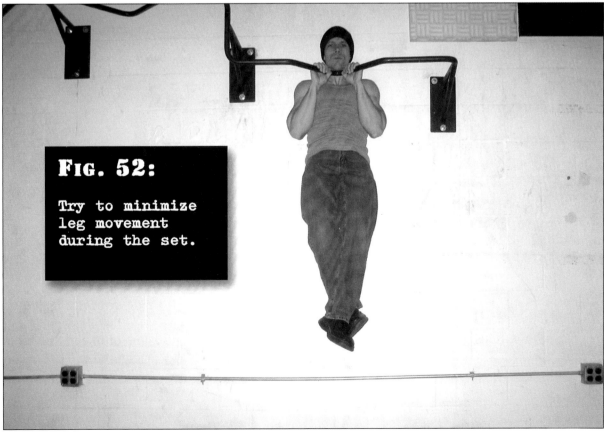

FIG. 52:

Try to minimize leg movement during the set.

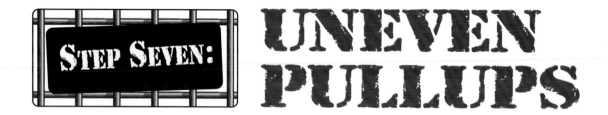

Performance

Grasp the horizontal bar with one hand. A side-on or underhand grip will be more comfortable than the classic overhand version. Now take hold of the wrist of the hand which is gripping the bar, using your free hand. The thumb of the hand holding your wrist should be just below your opposite palm, with the fingers below the back of your hand. Your feet should be off the ground, knees bent, with your ankles looped behind you. Your shoulder girdle should be flexed at all times. The arm that is holding the bar should be straight except for a slight kink in the elbow. Your other arm, due to its lower position, will be bent more acutely. Your elbows will be in front of your torso. This is the start position (fig. 53). Bend at the elbows and shoulders to smoothly pull yourself up until your chin is over the bar. This is the finish position (fig. 54). Pause at the top, before slowly lowering yourself back down to the start position. Pause again before repeating.

Exercise X-Ray

Uneven pullups go back centuries, but they were made instantly popular again when Sylvester Stallone performed them during the famous training montage of *Rocky II*. Due to the altered arm position, the arm gripping the bar has to do the majority of the work, preparing the athlete for the true unilateral pullup movements which follow in the series. The lats, biceps and back gain in strength as a result. The grip in particular gets a great workout.

Training Goals

- Beginner standard: 1 set of 5   (both sides)
- Intermediate standard: 2 sets of 7   (both sides)
- Progression standard: 2 sets of 9   (both sides)

Perfecting Your Technique

If you are strong enough to do *close pullups*, you should be able to do *uneven pullups*. The biggest difference is the fact that you have to hold your bodyweight with just one hand in this step. If you find this tough, devote some time to hanging one-handed after your pullups, to improve your grip.

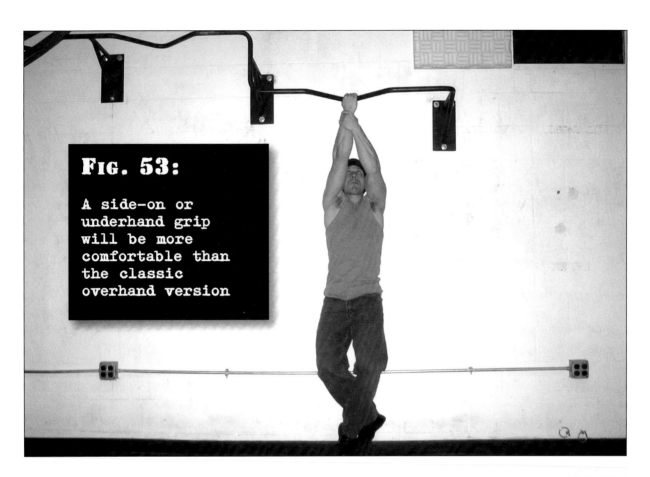

FIG. 53:

A side-on or underhand grip will be more comfortable than the classic overhand version

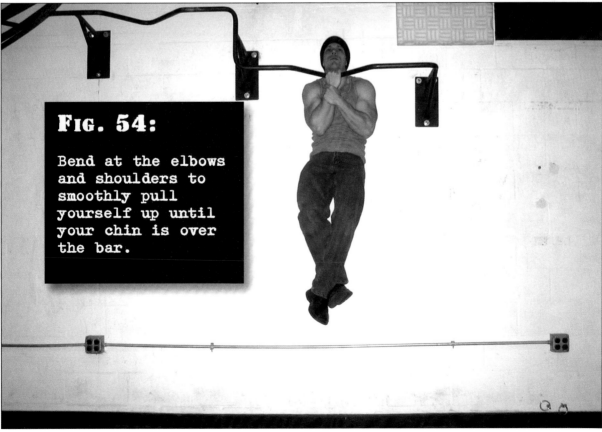

FIG. 54:

Bend at the elbows and shoulders to smoothly pull yourself up until your chin is over the bar.

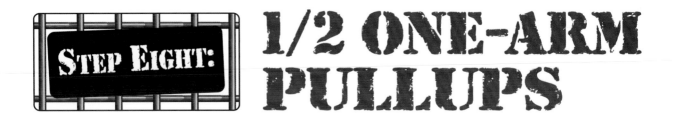

STEP EIGHT: 1/2 ONE-ARM PULLUPS

Performance

Grab an overhead bar with one hand, using your strongest gripping position. For some people, this will be an overhand grip; for others, side-on or underhand. Using a hanging ring is probably ideal for most people. Place your other arm anywhere that seems comfortable; most of my students like to leave it out to the side in mid-air, but I personally prefer placing it in the small of my back, as for *one-arm pushups*. Any position that doesn't interfere is fine. Set yourself (by jumping, kipping, using a chair, etc.) so that your lifting arm is bent halfway. The elbow should be at a right angle, with your upper arm parallel to the ground. Your feet should be clear of the floor and looped behind you as for previous steps. The shoulder of your lifting arm should be tightly braced, and your whole body flexed. This is the start position (fig. 55). Bend at the elbow and shoulder and smoothly pull your body up until your chin is over the height of the bar. This is the finish position (fig. 56). Pause at the top, before slowly lowering yourself back down to the start position. Pause at the bottom and repeat.

Exercise X-Ray

This is the first step in the series where the student pulls his total bodyweight with one hand. As well as teaching the balance and technical groove required for full *one-arm pullups*, it develops huge biceps and back power and builds big arms. It doesn't train the muscles in the stretched position though, so add a full-range motion such as *uneven pullups* or *close pullups* afterwards.

Training Goals

- Beginner standard: 1 set of 4   (both sides)
- Intermediate standard: 2 sets of 6   (both sides)
- Progression standard: 2 sets of 8   (both sides)

Perfecting Your Technique

The lower you descend, the harder pullups are. If you can't quite manage *half one-arm pullups* yet, focus on the top range of the motion, nearest the bar. Over time, add depth inch by inch until you can do this step properly.

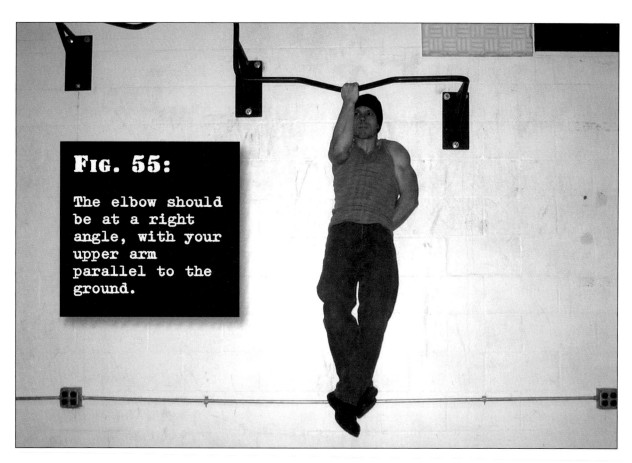

FIG. 55:

The elbow should be at a right angle, with your upper arm parallel to the ground.

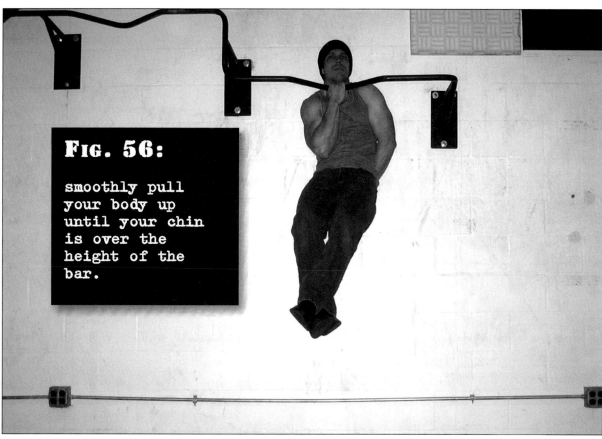

FIG. 56:

smoothly pull your body up until your chin is over the height of the bar.

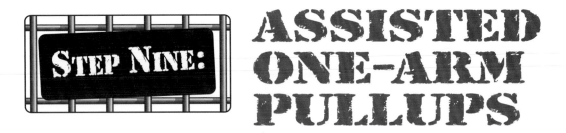

Performance

Throw a towel over a horizontal bar. Jump up and grasp the bar with your strongest grip so that the hanging towel is towards the inside of your hand. With your opposite hand, grab the towel as low as possible—around eye level is about right for most athletes. Bend the knees with the ankles looped behind the body. Keep the shoulders braced, and retain a slight bend in the arm which is holding the bar. This is the start position (fig. 57). Now begin to pull yourself up. For the first half of the movement—until the elbow of the arm holding the bar is bent at a right angle—assist yourself by pulling on the towel. Halfway up—when the elbow of the arm holding the bar is bent at a right-angle—release the towel, and continue pulling yourself up with just one arm until your chin is over the bar (fig. 58). Pause, before lowering yourself down using the power of your lone arm. When you reach the lowest position, grip the towel once again. Pause and repeat.

Exercise X-Ray

Assisted pullups are a specialized exercise. Their specific function is to help an advanced student "feel out" *one-arm pullups*, without getting stuck in the lowest position. This exercise slowly and safely builds the enormous levels of tendon strength required to correctly execute true one-arm pullups.

Training Goals

- Beginner standard: 1 set of 3   (both sides)
- Intermediate standard: 2 sets of 5   (both sides)
- Progression standard: 2 sets of 7   (both sides)

Perfecting Your Technique

The further your hand is down the towel or rope you use, the harder it is to provide assistance. If you have trouble getting five reps on this exercise, hold the towel nearer up to the bar. As you get stronger, hold the towel lower down. Eventually you will feel you are *pushing* down on the towel, rather than *pulling*. This is a great way to advance on *assisted one-arm pullups* and eventually prepare yourself for the Master Step—*one-arm pullups*.

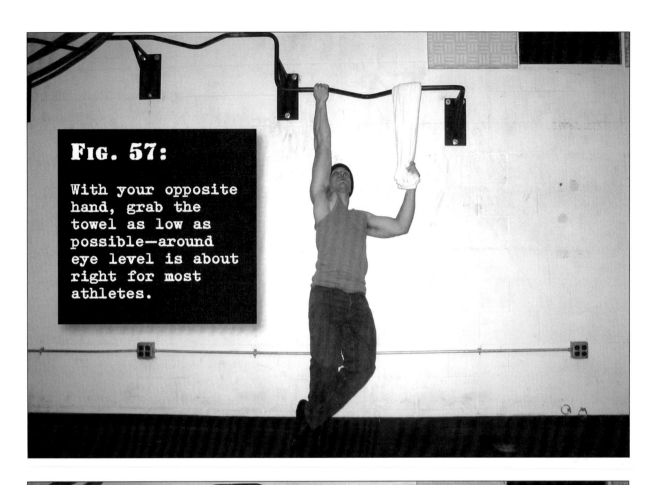

FIG. 57:

With your opposite hand, grab the towel as low as possible—around eye level is about right for most athletes.

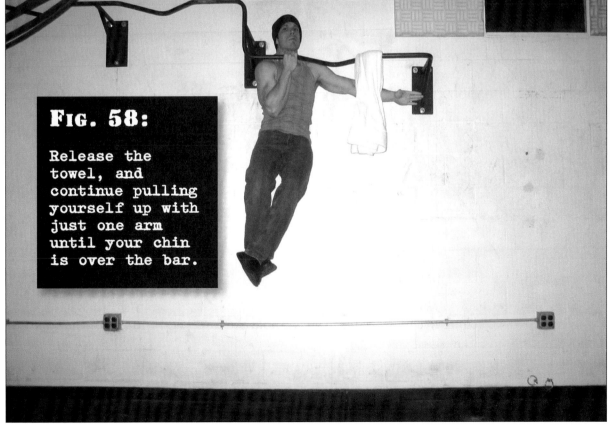

FIG. 58:

Release the towel, and continue pulling yourself up with just one arm until your chin is over the bar.

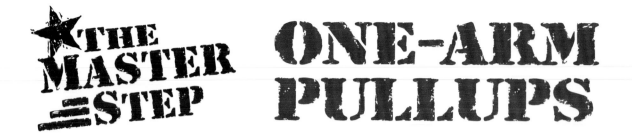

Performance

Jump up and firmly squeeze an overhead bar using your strongest gripping position. Your legs should be clear of the floor, with your knees bent so that your feet are behind you. Loop one ankle over the other to keep your legs still. Place your non-lifting arm in a comfortable position (you should have found your ideal position when you learned Step 8, *half one-arm pullups*). Your working shoulder should be set tight, and your body tensed for action. You are about to perform an advanced strength feat, and this should be reflected in your psychology. Your working arm should be virtually straight, with just a little kink in it to take the stress of the joints. This is the start position (fig. 59). Bend at the elbow and shoulder and pull your body up with as little momentum as possible until your chin is over the height of the bar. This is the finish position (fig. 60). Pause, and smoothly lower yourself back down to the start position. Pause at the bottom and repeat—if you can!

Exercise X-Ray

One-arm pullups, performed deeply and without "kipping" are the greatest back and arm exercise possible. They confer mighty strength *and* size. The master of this exercise will earn lats that look like wings and his upper back will be sprouting muscles like coiled pythons. Plus, he'll own a grip, arms and forearms *vastly* more powerful than the average gym rat—in fact he could probably rip a bodybuilder's arm off in an arm wrestling match.

Training Goals

- Beginner standard: 1 set of 1   (both sides)
- Intermediate standard: 2 sets of 3   (both sides)
- Elite standard: 2 sets of 6   (both sides)

Perfecting Your Technique

This is one *hell* of a hard technique, and although you *can* master it with dedication and effort, don't expect to do it overnight! Really take your time to milk the preliminary nine steps first. Initially, aim for just a single good rep, and practice *consolidation training* when you manage it (see page 268).

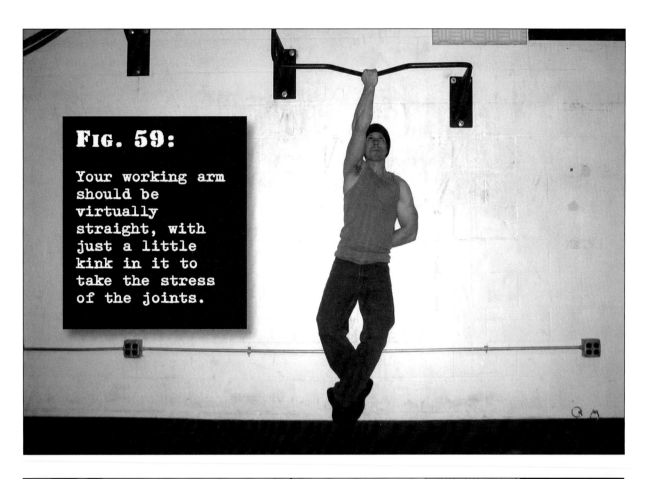

FIG. 59:

Your working arm should be virtually straight, with just a little kink in it to take the stress of the joints.

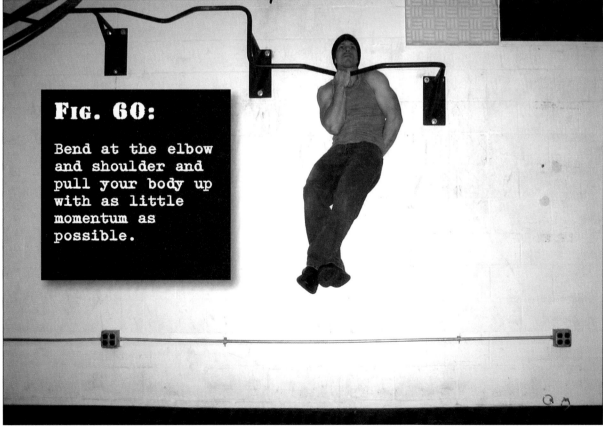

FIG. 60:

Bend at the elbow and shoulder and pull your body up with as little momentum as possible.

PULLUP SERIES PROGRESSSION CHART

STEP ONE	VERTICAL PULLS Pages 122–123	WORK UP TO: **3 SETS OF 40** Then Begin Step Two
STEP TWO	HORIZONTAL PULLS Pages 124–125	WORK UP TO: **3 SETS OF 30** Then Begin Step Three
STEP THREE	JACKKNIFE PULLS Pages 126–127	WORK UP TO: **3 SETS OF 20** Then Begin Step Four
STEP FOUR	HALF PULLUPS Pages 128–129	WORK UP TO: **2 SETS OF 15** Then Begin Step Five
STEP FIVE	FULL PULLUPS Pages 130–131	WORK UP TO: **2 SETS OF 10** Then Begin Step Six

PULLUP SERIES PROGRESSSION CHART

STEP SIX	CLOSE PULLUPS Pages 132–133	WORK UP TO: 2 SETS OF 10 Then Begin Step Seven
STEP SEVEN	UNEVEN PULLUPS Pages 134–135	WORK UP TO: 2 SETS OF 9 Then Begin Step Eight
STEP EIGHT	1/2 ONE-ARM PULLUPS Pages 136–137	WORK UP TO: 2 SETS OF 8 Then Begin Step Nine
STEP NINE	ASSISTED ONE-ARM PULLUPS Pages 138–139	WORK UP TO: 2 SETS OF 7 Then Begin Step Ten
MASTER STEP TEN	ONE-ARM PULLUPS Pages 140–141	ULTIMATE POWER: 2 SETS OF 6

Going Beyond

One-arm pullups are rare as all get out in gyms on the outside these days. They're practically extinct. But if you hang around a prison yard long enough, you might be lucky enough to still see this rare creature once in a while. You'll know when it happens; a kind of hush falls over the weights pit beforehand. Everybody who trains seriously knows the faces that belong of the masters of this technique, and they inevitably stop what they are doing to watch whenever these guys walk up to the pullup bar. Most of the weights guys—particularly the fat, ghetto bodybuilders—can only look on in awe and jealousy. Yep, one-arm pullups are considered an awesome feat of strength in any prison yard.

In fact, one-arm pullups are held in such high esteem in prisons—particularly West Coast penal institutions—that it almost feels like heresy to talk of *going beyond* the technique.

Once you've aced your first ever one-arm pullup—an amazing achievement in anybody's book—don't dance off looking for new back and biceps training techniques. Stay with the exercise and make sure you have a few reps under your belt first. To master the one-arm pullup for reps requires years of dedication, inherent talent and enormous proportional strength, not to mention maximum leanness. But it can be done. It's rare for bodybuilders to master the feat, however; their overemphasis on non-functional strength exercises and maximum body mass usually prohibits them from even getting past the intermediate stage of the pullup series. The ultimate master of one-arm pullups is probably India's Bhibhuti Nayak, and he's not even a strength athlete per se—he's a martial arts master. This sleek, unassuming-looking man recently astounded the world by performing *twenty-seven* perfect one-arm pullups in under a minute, smashing the world record as he did so. He gained his freakish power by training the way nature intended; not with machines or dumbbells, but by pulling his own bodyweight upwards.

If you can do more than two or three reps, and you are interested in experimenting with alternative methods, invest in a couple of hanging rings and look towards exploring traditional advanced gymnastics feats; techniques like the *iron cross*, the *Maltese cross* and the *front lever*. These might prove to be interesting and challenging new ways to move your bodyweight once you have mastered the one-arm pullups. They will teach you physical control, agility and extraordinary coordination, plus they look cool as hell. But if it's pure strength you're looking for, you really don't have to go beyond the one-arm pullups at all. It's the Big Daddy—everything you'll ever need.

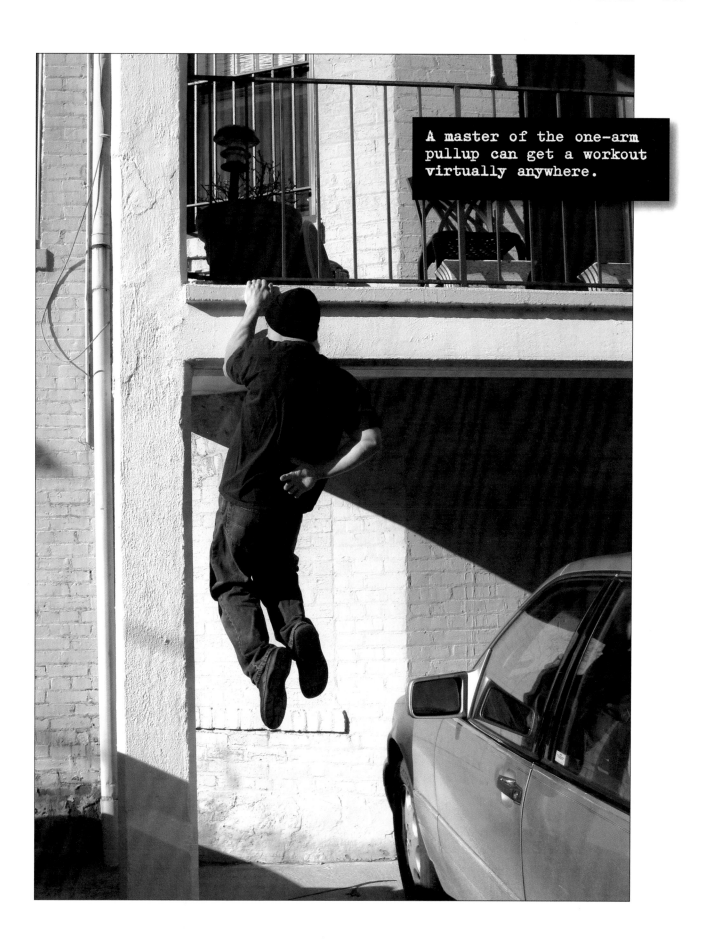

A master of the one-arm pullup can get a workout virtually anywhere.

Variants

When exploring alternative exercises to pullups, don't fall into the trap of using external loads such as free weights or back machines. External loads in motion lay the body open to injury and—particularly in the case of the pulling muscles—generate a kind of strength that is difficult to use in everyday life. Despite having less overall muscle mass than the legs, the back is the most complex bodypart. In muscular terms, it is usually divided into four quadrants: the spine (*spinal erectors, lumbar muscles*); the lats (the large *latissimus dorsi* along the side of the back); the upper back (*rhomboids, teres major* and *minor, mid-traps* between the shoulder blades, *rear deltoids,* etc.); and the upper traps (the large muscles of the neck/shoulder area). Rest assured that by the time you are doing both pullup and bridging movements in your program, *all* these muscles—and more besides—will be receiving maximum stimulation. No additional exercises are required. But if you want to add a new back exercise now and again for variety or when working around an injury, here are a few good ones to choose from.

Dips

Dips are usually considered to be an exercise for the pushing muscles, and it's true that they work the pecs and triceps hard. But because the arms strongly move downwards during the movement, the lats become significantly involved as well. In fact, I've met guys who get sorer lats from dips than from pullups. Grab some parallel bars—or position yourself between two chairs—and support your weight on straight arms. Bend at the shoulders and elbows until your elbows are at right angles, and pause for a moment before smoothly pushing back up. *Bench dips* (dips with the feet up on a stable surface) also work the lats, but to a lesser degree because the total bodyweight isn't moved.

Sentry Pullups

I'm a big believer that every student of bodyweight training should have at least one explosive movement in their arsenal for each bodypart. Sentry pull-ups are one of the best. Jump up to a chinning bar and do a full pullup. But don't stop at the top—keep lifting your torso up until it is over the bar, and then press your arms to lockout so that you are fully extended, with the bar at hip level. This should be performed as one fluid movement, and it will require some momentum to achieve. The explosive pullup works the back and biceps, and the circular transitional movement into a downwards press position very powerfully trains the elbows, wrists and forearms. The final part of the technique, the downwards press, works the same muscles as dips; triceps, pectorals and lats, mainly. Drop back down and repeat the exercise once your arms are straight. In the early days, you'll find yourself jumping hard to achieve the transition, but you'll do this less and less as you get stronger. In some circles, this exercise is called the *muscle-up*. In San Quentin, where I first learned this technique, the convicts called them "sentry pullups," although I've never heard the name anywhere else. I don't know for sure, but if I had to guess, I'd say that they were called this because it looks like the guy doing them is pulling himself up on something, to spy out into the distance. If I'm wrong and someone else knows the real source of the name, please write in and tell me.

Elbow Presses

This is an interesting, effective and little known exercise. Lie on your back on the floor, with your elbows down either side of you, a few inches out from your torso. Your forearms should be perpendicular to the ground, and your body must be locked straight, legs together. Now, if you push back hard through your elbows, you will—if you are strong enough—find that you can lift your body off the ground, holding your weight up only through your heels and elbows. At first, you will be barely able to clear the floor, but over time you'll be able to push your torso up to six inches off the ground. Your body must be held stiff, and only your elbows and heels should touch the floor as you rise. I've found that balling the hands into fists helps this movement for some reason. Lower yourself back down gently, and repeat for reps. Placing a couple of towels under the elbows will make the movement more comfortable. This exercise powerfully works the lats and mid-back, and the spine gets an isometric workout. It is essentially a rowing movement, but without the use of an external weight. Because nothing is held in the hands, only the back muscles move the load—the biceps and forearms are not involved. As a result, this is a brilliant exercise to use to keep your back muscles strong if you have injured an arm.

Bar Pulls

Convicts have been pulling on the bars of their cells to build strength for hundreds of years. If you are creative, you can use solid bars to give yourself a full body isometric workout. You might be surprised at what a versatile discipline bar pulling can be; I have a list of over a hundred bar pulling techniques in an old notebook somewhere. Bar pulls are an excellent method for training the back, so I'll limit myself here to a description of just one bar pulling workout for the back, consisting of a handfull of the best techniques:

Hulk pulls: Grab hold of two bars in front of your chest. Your forearms should be more or less parallel with the floor and your knuckles should be about six inches apart—the equivalent of one bar space. Your arms will be well bent so that your torso is only a few inches from the bars. This is the strongest bar pull position. Now pull as hard as you can, as if trying to pry the bars apart. This beauty works the arms and shoulders but especially the back muscles between the shoulder blades. When you get used to the position, you can generate a great deal of power in this pull. When you see the bars bending a little, you know you're heading in the right direction! Apply as much force as you can, breathing normally, for a count of five seconds. Take a ten second break, and repeat five more times.

Bow pulls: Grab hold of a single vertical bar with both hands. One hand should be approximately face level, the other chest level. Your arms should be nearly straight, but with a little bend at the elbow. As a result, your torso will be about two-thirds arm length from the bars. Now, push as hard as you can with the higher arm, whilst simultaneously pulling with the lower arm. The sensation is a little like the beginning motion of pulling back on a bow as in archery. Hold this push-pull tension for five seconds, before quickly reversing the dynamic; pull with your higher hand, push with your lower. Hold for five more seconds. Then take a ten second break before switching arms, so your lower arm is up highest, and the higher one is down lower. Repeat the above procedure. All this constitutes one cycle. Follow this process for another four cycles. The torque generated by the push-pull motion works the entire torso, and the varied arm position hits the lats nicely.

Crucifix pulls: Provided you have been working as hard as you can, by now your back will be sizzling. Time to deliver the final bullet to those aching muscles. Spread eagle your arms and grasp hold of the furthest bars you can comfortably grip. Press your chest up against the bars. Now—without moving at the elbows—pull directly backwards at the bars with all your might. In this position, the body won't be able to generate much force, but try hard anyway. If you're doing this right, you'll feel the small muscles of the back nearest your arms standing out, and cramping and burning. These muscles are the *rear deltoids*, and they are vitally important to strength in back training, as well as playing a major role overall shoulder stability. Hold this painful pull, squeezing the back muscles as hard as you can, for ten seconds. Pause for five seconds, before repeating. Do this exercise five times. Crucifix pulls are a brilliant finisher; although they will leave you sweating and in pain, they require no kit, and four cycles will take under a minute.

This is a good example of a compact isometric bar pull workout that hits the entire upper back. Isometrics can't replace calisthenics, but these techniques provide an interesting and productive change of pace once in a while. They go down like cold beer on a hot day. Once you get the hang of bar pulling, it's pretty easy to work out how to shift your grip positioning or body angle to work any muscle you want. Eventually you'll be able to pinpoint individual muscles with laser accuracy, giving them a specific, targeted training session any time you like. If you aren't locked into a cell with door bars, improvise. You can use window bars, the frame of a bunk, hot water pipes (wrapped with a towel), even doorframes or the corners of a room in some cases. If you aren't incarcerated, fences, railings and solid stair jambs are good alternative options.

8: THE LEG RAISE

A SIX-PACK FROM HELL

No muscle group in the fitness industry over the last twenty years has been paid more attention than the *rectus abdominis*—commonly known as the "six-pack." Just take a glance at the fitness section of any magazine stand; almost every cover of every magazine boasts of at least one article on how to get ripped abs. Turn on the TV and you'll be blasted with prolonged infomercials full of gadgets, all of which promise you a six-pack in *just four easy minutes per day!* or whatever.

Let me set out my stand right now; this kind of crap disgusts me. I have no interest in the kind of training and dieting that produces cute, defined little stomach muscles. I understand that this whole six-pack nonsense sells millions of dollars of equipment, books, magazines, training DVDs and such. But I despise it. I despise it because it represents everything that is wrong with physical culture today. It's about image over substance; it's about buying into some media letch's vision of what the male body should look like—slim and weedy, like an undernourished teenager; not rugged and muscular, like a man. It's about wasting what should be productive workout time doing silly, useless bloody exercises that do nothing more than tense your abs lightly, but produce no strength or health benefits.

All for the sake of vanity!

What is a Six-Pack from Hell?

This is the modern "vision" of the six-pack: a fluffy little set of abs and a skinny waist—preferably hairless and tanned. Do you know what that sounds like to me? The midsection of an underage Brazilian rent boy. If you are into that kind of thing, fair enough. But I'm not.

Your waist is about more than just appearance. It should be about much, much more. Let me introduce you to *my* vision of what a man's midsection should represent—not a pretty teeny set of abs, but a goddamn six-pack from hell!

A six-pack from hell consists of:

- An incredibly powerful midsection—highly trained not just in the central abdomen, but in *all* the muscles of the waist; the *obliques, transversus, psoas, intercostals* and *serratus*. A dynamite midsection that actually makes the *whole body* stronger.

- A supremely functional, flexible waist and hips that add power not only to the spine, but which can lift the legs up with incredible explosive force during jumping, kicking, climbing or any other gymnastic or athletic motions.

- A stomach wall so thick and well-trained that it can fend off blows to the breadbasket—muscles so strong that they will actually *hurt* an attacker to punch or kick!

- A lean gut that supports the internal organs so perfectly that even important functions like respiration and digestion become permanently efficient and healthy.

- Thick, scarily well-developed abdominal muscles that look more like bricks on a building than cute "fitness model" abs.

These are the qualities the convicts I know are looking for from their training. If you are only interested in six little, square abs that look like they belong to a young boy or a swimmer, skip this chapter and go back to the infomercials and guy's fitness magazines. If you want a six-pack from hell, keep reading.

Crunches and Other Modern Madness

If you really crave a midsection like the one I described above, the first thing you're going to have to do is forget everything you've learned about modern abdominal training methods. It might surprise you for example that the "ultimate" modern ab exercise—the one touted in all the gyms and muscle magazines—was never intended to develop the stomach muscles at all. This exercise is the *crunch* and all its variations; the *reverse crunch*, the *twisting crunch*, the *incline crunch*, etc.

Back before steroids, lifters all trained to develop six-packs from hell. They wanted thick, strong, masculine waists. The old school strongmen had better abs than any modern bodybuilders, but their *whole* waists were strong, and *functional* too. This ideal actually dates back to ancient Greece—the athletes of the era all did lots of powerful twisting motions like javelin and discus hurling, actions which built the oblique muscles on the side of the waist. The waists on classical statues aren't waspish little things; look at them and you'll see a cool, stocky, muscular look instead. More like a solid bull mastiff than a shivering greyhound.

Crunches only became popular after the steroid era of bodybuilding was in full swing. This happened because steroids don't only cause the arm, chest, back and leg muscles to grow—they also cause the stomach wall and the internal organs to swell in size. Whereas a drug-free athlete could *never* develop an oversized waist through training, many steroid-taking athletes from the seventies and eighties did, the result being an ugly, muscular paunch that is now known as a "roid gut." An even thicker, more powerful stomach wall was the last thing these guys wanted. So they stopped directly training their midsections with *effective* exercises, and the "crunch" was born—a pathetic isolation technique that is designed merely to tense and gently tone the front of the abdomen, to prepare this area to be posed during competition. The crunch is totally impotent to add any real athletic function, muscle or strength. But modern bodybuilders don't care—they are only desperate to reduce the size of their artificially bloated waists.

Unfortunately, because modern bodybuilders are now seen as the personification of the fitness scene, their futile ab training methods have become widely disseminated amongst the training public. No wonder you'll never see a real six-pack from hell in any gym near you.

Check out the midsections of Maxick (left) and Sandow (right). Two phenomenal six-packs—built in the century before "crunches" were invented.

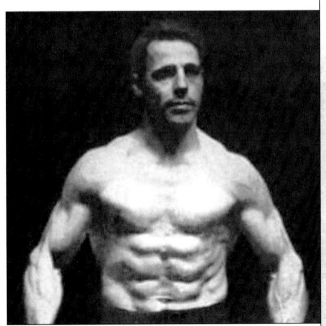

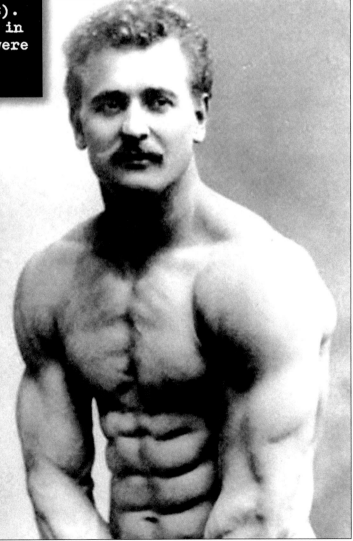

The idea that you need to perform multiple exercises to properly train your abdomen is another modern myth. You may have been told that in exercises where you raise the torso, the "upper" abs get worked, and that in exercises where you raise the legs or hips the "lower" abs get worked. Any trained anatomist will tell you that this is crap. The abdominal muscles are attached to the sternum at one end, and the pelvis at the other end. These muscles contract along their entire length *evenly*—you can't contract one end more than the other, no matter how you move. It would be like holding a length of elastic at each end and trying to pull one end to make it stretch more than the opposite side. You couldn't do it; the elastic would *stretch* evenly along its length, just as muscles *contract* evenly along their length.

Current training ideology is obsessed with the six-pack. This is another modern error in thinking. For athletic ability and true core strength, it's important to think in terms of the "midsection" or "waist" rather than just the abs. There are dozens of major muscles in the waist—the *rectus abdominis* is just one set. When training the midsection, never forget that it is just that—a *middle section*. It's not divorced from the upper and lower body; it exists to help them work together. For this reason, the best way to develop an all-round powerful waist is not by performing isolation exercises, crunches, or machine work—it's by using the body as an integrated unit. Punching, throwing, pushing, kicking, lifting the body around; all these activities combine to stimulate the waist muscles and bring about harmonious, balanced development.

Old School Ab Work: Sit-Ups and Leg Raises

The muscles of the midsection are firing to stabilize the body almost all the time. If they didn't, you would collapse. During strenuous movements—*any* strenuous movements—they fire proportionately harder. But if you really want to take your abdominal development to the next level, you need to specialize in training them with a *single* major movement. Really learn to master that movement, getting stronger and stronger over a long period of time until your waist possesses ungodly strength—that's the way to a six-pack from hell!

In the old days of training—before the nineteen-seventies—two exercises used to vie for the title of "ultimate" midsection exercise. These exercises were *sit-ups* and *leg raises*. Sit-ups and leg raises work the midsection in similar ways, but from opposite directions; in sit-ups, the abdomen contracts to lift the torso; in leg raises, the abdomen contracts to lift the lower limbs. Remember, you really don't *need* to do both—as I said earlier, there are no "upper" or "lower" abs. Either the abdomen contracts or it doesn't. So which of these two classics is best?

Both these "old fashioned" exercises are supremely effective, but in prisons leg raises have always been much more popular. There are three reasons for this:

a) **Hanging leg raises require less equipment than sit-ups.** This is a biggie, especially for convicts. To do sit-ups progressively, you need an adjustable sit-up board, or a Roman chair, or weights to hold onto; ideally, all three. To work up to hanging leg raises, all you require is something to grip—an overhead bar, a tree branch, stair railings, etc. Anybody can find something to hang from if they look hard enough.

b) **Hanging leg raises are more functional than sit-ups.** Sit-ups train the nervous system to push the torso forward at the hips; leg raises train the hips to lift up the legs. This second action is far more natural, and more useful in athletics; the legs must be lifted when kicking, jumping, running, climbing, etc.

c) **Hanging leg raises work more muscles than sit-ups.** Forcing the abs to work while the body is hanging causes many more muscles to come into play than during sit-up training. Hanging develops the grip, shoulders and lats, and forces the serratus muscles around the ribcage to work strongly as an intermediary link between the ribs and midsection. To keep the legs straight, the deeper muscle heads of the quadriceps also work hard during leg raises.

For these reasons, the *Convict Conditioning* system includes the leg raise as one of The Big Six: major movements. It really is the greatest single abdominal exercise known to man. It's all you'll ever need for maximum waist power, flexibility and muscle.

The Leg Raise Series

Most people who work out will be familiar with the *hanging leg raise*. It's fairly simple in execution—just grab a high overhead bar and let your feet hang down clear of the ground, before *slowly* raising your *straight* legs—*knees locked*—until they are parallel with the floor. Pause for a second before carefully lowering your legs again. Simple.

But just because an exercise is *simple*, it doesn't follow that it's easy. Despite it's simplicity, this classic waist exercise is extremely difficult. It requires stomach muscles of steel, extremely powerful, healthy hips, a strong spine, well-conditioned thighs and very flexible hamstrings and lower back.

The truth is, the hanging leg raise done slowly and with perfectly straight legs is beyond the ability of most people, even very agile athletes like martial artists and wrestlers. Don't worry though. You won't be expected to master this exercise immediately. As with all The Big Six: movements, you'll be taught how to develop the qualities you need gradually, by mastering a series of progressively harder exercises first. You'll begin with Step 1, *knee tucks*, a light exercise perfect for gently conditioning the abdominal muscles and strengthening the hips. From there, you'll head to the floor for a further four movements. When you have mastered the floor exercises, you'll graduate to hanging work. Another four preliminary hanging techniques will lead you to the point where you'll have a stronger midsection than 99% of athletes, and you'll be ready to tackle the *hanging straight leg raise* with confidence.

And you won't need to do a single crunch, blow up a Swiss ball, buy an ab machine, strap electrodes to your gut, or any of that other pathetic modern garbage.

Waist Training Ideas

It's difficult to give a strict list of technical pointers for the leg raise series, because some of the exercises are quite different—at least on the surface. But what I can do is pass on some general waist training ideas that have helped my students to develop their own midsection training philosophy. For example:

- The act of breathing tightens the abdominal muscles, as well as the intercostals around the ribs. Remember the last time you got sore abs just from laughing too hard? Inhale during the negative portion of the movement, and exhale fully at the top of your reps to maximize this effect. Take breaths between reps if you need to.

- The *transversus* is a thick layer of muscle deep within the waist that acts like a corset, holding the internal organs in place. When the transversus is weak, it can split under pressure, allowing some of the gut to bulge out. This is called a hernia. You should train your transversus by pulling the stomach in tightly during ab movements. It also helps to try to remember to retain by good posture by holding the stomach in throughout the day.

- Some people claim that leg raises can aggravate bad backs. If you build up to the movement slowly, this is not true. Sometimes, bad backs associated with leg raises are actually caused by strength imbalances—the abdomen is stronger than the lower back. To eliminate this imbalance, include exercises in your program that work the spinal muscles. Squats will do this, as will bridging.

- Ensure that your meals are well digested before performing abdominal movements. Leave at least two hours between eating and training abs, or your stomach will be distended and your technique will suffer.

- If you find *straight leg raises* very hard, this may be due to tight hamstrings. Stretching them out before training will ease the problem.

- The notion that lots of sit-ups will give you defined abs is an old wives' tale. Muscle definition is the result of leanness—absence of fat. Fat loss occurs proportionately over the entire body. You can't lose fat from one area just by working it excessively, so don't waste your time.

- If you want "ripped" abs, forget high reps. Stick with progressive strength work on leg raises to make your abdominal muscles thick and strong, and then diet off the fat to reveal the definition.

- Most modern abdominal programs include numerous isolation exercises such as *side crunches* and *cable twists* to work the abs "from all angles." These mini-exercises do nothing for fitness and don't effect your abdomen one iota. Comprehensive waist development comes from working progressively on multiple exercises which train the *whole body*. If you want a well-developed midsection, forget these teeny techniques and devote your energy to The Big Six:.

- Some bodybuilders believe that high rep twisting movements—with an empty bar or a broomstick—will reduce waist size. This is a myth. General over-training—such as running four marathons in a week—*will* cause muscle loss over the entire body, but specific exercises will not atrophy, or "wear down" a particular area, not matter how many reps you do. All high-rep twists will do is irritate your spine.

- Leg raises are much easier to do if you *swing*—use a little explosive momentum at the bottom of the movement. This is *not* what you want. If you can't do your techniques "clean" go back to earlier steps until you become powerful enough to use the correct form.

Okay, that's enough of the theory. Time to get to the meat of any program—the actual *techniques*. The ten steps of the leg raise series follow.

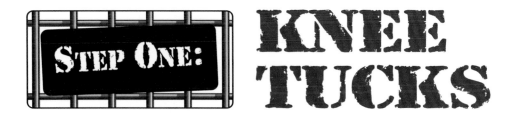

STEP ONE: KNEE TUCKS

Performance

Sit on the edge of a chair or bed. Lean back a little, grip the edge of the seat with your hands, and straighten your legs. Your feet should be together with the heels raised a few inches from the floor. This is the start position (fig. 61). Smoothly bring the knees up and in until they are approximately six to ten inches from your chest. Exhale as you draw the knees in. By the time the motion is complete, you should have exhaled fully and your abs should be tightly contracted. This is the finish position (fig. 62). Pause for a count of one before reversing the motion and finishing again in the start position. Inhale as you extend. Your feet should follow a straight line backwards and forwards, and should not touch the floor until the set is completed. Keep the stomach tucked in at all times. Resist the urge to pump out reps quickly. As with all waist techniques, take extra breaths between reps if you need to.

Exercise X-Ray

Knee tucks are an ideal midsection exercise for beginners. They cultivate good spinal posture, condition the abdominal muscles and strengthen the hip flexors. They are also relatively easy for most people and for this reason they present a great opportunity to start developing perfect technique for all your midsection exercises. Important elements to remember include smooth motion, correct breathing rhythm and keeping the stomach held in tightly.

Training Goals

- Beginner standard: 1 set of 10
- Intermediate standard: 2 sets of 25
- Progression standard: 3 sets of 40

Perfecting Your Technique

This exercise is equally hard in the start position—where the legs are stretched out—and in the finish position—where the knees are pulled towards the chest. To make the exercise a little easier, focus on a shorter range of motion between these two extremes. As your waist becomes stronger, gradually lengthen the range of motion until your form is perfect.

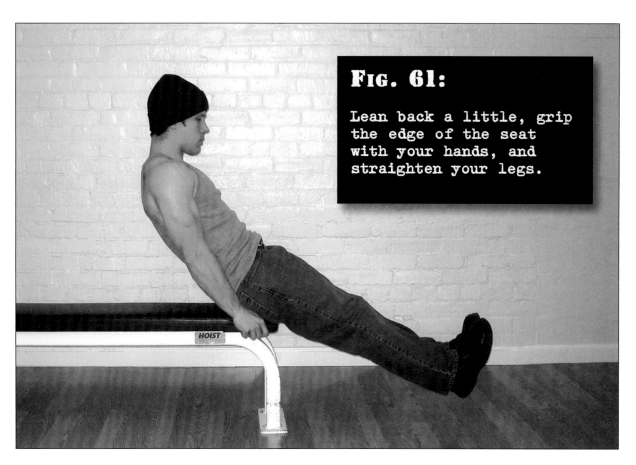

FIG. 61:

Lean back a little, grip the edge of the seat with your hands, and straighten your legs.

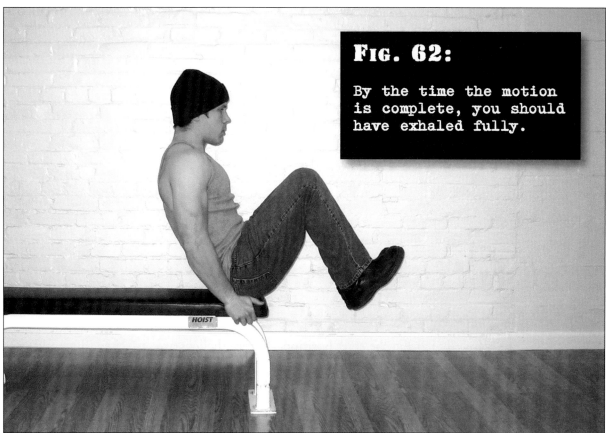

FIG. 62:

By the time the motion is complete, you should have exhaled fully.

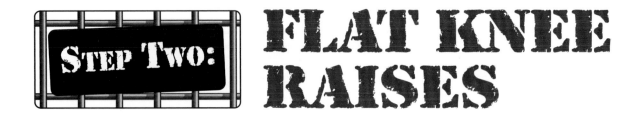

STEP TWO: FLAT KNEE RAISES

Performance

Lie flat on the floor, with your legs together and your arms by your side. Bend your knees so that they are at approximately ninety degrees (i.e., a right angle), with the feet an inch or two off the ground. Pressing hard on the floor with your hands will help keep your torso stable. This is the start position (fig. 63). Now smoothly bring your knees up over your hips, so that your thighs are perpendicular to the floor, and your calves are parallel to the floor. Keep the knees at a right angle throughout and exhale as you go, keeping your stomach muscles tight. This is the finish position (fig. 64). Pause for a count of one, before reversing the motion by extending your legs as you lower your feet. Inhale as you return to the start position. After you begin, at no point throughout the movement should your feet touch the floor.

Exercise X-Ray

This exercise continues where *knee tucks* leaves off, further strengthening the waist. *Flat knee raises* train the spinal muscles, abdominal muscles, obliques and transversus to function in a coordinated way. The muscles of the frontal thigh are also toned. The position on the floor requires increased hip flexor involvement, which will condition the athlete for the more intense floor and hanging exercises which come later in the leg raise series.

Training Goals

- Beginner standard: 1 set of 10
- Intermediate standard: 2 sets of 20
- Progression standard: 3 sets of 35

Perfecting Your Technique

One of the hardest elements of this exercise is keeping the feet off the floor with the legs outstretched. If this is causing you trouble, return your feet to the floor between repetitions. When you gain the strength to do reps while continuously keeping your feet off the floor, do so—even if it's only two repetitions—then as you tire complete the set by resting your feet on the floor between reps. Over time keep gradually adding reps with your feet clear of the floor.

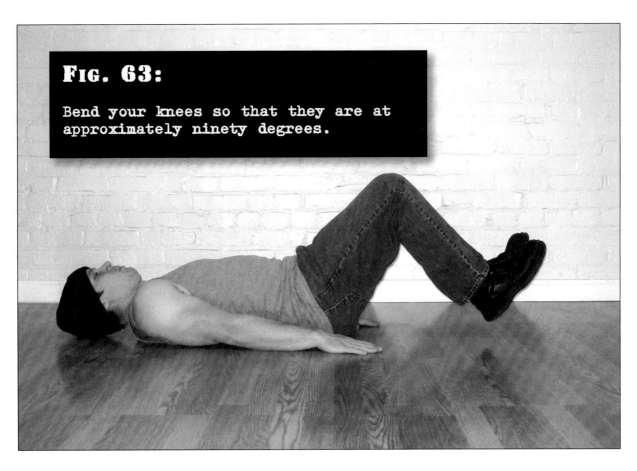

FIG. 63:

Bend your knees so that they are at approximately ninety degrees.

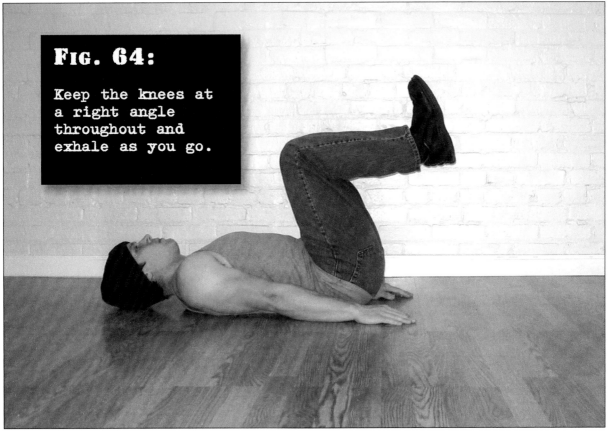

FIG. 64:

Keep the knees at a right angle throughout and exhale as you go.

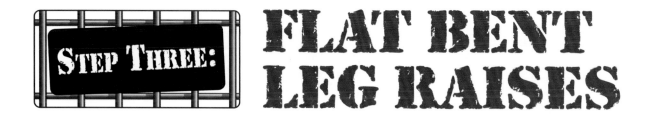

Performance

Lie on your back with your legs together and stretched out on the floor. Your hands should be by your sides, and also in contact with the floor. Raise your legs, bending them at the knee approximately forty-five degrees from the straight alignment. Your feet should be kept an inch or two off the floor. This is the start position (fig. 65). The positive portion of the exercise involves raising the legs and feet smoothly—over a count of two seconds—until the feet are directly above the pelvis (fig. 66). As you move, the angle of the knee should not change; it must remain "locked" in the same position. Pressing down on the floor with the hands will help you stabilize your torso throughout the movement. Pause at the top, before reversing the motion. Pause again in the start position before repeating as necessary. Exhale as the feet move up, inhale as they are moving down. Keep the stomach tight at all times. The feet should not touch the floor at all during the set.

Exercise X-Ray

The *flat bent leg raise* is a very simple continuation of the *flat knee raise*. Extending the knees places the feet farther away from the body, making the exercise harder due to leverage. This increases the stress on the hips and all the muscles of the waist and abdomen, building more strength and tone.

Training Goals

- Beginner standard: 1 set of 10
- Intermediate standard: 2 sets of 15
- Progression standard: 3 sets of 30

Perfecting Your Technique

Flat knee raises involve a ninety degree knee bend. *Flat bent leg raises* require a forty-five degree knee bend. The less the degree of bend, the greater the amount of leverage and the harder the exercise becomes. If you cannot meet the beginner standard, use more of a knee bend—a little less than ninety degrees. As you get stronger, start straightening your legs little by little, until you meet the forty-five degree criterion.

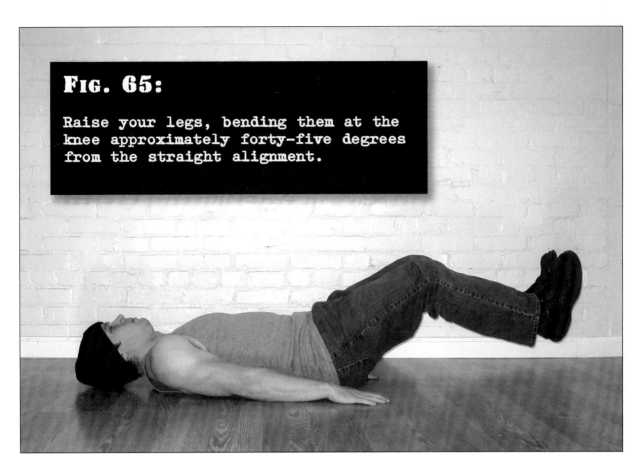

FIG. 65:

Raise your legs, bending them at the knee approximately forty-five degrees from the straight alignment.

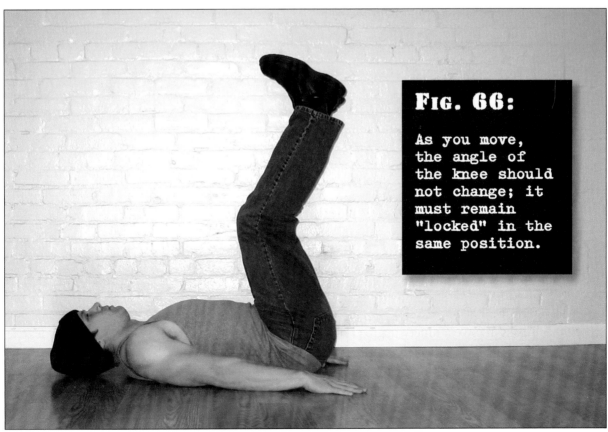

FIG. 66:

As you move, the angle of the knee should not change; it must remain "locked" in the same position.

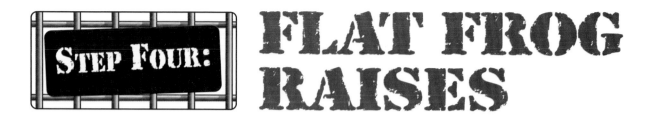

STEP FOUR: FLAT FROG RAISES

Performance

Perform the positive portion of Step 3, the *bent leg raise*, but instead of pausing at the top (fig. 66), straighten your legs out fully. They should be perfectly straight, and perpendicular to the floor, so that your legs and torso form a right angle. This is the finish position (fig. 67). You should exhale throughout this two-part motion. In most midsection work you would now reverse the movement; but not so here. Your muscles are stronger when *lowering* under resistance (because gravity helps), and *frog raise* techniques take advantage of this fact. Lower your legs, keeping them *perfectly straight* (fig. 68) until they are an inch or two off the floor (fig. 69). In most exercises you should take about two seconds to go up and two seconds to go down. But for this exercise count *four* seconds down, to allow your body more work in the stronger position. Inhale as your legs slowly descend. Repeat.

Exercise X-Ray

Whether they are performed in a flat or hanging position, the jump from *bent knee raises* to *straight leg raises* is a pretty big one because of the increase in flexible strength required. Frog raise techniques help athlete make this jump. They act as an ideal intermediary between bent knee raise and straight leg raise movements because they develop both strength and flexibility in the areas required, the hamstrings and back. Unfortunately frog raise movements are not very well known to the training public. They seemed to get lost after the sixties when leg raises became less popular and crunches took over.

Training Goals

- Beginner standard: 1 set of 8
- Intermediate standard: 2 sets of 15
- Progression standard: 3 sets of 25

Perfecting Your Technique

If you find this exercise difficult, focus your workouts on the top range—around the frog extension technique where the legs are up in the air. As you become stronger over time, slowly add depth until you are doing full reps.

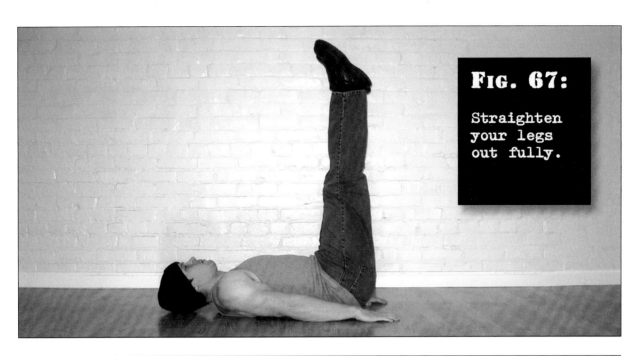

FIG. 67:

Straighten your legs out fully.

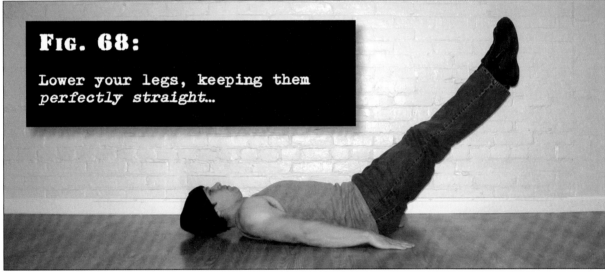

FIG. 68:

Lower your legs, keeping them *perfectly straight*...

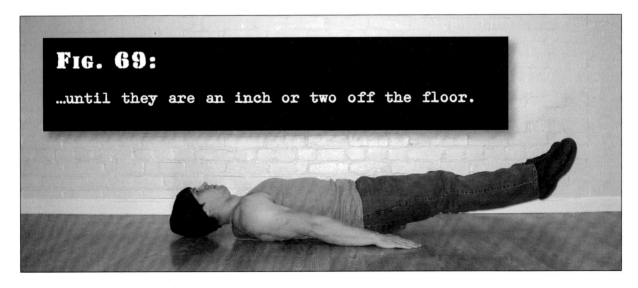

FIG. 69:

...until they are an inch or two off the floor.

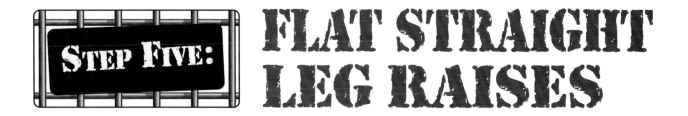

STEP FIVE: FLAT STRAIGHT LEG RAISES

Performance

Lie on the floor, face up. Your feet should be together, your legs should be straight, and your arms should be by your sides. Lift your feet an inch or two from the floor. Pressing down with the hands will help you keep your torso stable. This is the start position (fig. 70). Now, keeping your legs locked, raise your feet until they are directly above your pelvis. Exhale as you lift, keeping the stomach tight. It should take you at least two seconds to *smoothly* accomplish this—don't explode up. Your legs and torso will form a right angle at this point. This is the finish position (fig. 71). Pause briefly, before reversing the motion exactly, inhaling as you go down. Pause again in the start position and repeat. At no point should allow your knees to unlock, and your heels shouldn't touch the floor until the set is completed.

Exercise X-Ray

This exercise is a favorite in military training camps and martial arts schools alike, because it increases stomach and hip power and stamina, while promoting function and flexibility at the same time. It is deceptively easy, however; just bending the knees a fraction and "bouncing" the feet off the floor makes the exercise much easier. Unfortunately it also makes the exercise far less productive in terms of pure strength and conditioning.

Training Goals

- Beginner standard: 1 set of 5
- Intermediate standard: 2 sets of 10
- Progression standard: 2 sets of 20

Perfecting Your Technique

This exercise can be made a lot easier by bending the knees; but that's not an advisable shortcut because the major benefits of this exercise come from the fact that the legs are straight. If you can't meet the beginner standard, go back to *flat frog raises* (Step 4) and build up to 3 sets of 30 reps before trying again. If you still have problems, keep the legs straight but focus on shorter, top range reps and acquire more depth whenever you are able to.

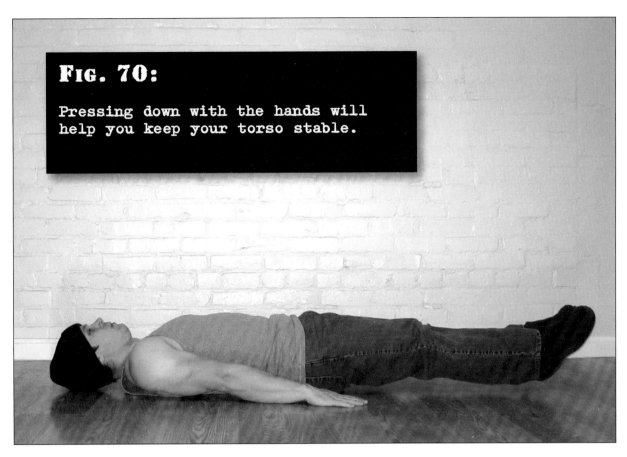

FIG. 70:

Pressing down with the hands will help you keep your torso stable.

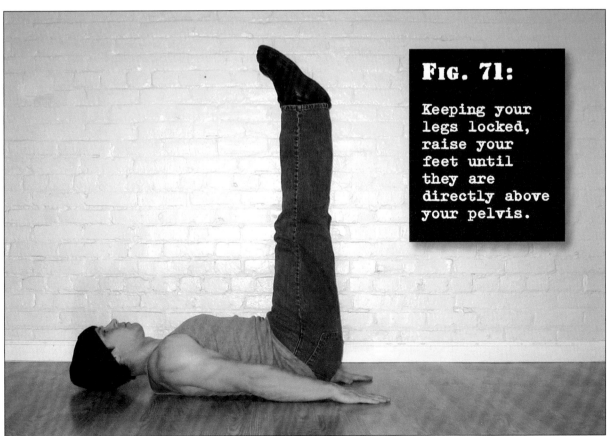

FIG. 71:

Keeping your legs locked, raise your feet until they are directly above your pelvis.

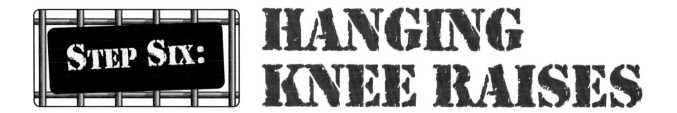

Performance

Jump up and grab an overhead bar. Your hands should be about shoulder width apart. The bar needs to be high enough that your feet hang clear from the ground, even if only by an inch. Your body should be in a straight line, and you must keep your shoulders "tight" (see page 117). This is the start position (fig. 72). Bring your knees up smoothly until they are level with your pelvis and your knees are at a right angle. Your thighs will be parallel with the floor. Exhale during this motion, keeping your stomach pulled in. This is the finish position (fig. 73). Pause for a moment, then reverse the motion until your body is fully extended, inhaling as you go. Repeat.

Exercise X-Ray

With this step, the athlete begins the harder hanging movements of the midsection series. While on the floor, the athlete was only partially fighting the forces of gravity; now he has to overcome gravity fully. The increased intensity amplifies hip and midsection strength radically, in a short space of time. In addition the bar hang element increases the activity of the important ribcage muscles (the *serratus* and *intercostals*) which function as intermediaries between the arms and abdomen. For this reason hanging ab work is vastly superior to ab work on parallel bars or similar devices.

Training Goals

- Beginner standard: 1 set of 5
- Intermediate standard: 2 sets of 10
- Progression standard: 2 sets of 15

Perfecting Your Technique

If you can't handle at least five good, strict reps of this exercise, reduce your range of motion. Focus on the top portion where the knees are in the finish position, and gradually add depth over time. Whatever you do, resist the urge to use momentum. Using smooth, controlled motions early on in the series will build a base of muscle and tendon strength which will prove invaluable if you wish to master later steps. Momentum won't help.

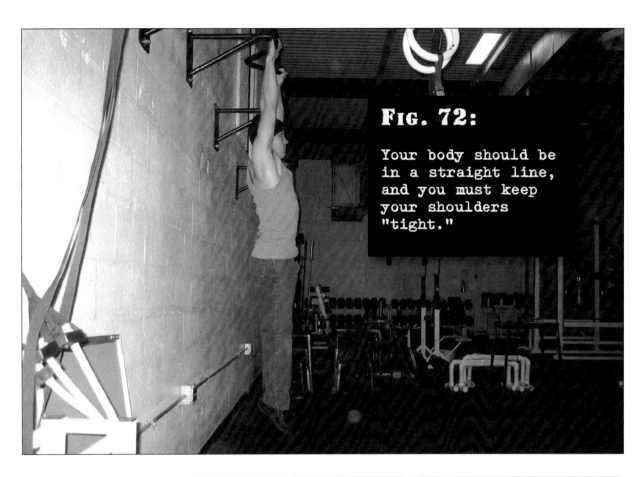

FIG. 72:

Your body should be in a straight line, and you must keep your shoulders "tight."

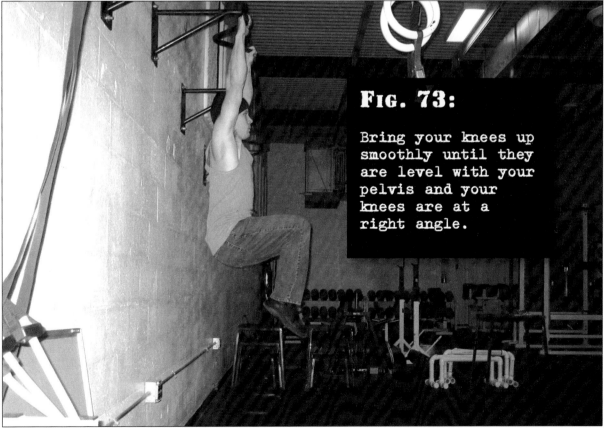

FIG. 73:

Bring your knees up smoothly until they are level with your pelvis and your knees are at a right angle.

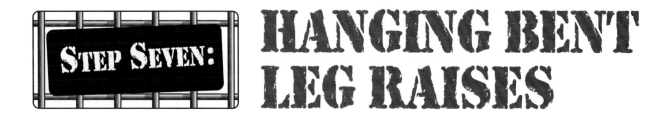

Performance

Grab an overhead bar so that your body is in a straight line and your feet are clear of the ground. Your hands should be approximately shoulder width, and your shoulders kept nice and tight. Now bend at the knees until your knee joints are angled off straight by around forty-five degrees. This will put your feet a few inches behind the rest of your hanging body. This is the start position (fig. 74). Smoothly raise your legs at the hips until your feet are opposite your pelvis. This is the finish position (fig. 75). Pause and reverse the motion, before repeating. Only move at the hips; keep your knee angle "locked" into place. Exhale as you raise your legs, inhale as you lower them. Keep the abs tense.

Exercise X-Ray

Hanging bent leg raises are a harder extension of *hanging knee raises*. In hanging knee raises, the knees are bent at ninety degrees, in hanging bent leg raises they are at forty-five. The increased leverage this provides makes the exercise the hardest in the series yet, and it develops the midsection accordingly. The abdomen, waist, serratus and hip flexors all get stronger.

Training Goals

- Beginner standard: 1 set of 5
- Intermediate standard: 2 sets of 10
- Progression standard: 2 sets of 15

Perfecting Your Technique

At first, you may find it difficult to keep your knees "locked" at the correct angle throughout the motion. There will be a tendency to straighten the legs out a little as you lower them. Try to avoid this, because resetting the correct angle as the legs are raised tends to impart momentum which leads to a swinging motion. If you have trouble with the exercise from the start, simply increase the angle of the knee bend from forty-five degrees to closer to ninety degrees. As you gain strength from workout to workout, gradually extend the legs until you meet your goal of forty-five degrees.

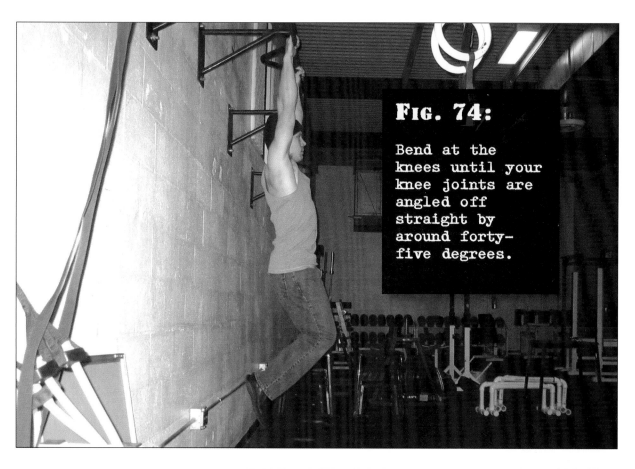

FIG. 74:

Bend at the knees until your knee joints are angled off straight by around forty-five degrees.

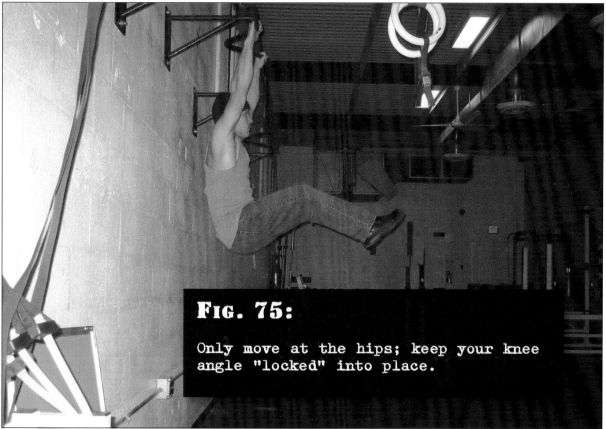

FIG. 75:

Only move at the hips; keep your knee angle "locked" into place.

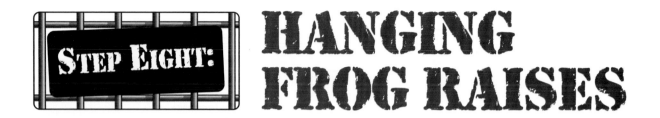

STEP EIGHT: HANGING FROG RAISES

Performance

Assume a start position identical to Step 7, *hanging bent leg raises* (fig. 74), and raise your legs just as you would for that same exercise. Once you reach the top position with your feet in line with your hips (fig. 75), extend your feet out in a line directly away from you, so that your legs are perfectly straight. This will put your locked legs level with the floor, and your upper and lower body at a right angle (fig. 76). Pause for a moment, but do not reverse the motion. Instead, lower your legs while keeping them locked out perfectly straight (fig. 77). Finish with your body fully extended (fig. 78) before assuming the start position again and repeating for the desired number of reps. Exhale as the legs are going up, inhale as they are going down, and keep the stomach tucked in at all times.

Exercise X-Ray

Hanging frog raises emphasize the fact that the finish position and negative (downwards) phase of leg raises are easier in terms of mechanics and leverage than the start position and positive (upwards) phase. By working hard with this exercise you can increase your strength and flexibility faster than would normally be possible, allowing you to more easily make the transition to straight leg variants of the leg raise (Steps 9 and 10).

Training Goals

- Beginner standard: 1 set of 5
- Intermediate standard: 2 sets of 10
- Progression standard: 2 sets of 15

Perfecting Your Technique

If you can meet the progression standard for *hanging bent leg raises*, five reps of *hanging frog raises* should be well within your capabilities. When students have difficulty moving from bent leg raises to frog-type movements, the issue is usually lack of flexibility rather than strength. This can be easily cured by bending forwards and stretching out the lower back and hamstrings for a few minutes before attempting this exercise.

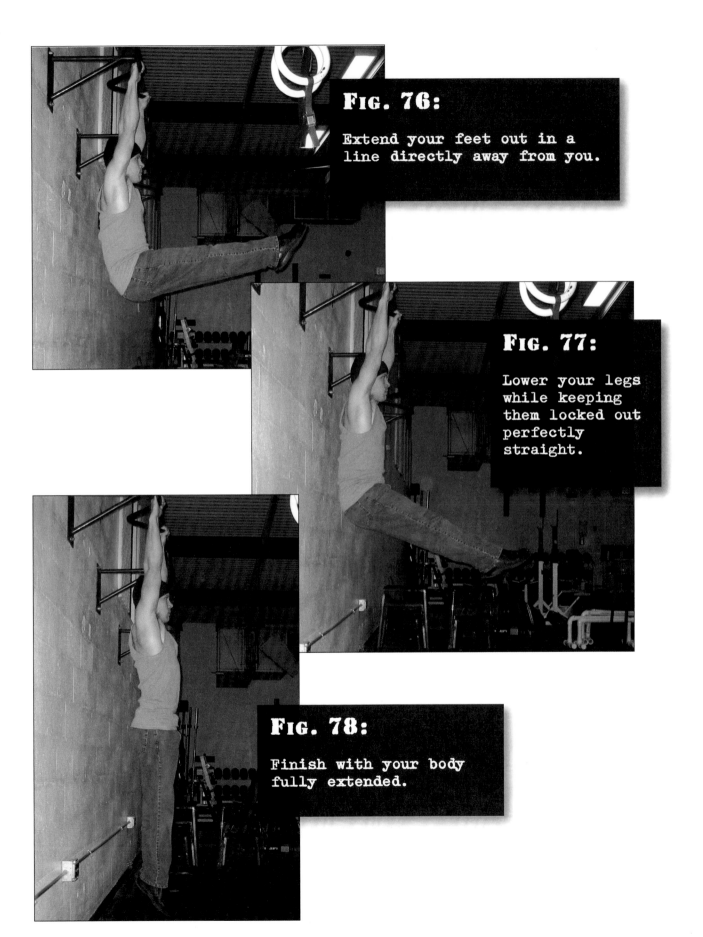

FIG. 76:

Extend your feet out in a line directly away from you.

FIG. 77:

Lower your legs while keeping them locked out perfectly straight.

FIG. 78:

Finish with your body fully extended.

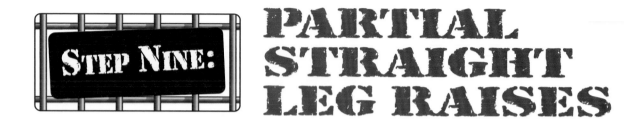

STEP NINE: PARTIAL STRAIGHT LEG RAISES

Performance

Hang from an overhead bar, with your body in a straight line and your feet off the floor. Tighten the shoulders. Lift the locked legs until they are at a forty-five degree angle, and hold. This is the start position (fig. 79). Keeping your knees locked straight, smoothly raise your legs until they are parallel with the floor. This is the finish position (fig. 80). Pause for a moment, before lowering the legs back to a forty-five degree angle. Repeat. Exhale as your legs move up, inhale as they move down. Keep the abs tight.

Exercise X-Ray

Straight leg raises, performed with locked knees and without momentum are an incredibly hard exercise—only perhaps one in five hundred serious trainees (maybe less) can execute them. One of the things that makes them so hard is the full range of motion—from the body straight all the way up to the jackknife right angle position. Once the athlete has developed the strength and flexibility required to perform the legs extended top position (as a result of *hanging frog raises*), hanging *partial straight leg raises* capitalize on this, by making the top position a little harder, and eliminating the rest.

Training Goals

- Beginner standard: 1 set of 5
- Intermediate standard: 2 sets of 10
- Progression standard: 2 sets of 15

Perfecting Your Technique

If you have met the progression standard for *hanging frog raises*, this means you will be able to hold the advanced legs extended position of the leg raise (fig. 80). If you find that *partial straight leg raises* are too hard, it must be because the range of motion is still too great for your strength levels. Focus on doing this exercise near the legs extended finish position, moving your legs down and back up, even if you can only move a few inches at first. Over time, your strength will increase and you'll be able to move your legs down to the full forty-five degree position and back up again.

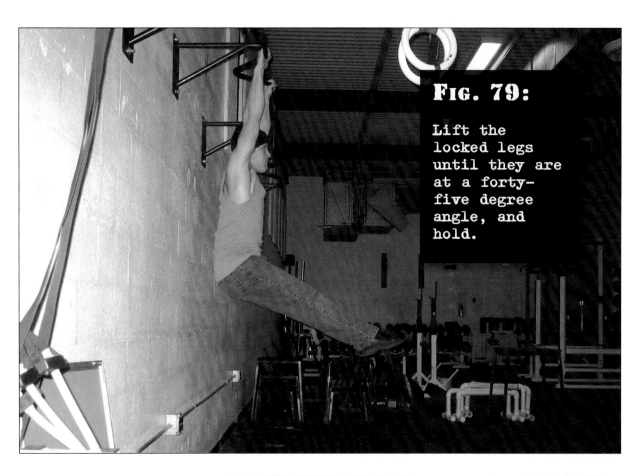

FIG. 79:

Lift the locked legs until they are at a forty-five degree angle, and hold.

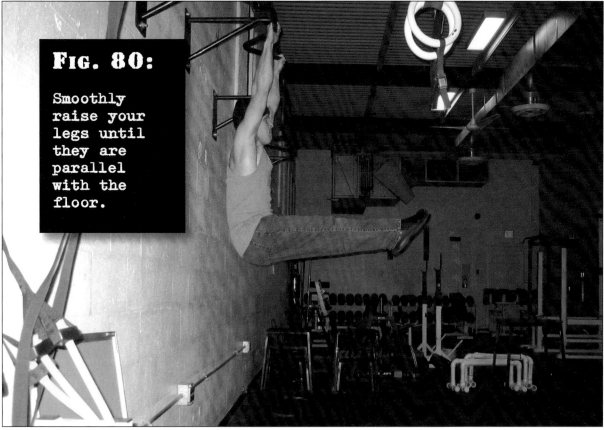

FIG. 80:

Smoothly raise your legs until they are parallel with the floor.

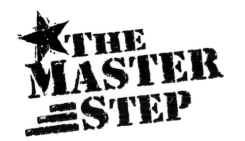

HANGING STRAIGHT LEG RAISES

Performance

You know the drill by now! Take hold of an overhead bar which is high enough to leave your feet a short distance from the floor when your body is extended. Your hands should be approximately shoulder width apart. Ensure that the shoulders are tight. This is the start position (fig. 81). Smoothly—over the course of *at least* two seconds—raise your legs until they are parallel with the floor. Exhale as your legs rise, blowing all the air you can out of your lungs so that the abdomen is fully contracted. This is the finish position (fig. 82). Pause, before reversing the motion perfectly for at least another two seconds until you are back in the start position. Inhale as you go. Remain "flexed," even in the start position. Your legs must stay locked at all times and you must use pure muscular control; no momentum allowed.

Exercise X-Ray

Hanging straight leg raises—performed strictly, according to the protocols given above—are the greatest all-round midsection exercise in existence. They blow crunches, machine work, and weighted sit-ups out of the water. By the time you can execute even twenty perfect reps of this exercise, your waist will be powerful and flexible, your obliques, serratus, transversus and intercostals will be carved out of solid rock and your abdominal muscles will be like plate steel. You *will* have a six-pack from hell!

Training Goals

- Beginner standard: 1 set of 5
- Intermediate standard: 2 sets of 10
- Elite standard: 2 sets of 30

Perfecting Your Technique

When you begin *hanging straight leg raises*, you should have already mastered hanging *partial straight leg raises*. If you haven't, go back and do so. If you *have* mastered the partial version, all you need to do is slowly increase your depth of motion from workout to workout—even by a fraction of an inch—and you'll be able to pull off this exercise before you know it.

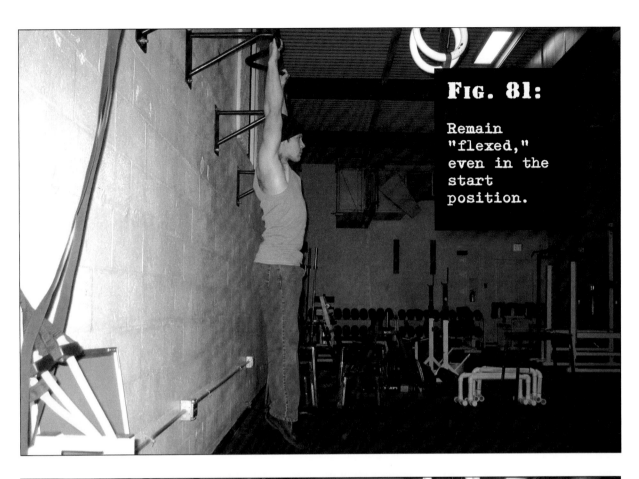

FIG. 81:

Remain "flexed," even in the start position.

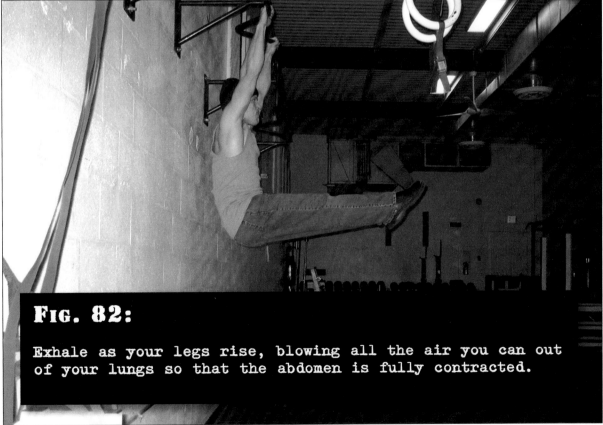

FIG. 82:

Exhale as your legs rise, blowing all the air you can out of your lungs so that the abdomen is fully contracted.

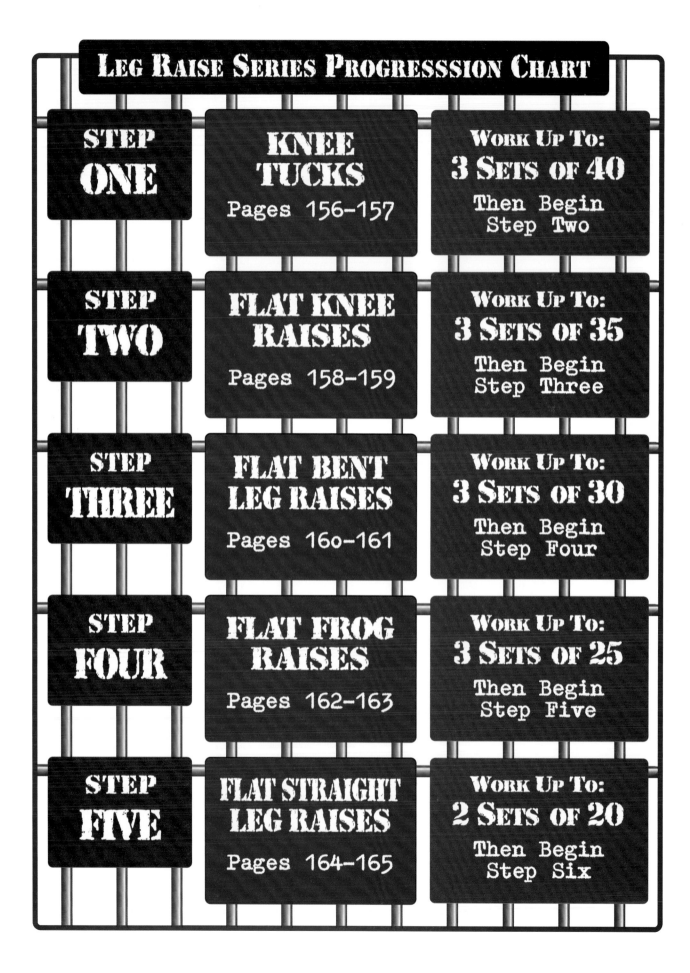

LEG RAISE SERIES PROGRESSSION CHART

STEP ONE — KNEE TUCKS — Pages 156–157 — WORK UP TO: **3 SETS OF 40** Then Begin Step Two

STEP TWO — FLAT KNEE RAISES — Pages 158–159 — WORK UP TO: **3 SETS OF 35** Then Begin Step Three

STEP THREE — FLAT BENT LEG RAISES — Pages 16o–161 — WORK UP TO: **3 SETS OF 30** Then Begin Step Four

STEP FOUR — FLAT FROG RAISES — Pages 162–163 — WORK UP TO: **3 SETS OF 25** Then Begin Step Five

STEP FIVE — FLAT STRAIGHT LEG RAISES — Pages 164–165 — WORK UP TO: **2 SETS OF 20** Then Begin Step Six

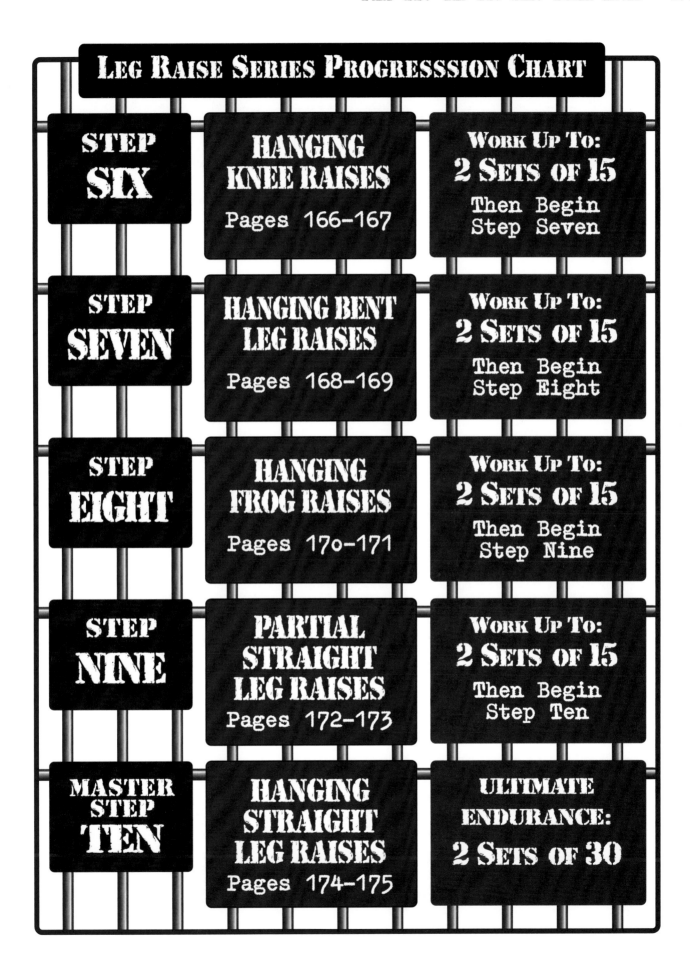

LEG RAISE SERIES PROGRESSSION CHART

STEP SIX	HANGING KNEE RAISES Pages 166-167	WORK UP TO: 2 SETS OF 15 Then Begin Step Seven
STEP SEVEN	HANGING BENT LEG RAISES Pages 168-169	WORK UP TO: 2 SETS OF 15 Then Begin Step Eight
STEP EIGHT	HANGING FROG RAISES Pages 170-171	WORK UP TO: 2 SETS OF 15 Then Begin Step Nine
STEP NINE	PARTIAL STRAIGHT LEG RAISES Pages 172-173	WORK UP TO: 2 SETS OF 15 Then Begin Step Ten
MASTER STEP TEN	HANGING STRAIGHT LEG RAISES Pages 174-175	ULTIMATE ENDURANCE: 2 SETS OF 30

Going Beyond

The leg raise series will give the vast majority of trainees—even very gifted athletes who can advance quickly—a great deal of scope for productive waist training. All the exercises in the series can be tweaked and altered (as per the descriptions in the *perfecting your technique* section), potentially turning each exercise into many different movements. The series will keep you getting stronger and stronger for a long time to come. By the time you reach the Master Step of *hanging straight leg raises*, you will truly have a six-pack from hell, but as you adapt, you can experiment with more volume. Try upping your reps—more than fifty hanging leg raises is a goddamned impressive goal, but not unheard of.

The average athlete should be incredibly proud of such an achievement, and there's absolutely no shame in leveling off your training at that point. It's an accomplishment *light years* ahead of what the average gym-trained zombie could ever attain. But some of you will want to go further. If you are one of this elite group, I would advise setting your sights to the most powerful midsection exercise possible—the *V raise*.

V raises are very rarely seen in gyms. You might witness the occasional expert martial artist performing them—they were a favorite of Bruce Lee—but they are usually the province of advanced gymnasts. They require a level of muscular strength, nervous power, coordination and flexibility that can only be cultivated through years of serious, progressive midsection work, specializing in only the hardest, most productive training techniques.

In classic leg raises, the legs are raised to a point of ninety degrees—they are perpendicular to the trunk in the top position. In V raises, the locked legs are raised much higher, so that the body forms a much more acute angle, like the letter "V" (hence the name). This sounds simple, but if you try it, you'll see that it's far from easy. It requires that the abdominal muscles have *enormous* contractile power, and this needs to be combined with iron hip strength. In addition, if the spine, glutes and leg biceps aren't extremely supple you won't have a hope of performing the movement.

You should only attempt V raises once you have attained the *elite standard* of the *hanging straight leg raise*. If you have, and you wish to master V raises, continue your training in leg raises, but work into V raises on a different day, when your stomach and waist muscles are fresh. After performing a warm up and some forward flexibility exercises, learn the movement while sitting on the floor. Supporting yourself on your hands and butt, lift your legs off the floor as high as you can. Allow yourself to tilt backwards until your thighs are close to your chest and you are in the "V" position. At first, this will be difficult, as your hips and abs just aren't used to being asked to contract so hard. As with all midsection work, use muscular control to perform your movements—momentum only makes you weaker. Once you've mastered the exercise, work for reps—build up to about twenty. When you can do twenty with your trunk tilted backwards, try again with your trunk totally vertical. This will be harder. By the time you have built up to twenty reps again, you will be used to the difficult top position, and you're ready to try for a greater range of motion.

Attempt the exercise again from between two chairs. Grab the chair backs and push your body up straight. From a position where your legs are straight with your feet resting on the floor a little way out in front of you, try the V raise again. Obviously your legs won't be hanging straight down—the chairs won't be high enough. But this intermediate version will teach you the middle range of the exercise. Slowly raise your feet from the floor, keeping your legs locked, up past the horizontal, until they are in the V position again. Work up to twenty reps like this.

Once you have mastered the top and middle ranges, you will be ready to try the full V raise exercise hanging from an overhead bar.

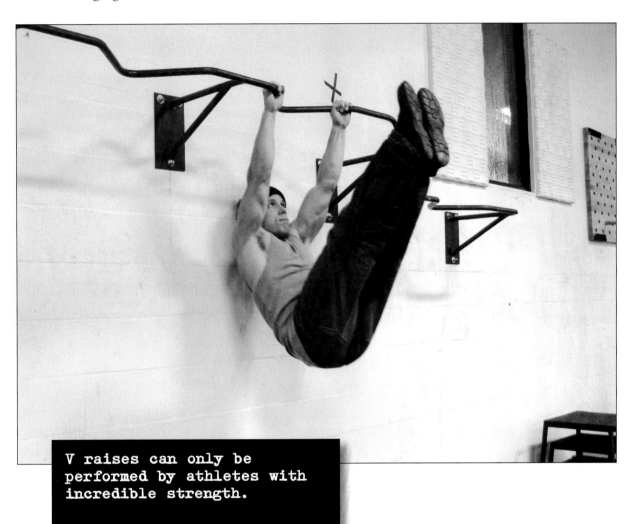

V raises can only be performed by athletes with incredible strength.

Variants

Virtually every fitness magazine you pick up from the newstands these days has an "ab training special" lurking within its pages. These articles are usually crammed with the least productive waist exercises known to man—the "crunch" and its sneaky variations. These variations include: *reverse crunches, twisting crunches, incline crunches, weighted crunches, Swiss ball crunches, side crunches*, and *cable crunches* as well as the various brands of *machine crunches*. These are all essentially isolation exercises, and pretty puny ones at that. They completely lack the power to transform the midsection into anything resembling a functional, athletic core. Avoid this nonsense. There *are* some useful midsection exercises you can throw into your routine from time to time, but they are usually quite old, and therefore considered to be archaic and antiquated by modern fitness writers who base their ideas on fashion rather than effectiveness. Here are a handful of techniques worth considering.

Sit-Ups

A classic yet simple exercise which works the entire midsection and hips. Lie on the floor, hook your feet under something sturdy and bend at the hips. The sit-up has got a bad rap as being dangerous for the spine, but if you bend well at the knees this is a total fallacy. Don't put your hands behind your head, or you can strain the ligaments in your neck. Instead, put your fists to your temples and come up until your elbows touch your knees. I've read a lot of garbage saying that sit-ups don't work the abdomen, but whoever writes this junk obviously isn't doing sit-ups. A few hundred reps of this beauty will make your abs deliciously sore the next day, from sternum down to pelvis. The real drawback to sit-ups is that you adapt to them quite quickly, so to increase strength people are usually forced to add weight. If you don't want to get into using weights, you can always progress over time to harder variations of the sit-up, like *Janda sit-ups, incline sit-ups* and *Roman chair sit-ups*.

Janda Sit-Ups

Janda sit-ups are named after the Czech scientist who invented them. They are identical to normal sit-ups, with the exception that you press down hard on the floor with the soles of your feet throughout the exercise, while clenching your glutes and hamstrings as tightly as you can. The thinking behind this says that doing your sit-ups this way takes the hip flexors out of the movement because the hip flexors are anatomically opposite the glutes and hamstrings. The underlying theory is called *reciprocal inhibition*. Proponents of this theory argue that if the glutes and hamstrings fire, the hip flexors *can't* fire—therefore the load is shifted onto the abdominals, which get stronger as a result. I'm pretty dubious about these claims. For a start, it's not actually true that contracting a set of muscles prevents the opposite set of muscles from contracting (the phenomenon known as *Lombard's Paradox*, is a good example; see page 78). Besides, why would you want your hips to stop working? The abdomen and hip flexors have evolved to work in *unison*, and if you develop one part of a system without simultaneously training the corresponding parts, you are asking for trouble. That said, Janda sit-ups *are* a useful addition to your training arsenal, not due to reciprocal inhibition, but because the isometric contraction required forces the muscles of the midsection work more intensely than they normally would. Once you can do more than fifty regular sit-ups, try Janda sit-ups.

Incline Sit-Ups

These require a board or platform you can elevate at one end. Hook your feet under the straps and do your sit-ups. As they get easier, lift the end of the board under your feet by a few degrees. This forces the midsection to work harder against gravity. If you have something high enough to secure the board on, you can keep going until you are almost vertical.

Roman Chair Sit-Ups

Roman chair training is a more intense modification of incline sit-ups. Hook your legs under something that will also support your thighs, so you can hang backwards with nothing supporting your torso or hips. Doing sit-ups from this position means that your midsection has to exert much greater force to control the trunk in the bottom position; you can also go back further than in regular or incline sit-ups, so the range of motion is increased. This exercise was a favorite in the golden days of American bodybuilding, from the thirties to the fifties. If you look back to photos of guys from those days—men like Zabo Koszewski or Leo Robert—you'll see that the lifters back then had incredibly well-built midsections, both tighter *and* more muscular than modern drug-built champs. The technique usually requires a special apparatus, but not always. In prison we would sit and lower ourselves sideways over a chair while another guy held our feet. I've seen guys in the ghetto jump up and hook their legs through a basketball hoop to do Roman chair work! I wouldn't recommend this, but it does go to show that where there's a will, there's a way. If you are resourceful, the whole world can be your gym.

Twisting Sit-Ups

This is the regular sit-up, but done with a twisting motion on the way up so that your elbow makes contact with the opposite knee, alternating the twisting direction with each repetition. A lot of bodybuilders (and boxers—who should know better) do this exercise in the hope of strengthening the obliques, the muscles at the side of the waist. Unfortunately there is very little force required to turn the torso during sit-ups, and as a result this variation adds little to the regular sit-up. Soviet trainers got wise to this fact decades ago and created a much more effective exercise for the twisting muscles of the waist; the *Russian twist*.

Russian Twists

Get into a Roman chair, or any position where your torso is horizontal and free of support. Grab a weight—in the gym a lot of guys use a 45 lbs. plate, but in the pen we liked a heavy book or water bottle in each hand—and incline your trunk slightly. Hold the weight at arm's length, and twist from left to right. Your arms (and therefore your waist rotation) only need to go from about the ten o' clock to the two o' clock position. You'll know when you get this movement right, because the muscles to the sides of your abs will start to burn like crazy. It's hard to make this exercise progressive, but it's a fun variation to throw into your workouts once in a while.

L-Holds

Sit on the floor with your legs locked out in front of you and your arms by your sides. Now press down hard though your hands, so that your butt and legs come fully clear of the floor. Your legs should remain at a perfect right angle to your torso. You'll need strong lats and arms to push your bodyweight clear of the floor, and your abs, hips and thighs need to contract hard or your legs will sag down. This exercise resembles the final position of the *hanging straight leg raise*, but it's not as effective for the abdomen because of the lack of motion. The absence of the hanging position also means the ribcage and serratus get less work than in the hanging exercises. It's a cool little trick though.

Medicine Ball Work

In the old days, athletes used to rely heavily on the medicine ball to train their waists, but this has largely gone the way of the dinosaur. It's a shame, because throwing and catching a heavy ball works all the internal muscles of the midsection, like the diaphragm and transversus. It forces the abs to contract quickly and powerfully in the way they need to fire when bracing for a fall or protecting the internal organs from a stout punch. You don't need a heavy authentic medicine ball, a basketball will do if you throw it hard enough. You don't even require a training partner—you can just shoot that sucker at a wall and catch it on the rebound.

Side Leg Raises

Lie on your side on the floor. Keeping your leg straight, raise your uppermost leg as high as you can. Ninety degrees is ideal, but this will be difficult at first as the side of the hips are usually pretty feeble unless you are into skating or martial arts. Once you have built up to fifty reps, try the same exercise standing, which is much harder. A weighted alternative to this technique is the *side bend* with a barbell behind the neck or with a dumbbell in one hand, but I wouldn't recommend using external weights while bending to the side as it puts the lower vertebrae in a precarious position. Modern books on exercise usually recommend side waist work, such as lateral crunch variations and twisting movements. In fact, the leg raise series works the entire waist including the obliques, and makes the hips good and strong. You really don't require extra "side" exercises if you work hard on the leg raise ten steps. But if you do wish to specialize this area for whatever reason, forgo all other exercises and gradually build up towards *twisting leg raises*.

Twisting Leg Raises

This is the ultimate specialist exercise for the flanks of the torso, but you need to be pretty strong to even attempt it. Build up to it with *side leg raises*, and by working your way through the regular leg raise series. Hang from a bar, and raise your legs. They should be fairly straight. At the top of the movement, turn one hip out to the front and twist the pelvis up as high as you can. Reverse the motion before repeating on the other side. One set of this exercise—when you are up to it—will do more than a thousand sets of side crunches or broomstick twists. It'll make your obliques stand out like fingers, and improve all your athletic twisting motions, taking your torque strength to stellar levels. This is because it's big, intense and painful. Like the man used to say, you can tap a stick of dynamite with a pencil a thousand times, and it won't go off. But hit it once with a hammer, and BANG! It'll detonate. The same is true of muscle cells. Just making them contract over and over won't make anything happen. They certainly won't become any bigger or stronger. That's why those electrical ab stimulation gizmos don't work—all they do is make the muscles contract repetitively. You need to *force* your muscles to respond. Hit those pesky muscle cells with a hammer—jump up and grab a bar for leg raises, son!

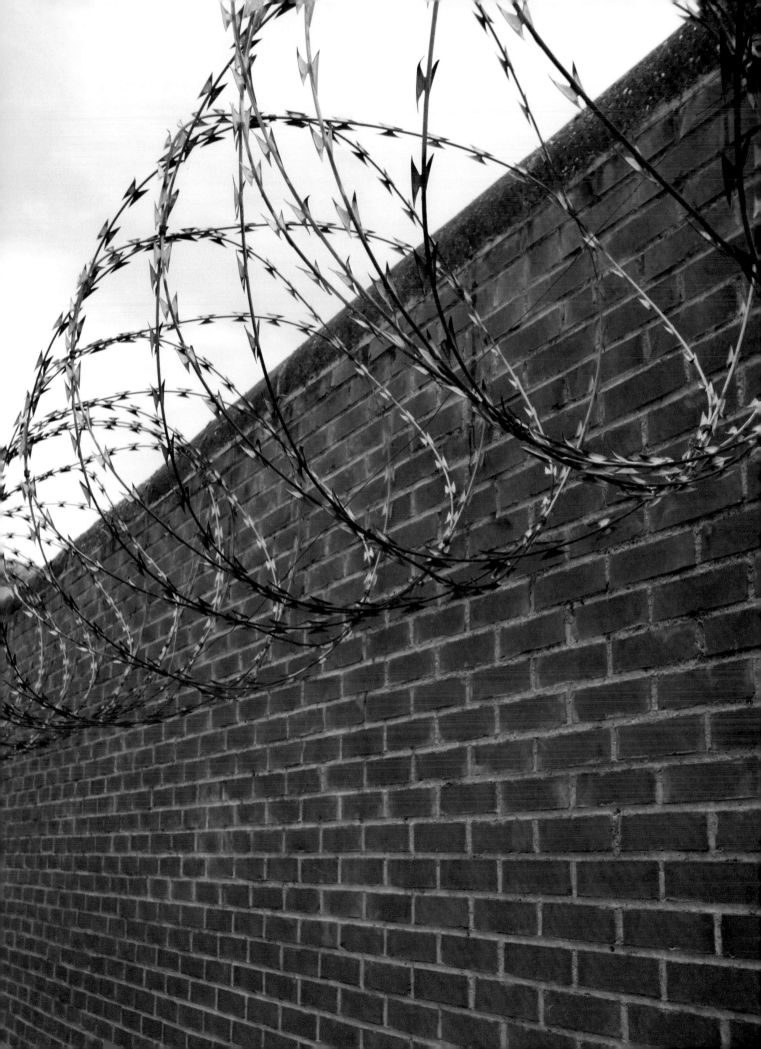

9: THE BRIDGE

COMBAT READY YOUR SPINE

If I had to name the most important strength-building exercise in the world, it would be the *bridge*. Nothing else even comes close.

Squats build big strong legs, pushups develop your chest, pullups create thick lats and biceps, and so on. There are any number of exercises that will build large, impressive muscles if you know how to perform them properly. There are hundreds of superficial, glossy books devoted to training the big, showy muscles of the body. But back bridging—the art of training the muscles of the *spine* for steel-like strength and elastic flexibility—is virtually unheard of. You won't see rows of guys in the gym, bridging. Fitness writers hardly ever waste any ink on this ancient exercise, preferring to focus on arm, ab and torso training. In fact, so few athletes know how to do bridging properly, that it's practically a secret technique!

Why is this? Most of it has to do with the modern culture of *appearance* over *ability*. Guys today have been brainwashed by bodybuilding philosophy. Nobody ever turns round and hits a "spinal muscles" pose. People today only care how big your arms are. When trainees get together and talk about muscles, the first question is usually *how big are your arms?* not *how strong are your spinal muscles?*

This is a real shame, because the spinal muscles are far more important for strength and athleticism than the biceps. In fact, your spinal muscles are the most important voluntary muscles in the body, bar none.

Training the Spine

The most important organ of the human body isn't a muscle. It isn't even the heart or lungs. It's *the brain*. The brain controls these secondary organs, just as it controls virtually every other structure and process in the human body. Our basic psychological identity is associated with the cerebral functioning of the brain; to a large degree, or brain is everything we are. When the brain dies, that's it. No more you.

The second most important organ of the human body is the *spinal cord*, because the spinal cord is the main means by which the brain communicates with the rest of the body. The spinal cord is a slim but incredibly complex tube of nerves, passing from the lower brainstem down the back of the body. No matter how powerful or healthy the brain is, if the spinal cord is damaged, it cannot communicate with the body and is effectively useless. Everybody remembers the tragic paralysis of *Superman* star Christopher Reeve following his horse riding accident in the mid nineteen-nineties. Reeve suffered no brain damage—the helmet he was wearing prevented it. But his brain was unable to influence his body because his *spinal cord* was horribly damaged.

The spinal cord is extremely delicate and, if unprotected, would be harmed very easily. Even a tiny amount of damage would have *disastrous* results on the functioning of the body. Fortunately, because of it's paramount importance for health and survival, the spinal column has been well-protected by evolution. It is encased in a thick pillar of flexible, articulated armor consisting of dense individual bones jointed by tough cartilage. These individual bones are the *vertebrae*, and the cartilage pieces are called *intervertebral discs*, or simply *discs* (as in the term "slipped disc"). The whole bony pillar is known as the *spinal column*. The spinal column is further protected by a network of connected ligaments and a sophisticated deep layer of muscles which control the movements of the spine. There are more than thirty pairs of *basic* spinal muscles. (Lack of space prevents me from listing them all and describing their functions. Interested trainees should pick up a copy of *Gray's Anatomy*.) Far from functioning separately, all these spinal muscles are molded into two thick, powerful, snake-like tubes bordering the spine. These muscle groups are called the *erector spinae*, or spinal erectors.

These twin pillars of muscle form the first line of defense against spinal injuries. In a very basic way, they function as a dense corset of flesh which protects the spinal column against accidents and danger from sharp or blunt objects. In a more dynamic sense, they also control the movement of the spine generally; they ensure that the vertebrae follow a range of motion that protects the spinal cord as well as dictating all spinal motions. Without the *erector spinae*, you couldn't walk, stand up, twist, or move the torso at all. You couldn't even turn your head.

The spinal erectors are absolutely crucial. But even they pale into insignificance next to the importance of the *spinal cord* which they help to protect. Impulses travel *down* through the spinal cord, so the higher an injury, the more devastating the effects.

- A complete injury to the lower spine (the *lumbar region*) will render the legs useless, and leave the victim incontinent and impotent.

- A similar injury to the middle portion of the spine (the *thoracic region*) will also leave the victim unable to control the muscles of the trunk.

- An injury to the highest third of the spine (the *cervical region*) will in addition paralyze the arms, shoulders, neck and—if high enough—the diaphragm which powers the lungs.

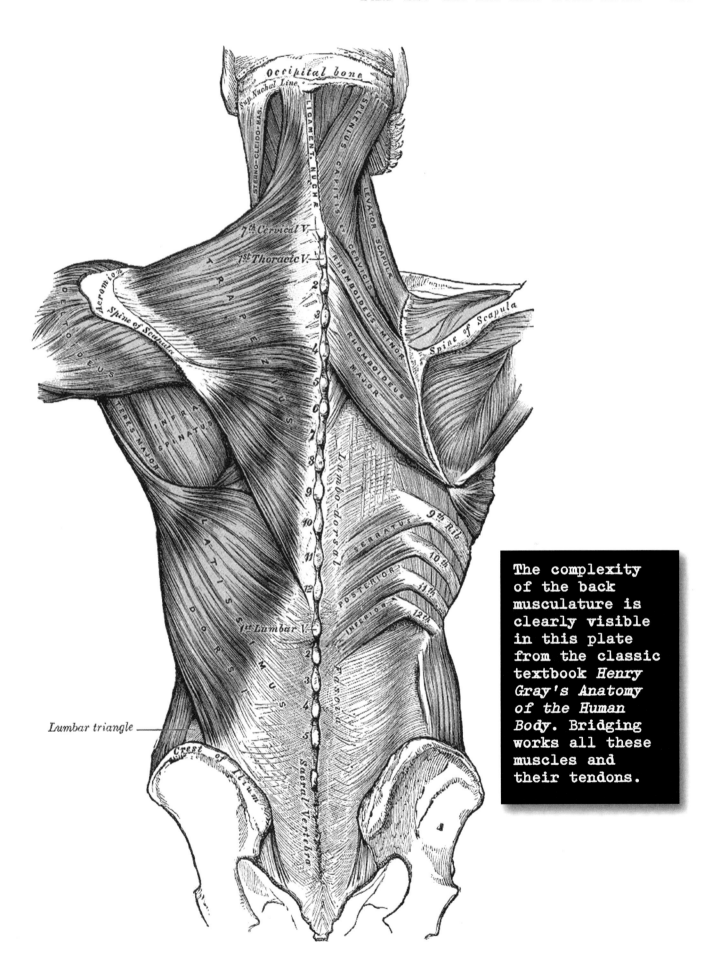

The complexity of the back musculature is clearly visible in this plate from the classic textbook *Henry Gray's Anatomy of the Human Body*. Bridging works all these muscles and their tendons.

Apart from these fundamental symptoms, spinal injuries are also associated with horrible side-effects including muscle atrophy, osteoporosis, neuropathic pain, and an inability to control basic physiological functions such as blood pressure, body temperature and heart rate. To make matters even worse, the nerve structure of the spinal cord is incredibly complex, and once it is damaged, the nerves only have a very limited ability to repair themselves. Christopher Reeve shattered the first and second vertebrae in his spine, in the neck, and as a result his functioning below the neck virtually disappeared. It took him many months of daily therapy before he was even able to breathe for short periods without a respirator.

The safety of the spinal cord is dependent upon the integrity of the spinal column. This in turn largely depends upon the health of the network of ligaments and muscles which support it. Once the spinal column is formed, the best way you can protect your spinal cord and keep it healthy is to maintain strong spinal erectors.

Perhaps short of breathing, eating healthily and sleeping regularly, when you invest time training to protect your spine, you are doing the most important thing you can do for your health. It's that simple.

The Spine and Athletic Qualities

If you are one of these guys who has a barbell set at home for fitness and strength, you would do well to sell it and buy a cushioned mat to train your spine on instead. I realize that this suggestion seems so far from the current bodybuilding-style culture of strength and fitness that it seems almost funny. But I'm not joking.

The spine is the equivalent of the universal joint on a motor car. Every piece of pressure generated by movement goes through it—from little motions of the head and neck, to very powerful forces such as those generated in a heavy football tackle. If your spine is weak, you can suffer all kinds of trauma from these actions—anything from an excruciating "slipped disc" to a compression fracture. You might even break your back. The more athletic movements you make, the more risk to your spine. The stronger your spinal muscles are, the more punishment your spine can take and bounce back smiling.

Apart from preventing sports injuries, the spinal muscles also play a fundamentally positive role in strength and athleticism. The spinal muscles are incredibly strong, and are involved in practically every major motion, from throwing and twisting to bending over and lifting. Without good, robust spinal muscles, *strength cannot exist*. It's impossible to use the limbs—whether curling, squatting, pressing or pulling—without using the spinal muscles. These muscles are used more than any other voluntary muscles. The stronger your spinal muscles, the better you will be at practically any athletic motion you can name.

Given this, it's ironic that the spinal muscles aren't the number-one priority of all athletes. It's downright *amazing* that most trainees don't seek to directly train their spinal muscles at all! Most of them just wouldn't know where to start. Is it really so surprising that lower back pain is the foremost plague of athletes the world over? Not at all. It's just a consequence of this neglect.

The Benefits of Bridging

There is a solution—an ultimate solution—to this neglect. *Bridging*. Bridging is a simple technique—you just arch your back off the floor by pushing up with your limbs—but if you bridge regularly you can eliminate the host of back problems associated with abuse of the human body. Unfortunately, this medicine is needed now more than ever. Human beings are at a spinal disadvantage to begin with; standing on two feet was the worst move our species ever made. Animals on all-fours rarely suffer spinal problems because they have to lean back frequently just to gain height. Unfortunately modern culture compounds this inherent disadvantage. The average person today leads a life which involves both disuse *and* misuse of the spine. They spend their days doing repetitive jobs slumped in front of computer screens or over desks with terrible posture which misaligns their spinal column; then they go home and slouch on the sofa in front of the tube. As a result, civilians are suffering more back problems and ever, and people are now getting disc degeneration in their thirties.

Bridging—even just once per week—prevents all these problems. It realigns the vertebrae into the correct position, and strengthens the deep muscles of the back responsible for proper posture. Even the *bones* become stronger over time, with the practice of the bridge. The discs in your back are made of cartilage, and like all cartilage, they have very little blood flow. Instead, they receive their nutrition from liquid in the joints, called *synovial fluid*. Because it's not associated with the circulation, fresh fluid can only reach the joints when those joints move around. Bridging removes waste and sends plenty of nutritious fluid to the discs, healing them, preventing degeneration and ensuring maximal health. Strong spinal muscles can reduce the likelihood of slipped discs, and even help fix the condition.

Aside from the above benefits, bridging will make all your athletic movements more powerful. Bridging is the *ultimate* exercise for the spinal muscles. The master of the bridge can be easily identified by two very cool pythons running up either side of the spine. But as well as being the primary exercise for the *erector spinae*, bridging develops practically every other muscle in the body. The arms and legs get work in pressing the body away from the ground, and the shoulder girdle and upper back get a *fantastic* workout in the process, too. The entire front side of the body—usually stubbornly tight in male athletes—gets a maximum stretch. Areas which particularly benefit are the knees, quadriceps, hip flexors, abdominals and chest. The unique overhead-and-back movement during bridging removes calcium deposits in the shoulders and makes the torso very supple. A lot of practitioners—including myself—believe that regular practice of the bridge can expand the ribcage and increase lung capacity.

Bridging bulletproofs the spinal column in preparation for heavy, explosive, or unexpected movements, allowing you to train harder, heavier, and faster. Because the spine is like a universal joint, strong spinal muscles unlock the power inherent in the waist, torso and limbs, power an athlete simply couldn't access if they had a weak back. The spine is constantly working during motion, so conditioned spinal muscles also result in extra endurance, both for sports and life generally.

I could go on, but I won't. In essence, the message is simple: bridging will do away with back pain, make you healthier, stronger, quicker, more agile, and increase your stamina. You should be bridging.

Bruce's Back

Many strength athletes perform barbell exercises for their spinal muscles, exercises like deadlifts and good mornings, where bar is placed on the shoulders and the athlete bows down. These techniques both work the *erector spinae*, but they load the spinal column at a fixed point, meaning that the deep muscles are worked unevenly. During bridges, the powerful spinal muscles are worked when the spine is arched *back*, which closes the joints. This is a very safe position, particularly if no external load is involved. Unfortunately, barbell exercises work the muscles with the spine rounded *forwards*, which opens the vertebrae, and puts the discs in danger of splitting or popping out. The leverage of the high external load as well as the convex opening of the vertebrae makes the back very vulnerable to injury during these barbell movements. The mighty Bruce Lee was performing barbell good mornings when he blew his back out badly in 1970. Doctors told him he would never perform kung fu again, but he trained himself back to full fitness—using calisthenics.

The Culture of Bridging

Bridging exercises are not widely practiced in the West. Perhaps this really *is* because our culture values appearance over ability, because in other parts of the world the bridge is highly esteemed as one of the greatest exercise techniques known—in the East, it is regarded as the "king" of exercises. Various forms of bridge are well known in Shaolin kung fu training, and are also practiced as part of the Taoist health arts like *k'ai men* and *tao yin*. But perhaps no country has devoted so much time to understanding the bridge as India, where it is called *chakrasana*—the wheel posture. In yoga, there are scores of bridging exercises, ranging from basic positions to highly advanced poses where the feet actually rest on the head. Indian physical culturists take the bridge so seriously because their understanding of the importance of the spine goes back thousands of years further than our own. Ayurvedic medicine (the ancient Indian philosophy of health) places so much importance on the spinal column that it is seen as possessing occult and even magical qualities.

Perhaps I'm maligning *Western* attitudes towards the bridge a little. Those disciplines where ability is more important than outward appearance still practice the bridge. Gymnasts practice the bridge, because their backs need to be strong and flexible for flips. Many advanced powerlifters practice the bridge, and swear by it. Wrestlers—as with many things—have been way ahead of the pack with their understanding of the importance of a strong back. As a result, bridging is a part of the basic training curriculum for all wrestlers, at all levels. One of the few times you'll ever see bridging performed at a high school in America would be during a wrestling class. What a pity. If it was taught to *all* our students from a young age, lower back pain and spinal disorders would be cut by 99% in a single generation.

The Four Signs of Perfection

A lot of athletes—and even yoga guys, who should know better—think that just because they can press their back off the ground, they can do a bridge. Not so. You should endeavor to perfect your technique in this important exercise. There are *four* signs of the perfect bridge:

1. **The spine should be convex.** It sounds obvious, but the back must be well-rounded during a bridge. If the deep spinal muscles are weak, the athlete will tend to lift his body using the limbs, and keep the back quite straight.

2. **The hips should be high off the floor.** The most obvious sign of a weak bridge is that the hips only just clear the floor. In the perfect bridge, your hips and butt should be even higher than the level of your head and shoulder blades. This will be hard to determine unless you get a photo taken of your technique from the side.

3. **The arms and legs should be straight.** It's relatively easy to straighten the arms during bridging, but straightening the arms *and* the legs requires a very high level of flexibility.

4. **Breathing should be smooth and deep.** This posture stretches the ribcage and puts the diaphragm under pressure, and can result in short, choppy breaths if the chest is stiff. Natural breathing is a sign of mastery of this pose. Never hold your breath during the bridge.

(These four signs relate to the *full bridge* (Step 6) and all the steps afterwards which include it as a part; they don't necessarily apply to the earlier steps, which may require different positioning. Sign number four applies to *all* bridging motions, however.)

A *perfect* bridge must include all four signs. A bridge which includes three can be counted as *good*. Any bridge with just two is *rudimentary*. A posture that includes one or none of the above technical signs is not a bridge at all, at least to a student of *Convict Conditioning*.

No matter how strong and supple you are, no athlete will be able to display all the four signs of the perfect bridge on their first attempt. It may take you months—or longer—until you get there. Don't worry about this. Even an imperfect bridge is better than no bridging at all, so keep on trying in confidence, knowing that every time you train you are getting better and doing something great for your body. If you persist in your efforts, one day your bridge will display all the four signs.

Mastering the Bridge

Just because bridging is an important exercise, it doesn't follow that you should launch into bridging right now if you are not used to it. In fact, this could be a hazardous thing to do. Very few athletes have the spinal power to do a bridge first time of asking. To make things worse the average body is usually completely unbalanced in terms of flexibility—even couch potatoes have to bend the spine *forwards* while sitting, to tie their shoes, or to pick up the remote control. But how often does the average person bend *backwards*? Not much, if ever—and the result is lopsided flexibility, which is always a dangerous thing. Combine a lack of muscular strength and control with this unsymmetrical flexibility, and you are asking for a muscle strain or worse if you just throw bridging into your training on a whim.

What you need is a *plan*. If you are new to bridging (or working out in general), I advise that you devote a good chunk of your time working on your fundamental strength. Lots of focus on squatting and leg raises will strengthen the muscles of the back and hips, and make the waist more supple. By the time you have mastered *close squats* (pages 94-95) and *hanging knee raises* (pages 166-167), you'll be ready to start tackling the bridge series of movements.

The first three steps of the bridging series represent the *therapy sequence*. They will ease old injuries, increase backwards flexibility, and loosen the tight hip flexors at the front. They will also awaken the deep layer of spinal muscles which you may not be used to using. You may feel these muscles begin to burn and ache as you progress. That's a good thing. The burning sensation means that your muscles have begun to build their glucose stores—it's these stores being utilized that results in the "burn." If you have built a base of strength with your leg raises and squats, these exercises will not pose much of a problem. But don't be in a rush. Build on your training momentum, don't destroy it. Take your time with these exercises more than any other; your spine is precious. Be kind to it.

The next three steps will gradually lead you to the *full bridge*. At this level, strength and flexibility will develop hand-in-hand. Once you have got to grips with the full bridge (Step 6), make sure to spend some time on it—a good few months at least. Be aware that there is a *good* bridge, and a *bad* bridge. There are good and bad versions of all exercise techniques, but this is particularly true when it comes to bridging. In a good bridge, the hips are high, the limbs straight, and the back nicely arched to display great flexibility. It appears effortless. A bad bridge is sloppy; the limbs are bent, the body isn't far of the floor, and the spine looks stiff as a board. It looks like a strain, which it is. If you have followed the earlier steps faithfully, once you get to this stage your body will become accustomed to the bridge very quickly—and this will be an excellent time to really get to know the technique. Some of my students used to say that they could actually *feel* their bridges getting noticeably better every time they practiced. This adaptation happens quickly—even in older guys—because in most men the deeper spinal muscles are "virgin territory." They are not used to being asked to produce high levels of contraction, and they learn fast.

Once you have got to the stage where you can do a good basic bridge, you can pat yourself on the back. Your back will feel better than ever, and your spine will be stronger and more flexible than the next ninety-nine athletes—"like a steel whip" as one of my ex-students put it. He was a martial artist, and knew the value of owning a spine like that. But the journey isn't done yet—you're going to get even better. So far, you will have started your full bridges lying flat on the floor. The remaining four steps will teach you advanced tactics for getting into the bridge, until eventually you can do the *stand-to-stand* bridge. This involves standing up straight and bending over backwards into a bridge, before smoothly reversing the movement and standing up straight again. This motion is the Master Step of the bridging series of movements. Good luck finding anybody who can do ten good reps of this beauty! Not only will this give you incredible power and flexibility in your spine and waist, it produces total-body strengthening benefits, and it looks damn cool, too.

Now, onto the ten steps. Feel free to read about these movements, but remember—you are advised not to actually attempt these exercises until you can do Step 6 of both the squatting and leg raises series.

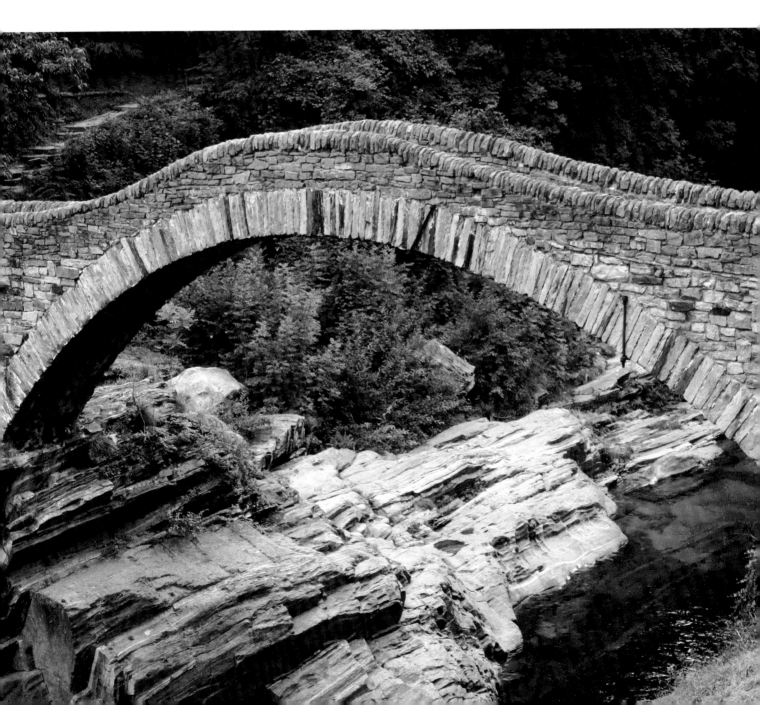

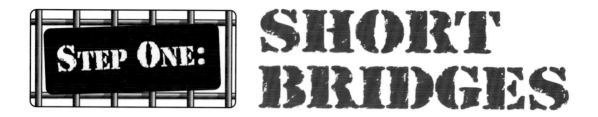

Performance

Lie on your back, with your legs stretched out and your hands crossed on your stomach. Draw your feet in, bending the knees until your shins are nearly parallel to the ground and your feet your feet are flat on the floor. The feet should be shoulder width apart or a little less, depending upon your frame. Your heels will be around six to eight inches from your buttocks. This is the start position (fig. 83). Press down through the feet, lifting the hips and back clear of the ground until only the shoulders and feet are supporting the bodyweight. At this point, your thighs, trunk and torso should form a straight line, with no sagging of the hips. This is the finish position (fig. 84). Pause in the top position for a moment, before reversing the motion, lowering your body back to the start position. Repeat the exercise for your target repetitions, exhaling as you go up, inhaling on the way down.

Exercise X-Ray

Short bridges involve pushing through the lower limbs, and are the gentlest way to begin spinal training because in everyday life we usually activate the spinal muscles via the legs. We do this simply by moving around, bending down, etc. The act of keeping the trunk straight at the top of the short bridging movement stimulates the spine and hip muscles with hardly any pressure running through the vertebrae. As a result this exercise is wonderful therapy for those who have suffered disc injuries.

Training Goals

- Beginner standard: 1 set of 10
- Intermediate standard: 2 sets of 25
- Progression standard: 3 sets of 50

Perfecting Your Technique

Most people should be able to do *short bridges* without much difficulty. If you are recovering from a back injury and this exercise poses a problem, simply reduce the range of motion by performing the technique with a few pillows or cushions under the hips.

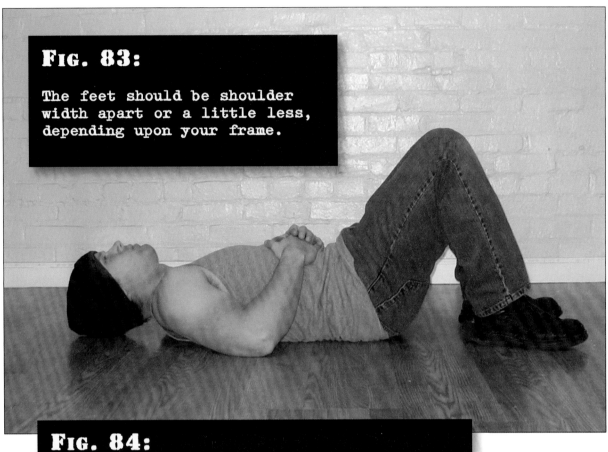

FIG. 83:

The feet should be shoulder width apart or a little less, depending upon your frame.

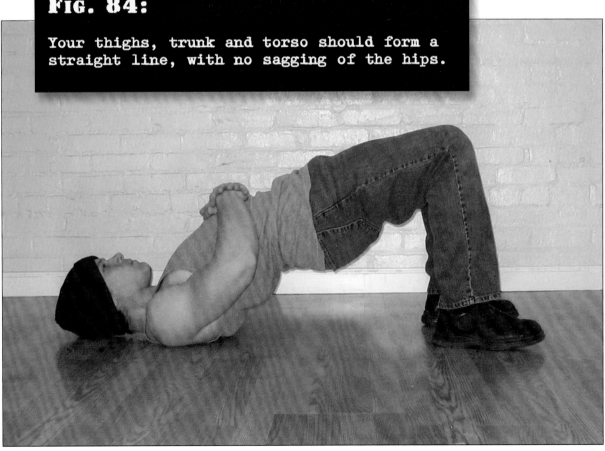

FIG. 84:

Your thighs, trunk and torso should form a straight line, with no sagging of the hips.

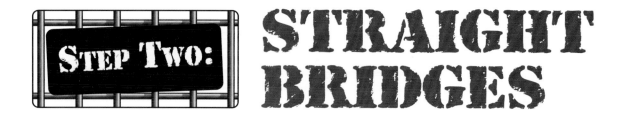

Performance

Sit on the ground with your legs stretched out in front of you. Your knees should be straight, with your feet about shoulder width apart. Place your palms on the floor on either side of your hips, with your fingers pointing towards your toes. Sit up straight. Your body will now form a right angle, with your trunk perpendicular to your legs. This is the start position (fig. 85). Press down through the hands, tensing the arms as you simultaneously push your hips upwards until your legs and torso form a straight line. Draw the chin up and look towards the ceiling. At this point your bodyweight will be passing through your palms and heels. This is the finish position (fig. 86). Pause before reversing the motion and repeating as necessary. Exhale as you press yourself up, inhale as you go down.

Exercise X-Ray

Short bridges require you to activate the spinal muscles mainly by pushing through the legs; *straight bridges* require pressure through the arms also. It's this factor, combined with the elongated body position, that makes straight bridges slightly more difficult. The movement not only tones the arms, it also loosens the torso and strengthens the muscles between the shoulder blades that are crucial for performing harder versions of the bridge.

Training Goals

- Beginner standard: 1 set of 10
- Intermediate standard: 2 sets of 20
- Progression standard: 3 sets of 40

Perfecting Your Technique

If the *straight bridge* described is too difficult, you can make the exercise easier by reducing the leverage. Instead of performing the technique with the legs straight, do it with the legs bent, as they are in *short bridges* (fig. 84). If this is still too difficult, simply perform the exercise kneeling down, leaning back and pressing the buttocks a few inches up and away from the calves. Continue using this partial motion until you get strong enough to try again.

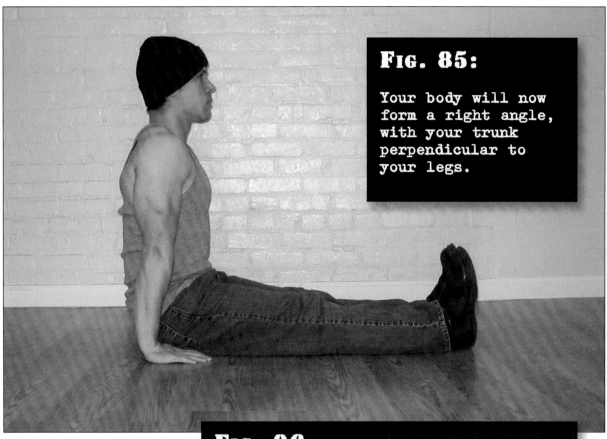

FIG. 85:

Your body will now form a right angle, with your trunk perpendicular to your legs.

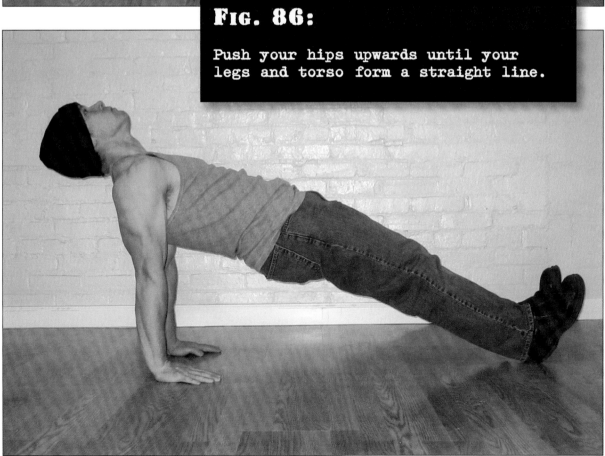

FIG. 86:

Push your hips upwards until your legs and torso form a straight line.

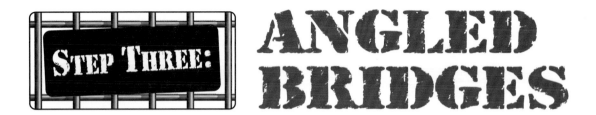

Performance

Angled bridges require an object which is about knee height or a little higher. In prison, a bunk is perfect. The average bed in an American home is a bit taller, but still acceptable for our purposes. Sit on the edge of the bunk or bed, and lie back with your feet flat on the ground. They should be approximately shoulder width apart. Shuffle forwards a little so that your hips are off the bunk, and place your hands either side of your head, with your fingers pointing towards your feet. This is the start position (fig. 87). Press down through the hands, straightening the elbows and pushing the hips up, arching your back as you do so. Continue smoothly pushing as far as you can, at least until your head and body are entirely clear of the bunk. The arms don't need to be fully extended; the elbows will be bent. You may only lift up a few inches. That's fine. Allow your head to tilt back under control, so that you can see the wall behind you. This is the finish position (fig 88). Reverse the motion, lowering yourself until your torso and head are resting completely on the bunk again. Repeat as necessary, breathing normally.

Exercise X-Ray

Angled bridges are the first exercise in the bridging series to utilize the full "hands alongside head" position used in advanced bridging. This position will strengthen the wrists and open up the shoulders and chest in preparation for later exercises. This motion also requires greater flexibility and contractile strength in the upper spine than the earlier steps.

Training Goals

- Beginner standard: 1 set of 8
- Intermediate standard: 2 sets of 15
- Progression standard: 3 sets of 30

Perfecting Your Technique

Bridging is easier the shallower the angle—i.e., the higher your head and hands are. If an *angled bridge* off a bunk is too hard, try it against something higher—maybe a table or desk—until you can manage the lower surface.

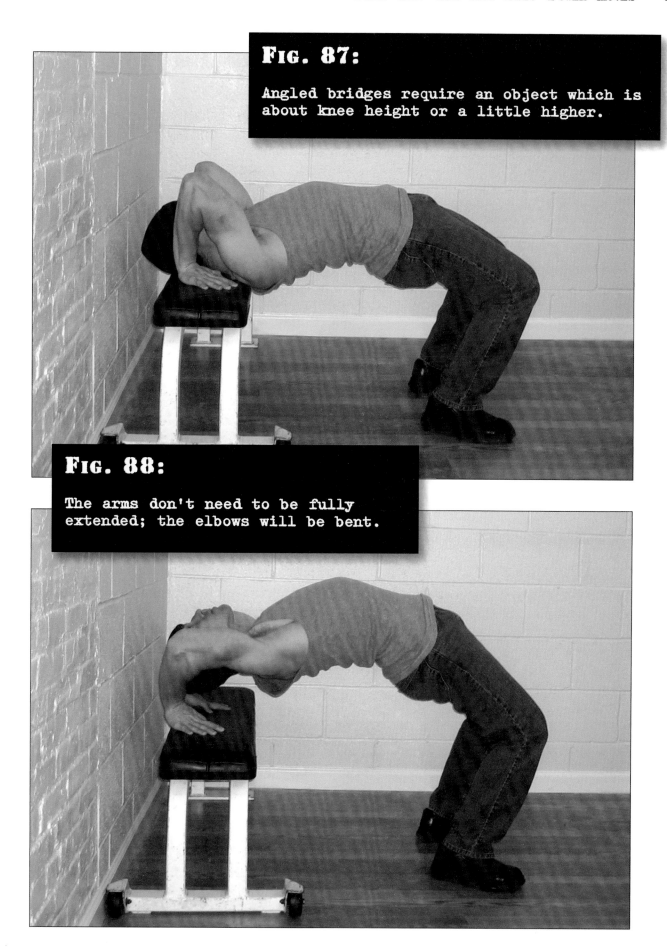

FIG. 87:

Angled bridges require an object which is about knee height or a little higher.

FIG. 88:

The arms don't need to be fully extended; the elbows will be bent.

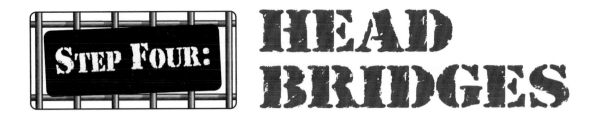

STEP FOUR:

HEAD BRIDGES

Performance

Lie with your back on the floor. Draw your feet in, bending the knees until your heels are approximately six to eight inches from your glutes. The feet should be shoulder width apart or slightly closer. Place the hands alongside the head, with the palms flat on the floor and your fingers pointing towards your toes. Your elbows should be angled towards the ceiling at this point. Now push the hips as high as you can, lifting the body from the floor. Continue pushing through your arms and legs until your back is well arched, and your hips are high. The head should be tilted down, with the crown of your skull pointing towards the floor. This is a *bridge hold*. Retain this position momentarily, before bending at the arms and legs until the top of your skull very gently touches the floor. This is the start position (fig. 89). Pause again briefly, before pushing yourself back up to the bridge (fig. 90). This is the finish position. Go carefully, so that you don't bang your head. Maintain the deep arch in the back all the way throughout the set, breathing as normally as possible all the way through. When you have finished all your reps, smoothly lower your shoulders, back and hips to the floor.

Exercise X-Ray

Unlike yoga, which trains the back with static holds, old school calisthenics focuses on dynamic (or moving) strength. This short-range technique is only a preliminary step towards learning complete bridging movements.

Training Goals

- Beginner standard: 1 set of 8
- Intermediate standard: 2 sets of 15
- Progression standard: 2 sets of 25

Perfecting Your Technique

If you have some difficulty getting into the initial *bridge hold*, begin by lying with something under the small of your back—two or three cushions or pillows should do the trick. If you can't touch your head to the floor, just use a shorter range of motion and go lower from workout to workout.

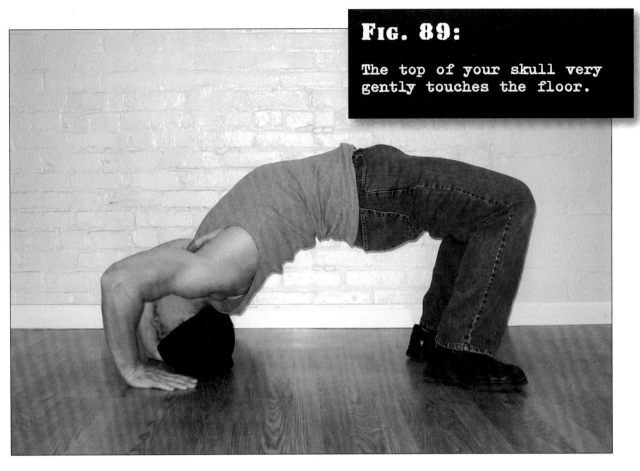

FIG. 89:

The top of your skull very gently touches the floor.

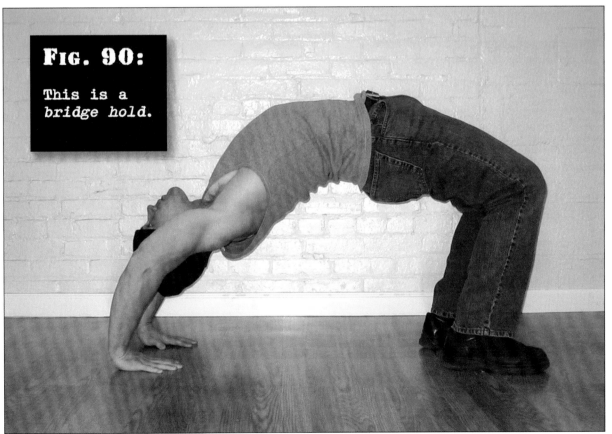

FIG. 90:

This is a *bridge hold.*

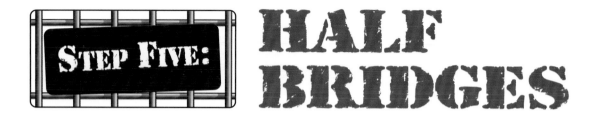

Performance

This exercise will require a basketball or soccer ball to monitor your form. Sit down on the floor, placing the ball on the ground right behind you. Lay back so that you are lying down with only your shoulders and the soles of your feet on the floor. The feet should be shoulder width apart or a little closer, and the ball should be supporting the small of your back. If you find this position uncomfortable, lay a folded towel or cushion over the ball before you begin. Place the hands alongside the head, with the palms flat on the floor and your fingers pointing towards your toes. Now press through the hands, pushing your shoulders and head off the floor so that only the soles of your feet, the ball, and your palms are supporting your bodyweight. This is the start position (fig. 91). From here, push the hips as high as you can, extending the arms and legs and lifting the back up until it is well clear of the ball. Keep going until your back is fully arched. This is the finish position (fig, 92). Pause for a moment at the top, before lowering yourself slowly to the start position. After starting the set, only descend until the small of your back lightly touches the ball—don't rest your bodyweight on it. Repeat, breathing as normally as possible.

Exercise X-Ray

This movement constitutes the top half of the range of Step 6, the *full bridge*. By the time you can perform this motion for the reps listed under the *progression standard*, your spinal muscles will be powerful and lithe enough to start including the more difficult lower half of the bridging movement.

Training Goals

- Beginner standard: 1 set of 8
- Intermediate standard: 2 sets of 15
- Progression standard: 2 sets of 20

Perfecting Your Technique

As with most bridging movements, if you have trouble performing the reps as described, start shallow and build up your range of motion over time.

FIG. 91:

The feet should be shoulder width apart or a little closer, and the ball should be supporting the small of your back.

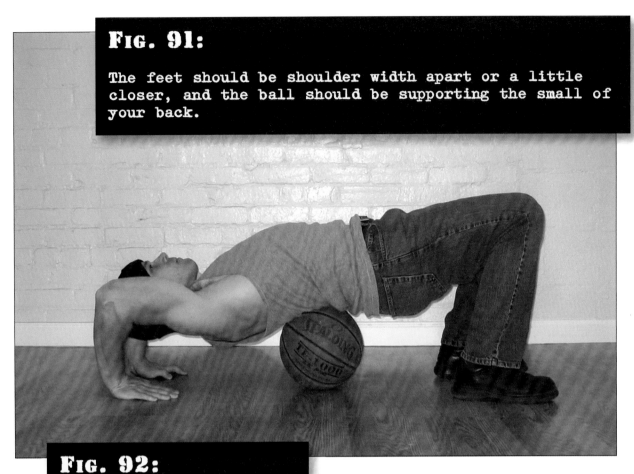

FIG. 92:

Keep going until your back is fully arched.

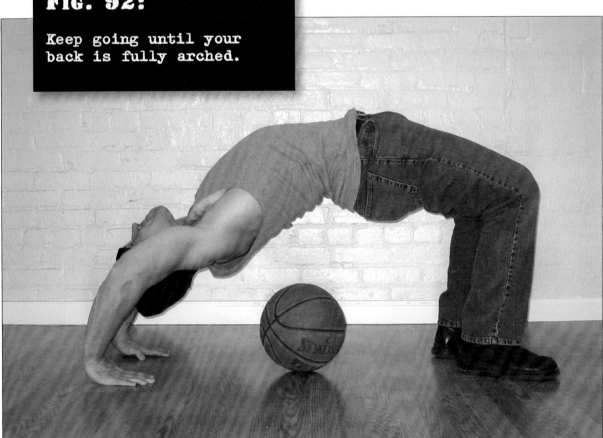

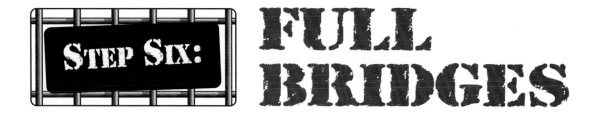

STEP SIX: FULL BRIDGES

Performance

Lie on your back. Draw your feet in, bending the knees until your heels are approximately six to eight inches from your glutes. The feet should be shoulder width apart or slightly closer. Place the hands alongside the head, with the palms flat on the floor and your fingers pointing towards your toes. Your elbows should be angled towards the ceiling at this point. This is the start position (fig. 93). Now push the hips as high as you can, lifting the body from the floor. Continue pushing through your arms and legs until your back is well arched, and your hips are high. In the perfect bridge, your arms will be totally straight. Allow the head to tilt backwards between the arms, so that you can look at the wall behind you. This is the finish position (fig. 94). Hold this top position for a moment, before reversing your motion. Control your descent—you will gain more benefit from the exercise if you lower yourself smoothly than if you simply collapse. Continue going all the way back down until your hips, back and head are resting completely on the floor again. This sequence constitutes one rep. Push yourself back up again for your target reps, breathing normally throughout.

Exercise X-Ray

The *full bridge* is a phenomenal exercise. As well as preventing and curing many back problems, it increases total-body flexibility, adds power to the deep muscles of the spine, expands the ribcage, limbers up the shoulders, tones the arms and legs, improves circulation and even aids the digestion.

Training Goals

- Beginner standard: 1 set of 6
- Intermediate standard: 2 sets of 10
- Progression standard: 2 sets of 15

Perfecting Your Technique

Attaining the ideal bridge—particularly the full extension of the arms and legs—is difficult and requires patient practice. When you begin, simply push your body as high as you can. Perfection will come with time.

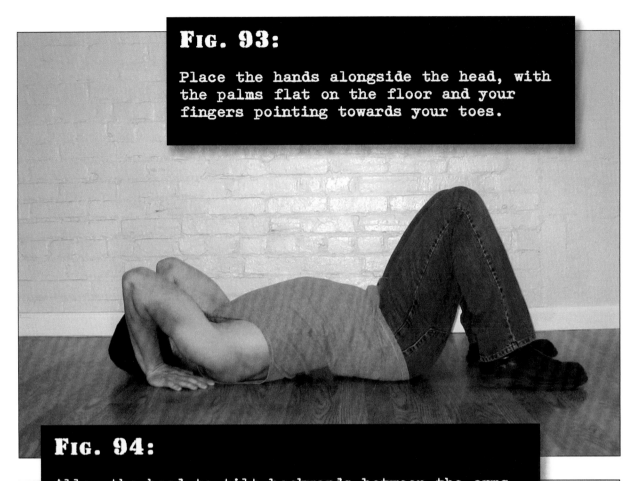

FIG. 93:

Place the hands alongside the head, with the palms flat on the floor and your fingers pointing towards your toes.

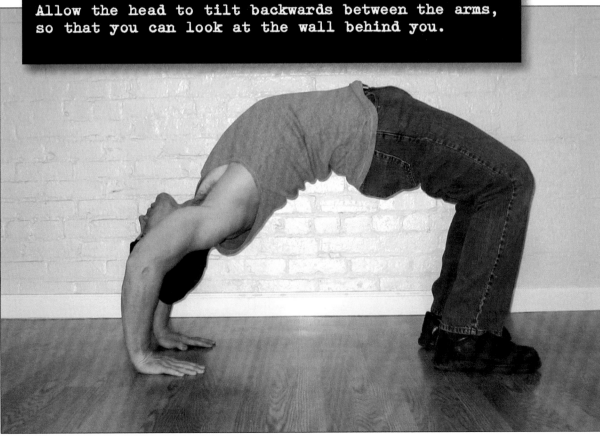

FIG. 94:

Allow the head to tilt backwards between the arms, so that you can look at the wall behind you.

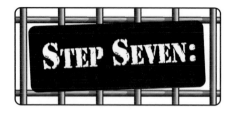

WALL WALKING BRIDGES (DOWN)

Performance

Stand approximately one arm's length from a wall. If in doubt about your positioning, it's better to stand closer to the wall than further from it—you can more safely adjust your position this way. Your feet should be about shoulder width apart. Push the hips forwards and begin bending backwards. Raise your chin, tilting your head back as far as is comfortable. Continue smoothly bending back until you can see the wall behind you. As soon as you can see the wall, raise your hands, moving them over your shoulders and placing the palms flat on the wall, fingers pointing down, level with your head. This is the start position (fig. 95). Shift some of your bodyweight back through your hands, and lower one by a few inches, before placing it securely on the wall again. Now follow suit with your opposite hand, lowering it even further on the wall. Keep bending backwards as you "walk" down the wall with your hands (fig. 96). As you move downwards, you will need to move slightly away from the wall to accommodate your body bend. Do this by taking mini-steps forwards any time you feel the need. Continue alternating this movement until you run out of wall. When this occurs, place your hands flat on the floor. At this stage you will be in a full *bridge hold* next to the wall. This is the bottom position (fig. 97). From here, simply lower your backside to the floor, and stand up. Return to the start position, and walk back down again. Breathe regularly as you go.

Exercise X-Ray

Walking down the wall is easier than walking up it. Master this step first.

Training Goals

- Beginner standard: 1 set of 3
- Intermediate standard: 2 sets of 6
- Progression standard: 2 sets of 10

Perfecting Your Technique

Very few people manage to walk fully down the wall their first time. Just try to go lower every time you train. Smaller "steps" will make things easier.

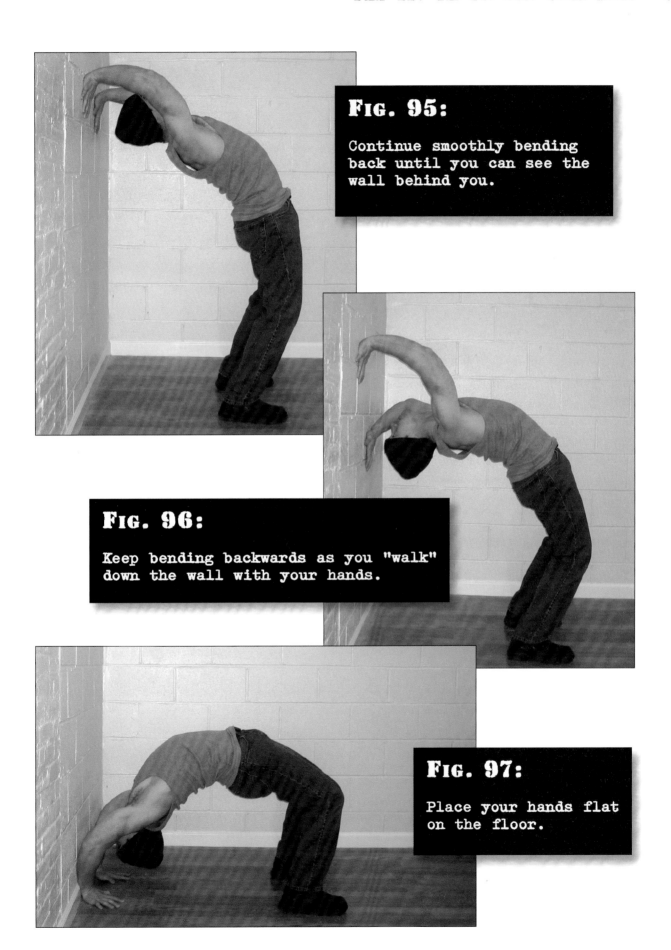

FIG. 95:

Continue smoothly bending back until you can see the wall behind you.

FIG. 96:

Keep bending backwards as you "walk" down the wall with your hands.

FIG. 97:

Place your hands flat on the floor.

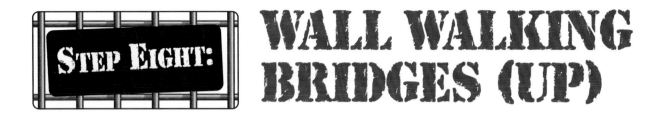

Performance

This step begins when you are standing totally clear of the wall, with your back to it. From here, assume the start position you learned for walking down; bend backwards with your hands over your shoulders making contact with the wall (fig. 95). Then walk down the wall as described in Step 7, until you are in a full *bridge hold* next to the base of the wall (fig. 97). Now it's time to go back up. This is done by reversing the movement. Place one palm back on the wall, pushing through it. Next, place your other palm above it (fig. 98). This transition whereby your palms go from the floor back onto the wall is the hardest part of the technique. Now simply place one palm above the other repeatedly as you go back up the wall. As your body straightens, you will probably have to take mini-steps back towards the wall to keep a healthy pressure going through your palms. Continue walking upwards until you are nearly straight (fig. 99). From here, push gently away from the wall until you are standing totally clear from it again (fig. 100). This cycle—standing, walking all the way down, walking back up, and standing free again—constitutes one single repetition of this exercise.

Exercise X-Ray

Once you have the flexibility and strength to walk *down* a wall, it's time to master this step and walk *upwards*. This doesn't require any extra flexibility, but it does require extra strength because you are moving against gravity.

Training Goals

- Beginner standard: 1 set of 2
- Intermediate standard: 2 sets of 4
- Progression standard: 2 sets of 8

Perfecting Your Technique

As with Step 7, the key to perfecting this exercise lies in progressively increasing range of motion. When you first try it, only go down the wall to a point where you are sure you can hand walk back up. Mark this level with a piece of chalk if it helps. Simply increase the depth over time.

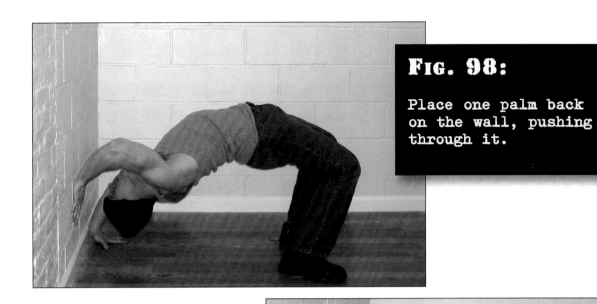

FIG. 98:

Place one palm back on the wall, pushing through it.

FIG. 99:

Continue walking upwards until you are nearly straight.

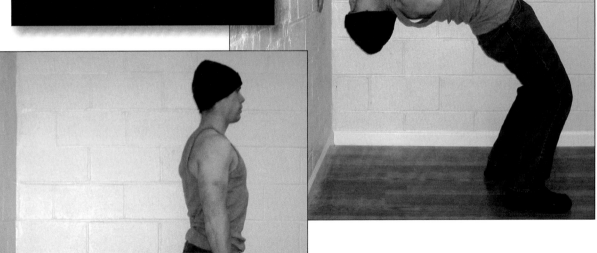

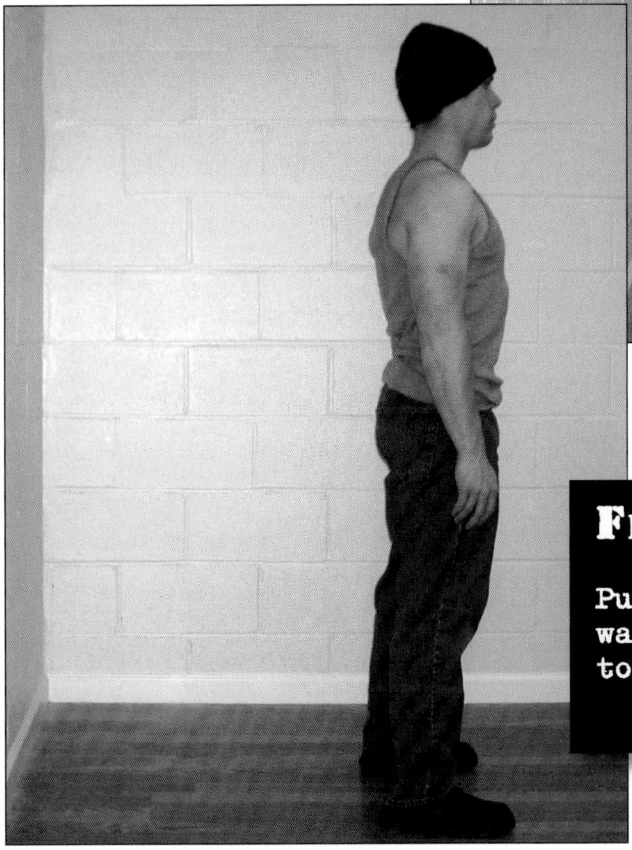

FIG. 100:

Push gently away from the wall until you are standing totally clear from it again.

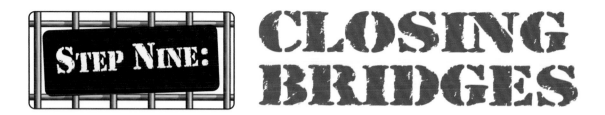

Performance

Stand up straight with your feet approximately shoulder width apart. The space behind you should be clear of objects for at least the distance of your height. This is the start position. Place your hands on your hips and begin pushing your pelvis forwards (fig. 101). When your pelvis is as far front as it will go, begin bending your knees as you simultaneously arch your spine backwards. Tilt your head back and look behind you as you go. This must all form one smooth movement. Continue this arching motion until you can see the ground a few feet behind you. As soon as you see the floor, take your hands off your hips and pass them back over your shoulders, beyond your head (fig. 102). This moving posture requires considerable flexibility, but you will find that the forwards shift of your hips combined with the bend in the knees prevents you from falling backwards. Extend your arms as you keep the movement going, until your palms are resting on the floor. This is the finish position, the full *bridge hold* (fig. 103). From here, bend the arms and legs until your back is on the floor. Now stand up into the start position again to begin your second repetition. Breath normally throughout the set.

Exercise X-Ray

This movement is the hardest bridging technique so far. It comprises the "eccentric" or negative phase of the Master Step, *stand-to-stand bridges*.

Training Goals

- Beginner standard: 1 set of 1
- Intermediate standard: 2 sets of 3
- Progression standard: 2 sets of 6

Perfecting Your Technique

At first, you will probably fall backwards over the last third of the movement, landing on the palms if you are lucky. This is unacceptable—you must continue practicing until you can gently *place* your palms on the floor. One trick that can help is reaching back onto stairs. Reach back onto lower steps each time you train until you are placing your palms on the ground.

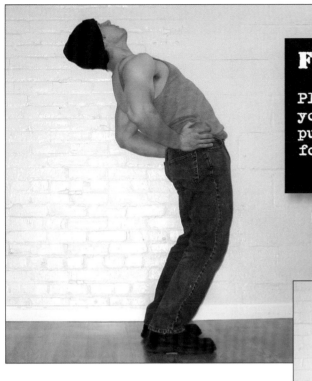

FIG. 101:

Place your hands on your hips and begin pushing your pelvis forwards.

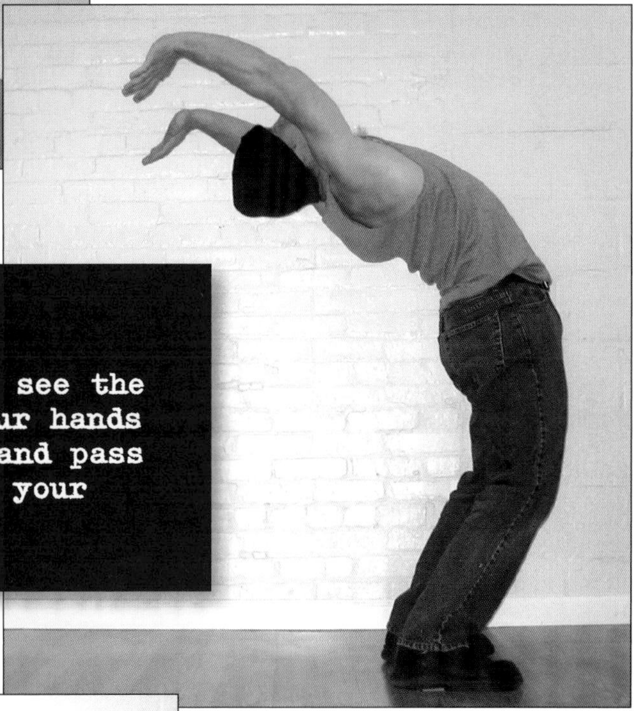

FIG. 102:

As soon as you see the floor, take your hands off your hips and pass them back over your shoulders.

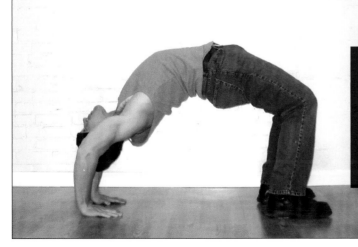

FIG. 103:

Extend your arms as you keep the movement going, until your palms are resting on the floor.

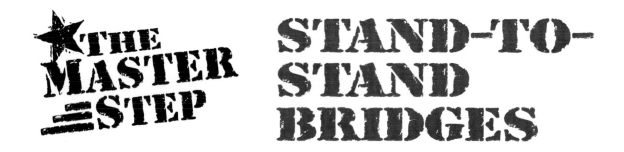

Performance

Stand up straight and perform a *closing bridge* (Step 9) into a full *bridge hold* (fig. 104). From this position, shift your weight forwards through the thighs, and bend the knees as you straighten your arms. Continue gradually shifting your weight forwards as your press through the hands and finally the fingers, lifting the palms off the floor. At this point, provided your back is flexible enough to maintain a high arch, and your stomach is powerful enough, your fingers will leave the ground as you start to straighten yourself up (fig. 105). This upwards motion should be the consequence of a smooth forwards transfer of your bodyweight, *not* the result of an explosive push off the floor with the hands. Continue the movement, drawing your hands back over your shoulders and pivoting the neck up in line with the body. Finally, pull the hips in until you are standing straight with hands by your sides. This is the finish position (fig. 106). Going from standing up, down to a full bridge hold, then straightening yourself back up to the standing position again constitutes one full repetition. Repeat the exercise, breathing normally.

Exercise X-Ray

This is the ultimate bridging technique of the series. It requires incredible flexibility, strong joints, powerful muscles, balance and coordination. When performed regularly, *stand-to-stand bridges* increase agility, massage the internal organs, align the spine and muscular system and increase energy. When worked for high repetitions, they supercharge the metabolism.

Training Goals

- Beginner standard: 1 set of 1
- Intermediate standard: 2 sets of 3
- Elite standard: 2 sets of 10-30

Perfecting Your Technique

Just as with *closing bridges* (Step 9), you can use stairs to increase your depth in this movement over time. Employing a very wide foot position will also be of help. Strive to use a shoulder width stance eventually, however.

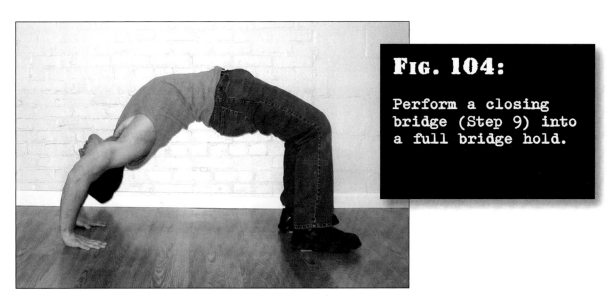

FIG. 104:

Perform a closing bridge (Step 9) into a full bridge hold.

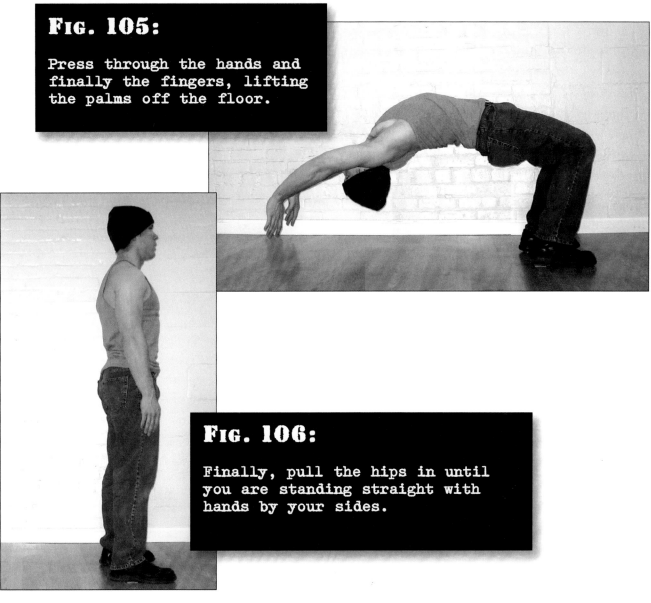

FIG. 105:

Press through the hands and finally the fingers, lifting the palms off the floor.

FIG. 106:

Finally, pull the hips in until you are standing straight with hands by your sides.

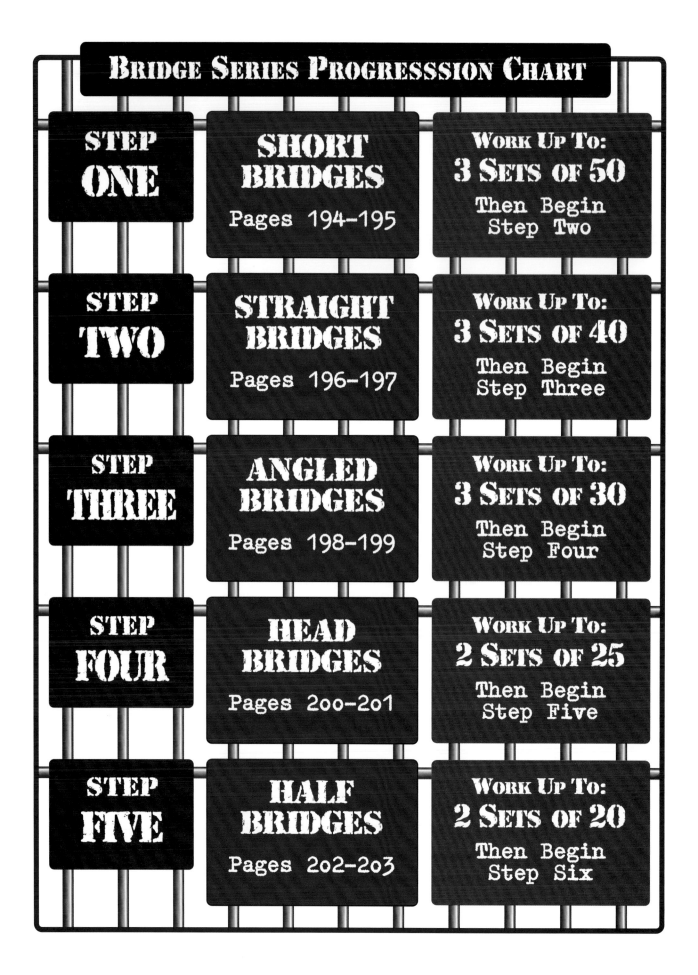

BRIDGE SERIES PROGRESSSION CHART

STEP ONE	SHORT BRIDGES Pages 194–195	WORK UP TO: 3 SETS OF 50 Then Begin Step Two
STEP TWO	STRAIGHT BRIDGES Pages 196–197	WORK UP TO: 3 SETS OF 40 Then Begin Step Three
STEP THREE	ANGLED BRIDGES Pages 198–199	WORK UP TO: 3 SETS OF 30 Then Begin Step Four
STEP FOUR	HEAD BRIDGES Pages 2oo–2o1	WORK UP TO: 2 SETS OF 25 Then Begin Step Five
STEP FIVE	HALF BRIDGES Pages 2o2–2o3	WORK UP TO: 2 SETS OF 20 Then Begin Step Six

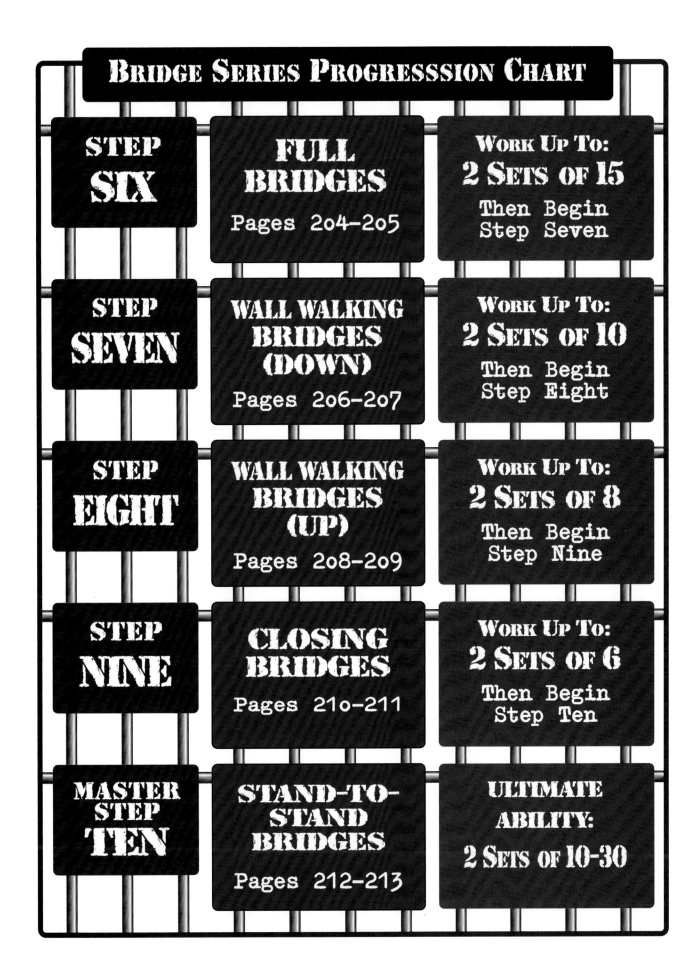

BRIDGE SERIES PROGRESSSION CHART

STEP SIX	FULL BRIDGES Pages 204-205	WORK UP TO: 2 SETS OF 15 Then Begin Step Seven
STEP SEVEN	WALL WALKING BRIDGES (DOWN) Pages 206-207	WORK UP TO: 2 SETS OF 10 Then Begin Step Eight
STEP EIGHT	WALL WALKING BRIDGES (UP) Pages 208-209	WORK UP TO: 2 SETS OF 8 Then Begin Step Nine
STEP NINE	CLOSING BRIDGES Pages 210-211	WORK UP TO: 2 SETS OF 6 Then Begin Step Ten
MASTER STEP TEN	STAND-TO-STAND BRIDGES Pages 212-213	ULTIMATE ABILITY: 2 SETS OF 10-30

Going Beyond

There are a lot of pumped up guys in gyms today who have pretty strong limbs and torsos—pretty strong, that is, for lifting weights in the gym. But that's the only qualities they've got. Have no doubt about it, once you have achieved the Master Step of the bridging series, you will possess incredible spinal strength, not just in the superficial muscles of the back, but also in the deepest layers of tissue usually untouched by heavy weightlifting techniques. Likewise, I've met a lot of martial artists who thought they were flexible, but when you train with them, they are only really flexible in forwards bending positions—ask them to bend over backwards and touch the floor and they inevitably land on their asses.

The bridging series will grant you an incredible combination of strength paired with flexibility. If this was all the bridge offered you, it would be well worthwhile including it in your routine. But completing the bridge series will give you more—more than practically any other exercise on earth. Much, much more. It fixes old back injuries and prevents new ones, like slipped discs; it tones the stomach, deltoids, legs and arms; it expands the chest and loosens the shoulders; it renders the entire body agile and coordinated; it improves balance and promotes healthy digestion. I could go on and on.

When the time comes that you reach the Master Step and you are wondering how to further your training, it's wise to bear these facts in mind. Bridging is more than just a strength exercise or a flexibility technique—it stands alone as a *total* training method that facilitates development in practically every area of fitness and health. For this reason, don't think just in terms of strength or flexibility when you are looking to go beyond stand-to-stand bridges.

Certainly, you can improve your strength in the bridge; one way is to return to full bridging and add weights—perhaps in the form of a weighted training vest. I knew one very large powerlifter in San Quentin who used to hold a full bridge with his two hundred pound buddy sitting on his stomach! You wouldn't believe that such a large man could perform such a lithe feat—he was well over three hundred pounds, and not all of it was muscle. Yet years of bridging made him astonishingly limber. Although I find weighted bridges impressive, I'm always wary of adding heavy weights to *any* spinal exercise; trying such things once or twice is one thing, but if you practise it over years—which you need to if you are going to keep feeling the benefits—it'll come back to bite you in the end.

You can also continue increasing your *flexibility* fairly easily if you want to. This simply involves focusing on your extreme range of motion while holding the bridge, and attempting to bring your head closer to your toes each time. The ultimate human level of flexibility in this movement would involve placing the soles of the feet on the head—a pose known in yoga as *the scorpion*. You might have seen contortionists perform this trick—watching others is certainly the closest I've ever got to it! Unless you begin gymnastics at a young age, and are female, your chances of getting to this level are practically nil. It's very rare for adult males to be able to do this technique unless they have the medical condition of *hypermobility*, which is sometimes (wrongly) called being "double-jointed." Flexibility is important but there are safer and more efficient ways to get good back suppleness, so I wouldn't advise you to focus on this kind of training.

If you are looking to go beyond stand-to-stand bridges, there are two avenues I'd suggest. First off, I'd look towards *integrating* your bodyweight skills—in particular, synthesizing handstand pushups with bridges. When you are in a bridge, instead of pushing up with your *hands*, kick up with your *legs*, holding the handstand position when you become vertical. This is takes a little practice but it's actually one of the coolest ways to get into a handstand. Once you can do this, try the reverse—from a handstand, lower your feet until you drop into a bridge. (Make sure you put something out to cushion your fall the first time you try this.) When you can perform both of these transitions smoothly, you'll be able to combine them; flip into a handstand, then down to a bridge, and kick back up to a handstand again. This kind of advanced two-part technique requires iron strength and whip-like flexibility in every muscle in the body. It's fantastic for total-body control, and it's wonderfully satisfying to learn. It goes without saying that you should only ever even *attempt* this kind of chain of exercises once you have mastered stand-to-stand bridges along with at least Step 4 of the *handstand pushup* series (see pages 236-237).

If this brand of strength-gymnastics just isn't your shot of whiskey, try your hand at *platform bridging*. Using a platform is a little-known way to make stand-to-stand bridges harder and increasingly more explosive without adding any external resistance. Stand up straight on a raised platform. A step would be a good option. Now bend backwards, ultimately dropping into a bridge. If you can, push yourself back up to standing position. The altered angle means that this will require enormous body power. This is probably the ultimate way to move beyond stand-to-stand bridges, but start slowly and be careful, as platform bridging can be hard on the wrists.

Variants

Bridging is an incredibly comprehensive exercise, and for this reason there are very few true variants you can perform in place of it. Some of the exercises that follow—the *camel hold* is a good example—go some small way towards mimicking the bridge, because they require the twin qualities of spinal strength *and* flexibility. Others, however—such as the hyperextensions—merely strengthen the spine and hips with minimal effect on the elasticity of the trunk. As a result, these are good exercises to use to retain your back strength if you can't do genuine bridging exercises for some reason, such as an arm injury, etc.

Bow Hold

This is a classic spinal exercise that will develop the contractile ability of your back, as well as training the vertebrae and their surrounding ligaments. Lie face down on the floor. Bend your knees, bringing your feet up over your buttocks, and reach back to grasp your ankles with their corresponding hands. This in itself will provide a stretch, but we're not done yet. Using pure spinal power, simultaneously lift your chest and knees as high off the ground as you can. Hold the position for between ten and thirty seconds. Once you are comfortable in the *bow hold*, you can try the *camel hold*.

Camel Hold

Kneel on the floor with your knees a few inches apart. Rather than sitting down on your calves, raise yourself up so that your hips are straight and your body forms an "L" shape. From this position, slowly arch your spine back and reach behind you to grasp your ankles. Once you have hold of them, push your hips forwards, maximizing the bend in your spine. Although this sounds easy, it requires some strength in the deeper spinal muscles to complete the position. Hold for ten to thirty seconds. I learned this nifty stretch from a yoga guy living on the West Coast. Nobody seems to know why it's called the "camel"—looks nothing like a camel to me.

Gecko Bridges

These are a slightly harder variation on the full bridge. Simply get into the full *bridge hold* (fig. 90), and lift one hand and the opposite foot from the floor, pointing these limbs out horizontally. Hold the position briefly, before supporting yourself with all your limbs again, and alternating the position with the other hand and foot. This requires more limb strength than regular bridge holds, and also firms up the lumbar muscles which have to tense very strongly to maintain balance.

Hyperextensions

This is one of the few exercises I advocate which requires a training partner. Lie face down on a table, desk or high bench, so that your legs are resting on the surface up to your pelvis, but your torso is hanging straight down. Your trunk and legs will form a right angle at the hips. To maintain this position, you'll need somebody to push down on your ankles so you don't fall off. A cushion or wrapped up towel under your hips is also a good idea to prevent the edge of the table from cutting into you. Place your hands behind your head, and raise your torso until it is level with your legs. Hold this position for a moment before lowering yourself back down again and repeating for high reps. Hyperextensions work the hamstring complex, the glutes, the hips and spinal muscles. It's a handy exercise to know, because it trains all these muscles without transmitting any pressure down through the spinal column. Guys who have ruptured or partially dislocated their discs by doing heavy deadlifts and squats will be able to train their back muscles with this exercise without aggravating their existing injuries.

Reverse Hyperextensions

Hyperextensions involve keeping the legs stable and lifting the torso, with the hips being the major axis, or pivot. It stands to reason that you can work similar muscles by reversing this dynamic, by keeping the torso stable and lifting the legs, with the hips once again being the pivot point. To do this, you'll have to lie face down over a table or desk—width-wise is usually best—with your torso and face on the desk and your legs off the end. (Because the legs are longer than the torso, they will probably touch the floor. That's fine.) Grab the table whichever way you can to keep your torso secure, and raise your legs up behind you until they form a line with your trunk. Keeping your legs as straight as possible will make the exercise harder. Hold the position at the top briefly, before allowing your feet to descend under control. Repeat for high reps. I have found that big, couch-style armchairs make an excellent reverse hyperextension unit—drape your-self sideways over the chair, with your hips over one padded arm and your chest on the other, as you reach down to hook a hand under the chair for stability. Try this if you have a comfy chair at home—unfortunately bunks and beds just aren't high enough to make the technique worthwhile. Reverse hyperextensions confer all the benefits of regular hyperextensions with the added plus that this variation doesn't require a partner. The exercise is of real therapeutic value to athletes with bad backs, because it increases circulation and tone in the lower back without the usual accompanying strain.

Prone Hyperextensions

Lay face down on the floor with your feet close together and your hands behind your head. Simply lift your chest and feet as high as you can, without bending the knees. In reality you will only be able to move your extremities a few inches, but this is an excellent exercise for the spinal muscles. Repeat for high reps, or go for ten to thirty second holds—whatever floats your boat. Because of the minimized leg motion in this version of the hyperextension, the hamstrings, gluteal muscles and hips don't get nearly as much work as the spinal erectors. I've personally found this to be a very therapeutic exercise for working out those little kinks in the mid-back region we all get from time to time. This is also a brilliant exercise to refresh the back if you have to hunch over a desk at work, and because it's quite gentle it can be done several times a day if you like. Placing your arms straight out in front of you (as if you were flying) will make the exercise slightly more difficult, due to leverage.

Back Handsprings

It seems inevitable. At some point during the bridging series, as your back gets more flexible and you become adept at bending over backwards, you will probably begin to wonder if you could make a back handspring. You know the stunt—you've probably seen it in movies often enough. Jump up and flip back, briefly planting your hands on the floor before landing on your feet, agile as a cat. How cool is that? In fact, the urge to explore this move is no bad thing; as well as look-ing damn sweet, the back handspring is in many ways the plyometric counterpart of bridging—it allows you to train your spinal muscles, hips and legs in a more explosive manner than bridging does, and it has the benefit of forcing the entire body to act in a rapid, athletic fashion. Actually, once your hips and spine are loosened up from bridging, learning the back handspring isn't all that hard. Provided you are fast and follow through, even heavy guys can pull it off. I've seen chubby martial arts star Sammo Hung perform the technique many times, well into his forties. The real key to the move is *confidence*. The first time I ever tried to do a back handspring, I nearly brained myself because I chickened out half way through. This was on concrete, and the experi-ence drained my confidence even further. When you first learn, it's a good idea to practice on thick foam mats if you get the chance. Back handsprings are a lightning fast move that need to be expe-rienced to really be understood, so describing how to do them is kind of artificial, but I can at least give you a few pointers. Jump hard, but don't jump *up*; jump up *and* back. Coordinate your arms with the movement, swinging up, overhead and back as fast as you can. Arch your back tight and keep your head back between your arms, looking for a place to plant your hands. When you find one, continue swinging your legs as momentum carries you over. Once you have mastered the back handspring, you might want to try the *backflip*—which is the same move, but without placing the hands on the ground (see the photo below). This requires much more explosive leg and spine power, as well as powerful abs to tuck the knees up and over. It's a brilliant exercise which will lead on to other tricks like *wall flips, flash kicks* (i.e., *overhead flip kicks*), *twisting flips* and so on, if you wish to explore these kind of moves in your training.

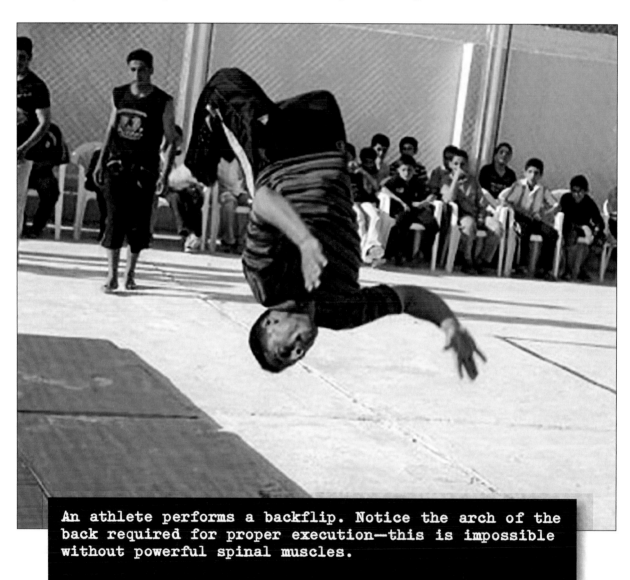

An athlete performs a backflip. Notice the arch of the back required for proper execution—this is impossible without powerful spinal muscles.

10: THE HANDSTAND PUSHUP

HEALTHY, POWERFUL SHOULDERS

I t's hard to think of any body part more associated with pure masculinity than the *shoulders*. Since Atlas held the heavens aloft on his, men have inherently understood the connection between shoulders and strength. The primary muscles of the shoulder, the *deltoids*, transmit the force of the major torso muscles in virtually all powerful arm movements—therefore, if the shoulders are weak, the whole upper body is weak by default. Broad shoulders project an image of power and physical superiority unmatched by any other visual quality a physique can possess.

Sounds great. But there is a problem associated with modern shoulder training methods.

And it runs *deep*.

Those Aching Shoulders

Tragically, shoulder pain and strength training methods seem destined to go together like ham and eggs. Abbott and Costello. Love and marriage. It doesn't matter what form of training you favor—bodybuilding, powerlifting, Olympic weightlifting, machine training, dinosaur training, whatever. Shoulder injuries are everywhere in strength training. The two are practically synonymous. If you have been training with weights or resistance machines for over six months, the chances are that you will have already experienced some kind of nagging shoulder pain, however minor. If not, you are one of the very lucky minority, and the chances are that if you continue training, you *will* suffer injury.

The vast majority of these injuries are to the *rotator cuff*. You may have heard this term. It's thrown around like a buzzword in any discussion of sports injuries these days—it's right up there with the ACL as a trouble spot for athletes. Unfortunately, although the word is well-used, many trainees aren't really aware of what the rotator cuff *is*, or what it *does*. For a start, the rotator cuff is not a muscle. It is a *group* of muscles which stabilize the humerus, the arm bone, in the shoulder socket. For those of you interested in anatomy, there are four rotator cuff muscles; the *supraspinatus, teres minor, infraspinatus* and *subscapularis*. The deltoid—the large muscle of the shoulder cap—takes care of the *major* movements of the arms. Working in synergy with the *latissimus dorsi* (side), *teres major* and *trapezius* (back) and *pectorals* (chest), the deltoids bring the arms down, back, forwards and up. But, as the name suggests, it's the rotator cuff muscles that control the *rotation* of the upper arm forwards and backwards.

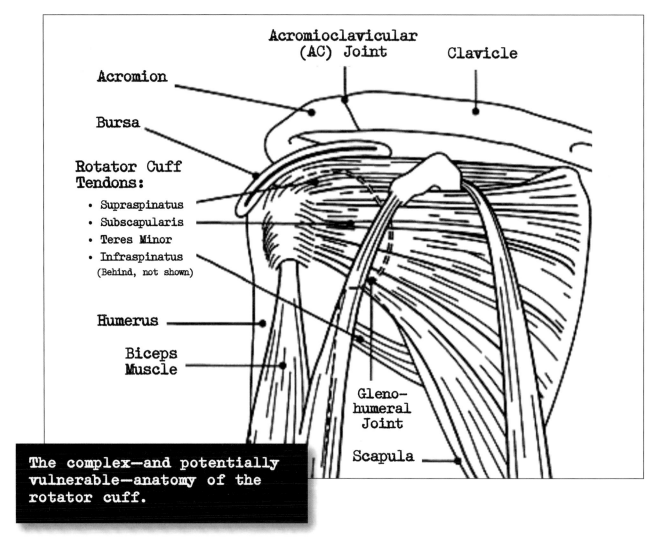

The complex—and potentially vulnerable—anatomy of the rotator cuff.

This is an important job, for two reasons. Firstly, it's important because the arms are constantly rotating during motion. Even during movements which seem fairly straight—like presses or rows—the humerus is rotating forwards or back to complete the motion. The greater any given movement, the greater the rotation; exaggerated movements cause the humerus to twist significantly in its socket. This rotation is crucial. The arms are connected to the clavicles by a ball-and-socket joint, and if the humerus couldn't rotate, your upper arms would pretty much be paralyzed. The second reason has to do with *safety*. The engineering of the ball-and-socket joint gives it remarkable mobility, but that mobility comes at a price—a corresponding vulnerability. The shoulder is weak and highly susceptible to trauma along its rotational axis. When the humerus is strongly twisted, the rotator cuff is particularly vulnerable to injury. The end result is that during heavy barbell work—presses in particular—the rotator cuff muscles are forced to cope with a great deal of pressure. The larger surrounding muscles—the delts, pecs, lats, etc.—are big, strong, and their functioning is pretty straightforward. They can take a lot of work, and repeated heavy loads. But the smaller, more complex rotator cuff is just not designed for the kind of beating weight-training dishes out.

The rotator cuff can become irritated after as little as *one* barbell workout. Virtually all dedicated weight-trainers receive their share of shoulder pulls and injuries. At first, these are usually minor. The rotator cuff and associated tendons become tender and inflamed; there may be shoulder strains. Spurred on by their gains in muscle and size, dedicated athletes continue lifting weights. This actually causes further problems, because the larger muscles surrounding the rotator cuff become big and strong much quicker than the cuff can keep up. This leads to a mechanical disadvantage within the muscle, and the rotator cuff is forced to undergo further stress. The bench presses and military presses get heavier and heavier, and the chronic damage to the shoulders adds up. The athlete learns to use his shoulders less when he's not in the gym, because they are constantly inflamed; they're sore to move. They crack and pop. This decrease in daily movement leads to an eventual reduction in flexibility and deep blood flow, which further aggravates the problem. The end result is consistent ailments like *tendonitis, impingement, bursitis* and *frozen shoulder*. By the time weight-lifters have reached an advanced level, virtually all of them live with shoulder pain. Advanced gym rats may *look* really big and even be very strong, but you can bet that their shoulder health is terrible—when you examine the internal anatomy of a bodybuilder's shoulder during an arthroscopy, it often looks like a bomb's gone off inside! Most senior lifters who have been working out consistently for over ten years will suffer *some* form of shoulder arthritis. The unlucky ones will eventually suffer complete tears of one or more of the rotator cuff muscles, and surgery will be required. Pain will become a way of life for them, whether they continue with the daily medication and physiotherapy or not.

Authentic and Artificial Shoulder Movements

Many strength athletes believe that there's only one way to confront shoulder pain—and that's to learn to live with it. I think that's terribly sad. I'm here to tell you that it's also *untrue*. Believe it or not, there's a way you can develop massive, powerful, functional deltoids, without damaging your shoulders in the first place. But in order to understand how, you have to appreciate what's going wrong in the first place.

Because something *is* going wrong. Pain is *not* something we have to learn to live with as a result of our training. In fact, I'm a strong believer in the notion that if your training isn't gradually *lessening* the pain in your life, you're doing something wrong.

So why do weight-training movements cause so much shoulder pain? The knee-jerk reaction might be to say that the problem has to do with heavy weights. The reason actually has nothing to do with the weights used during exercises. The human body can reach awesome levels of strength with no joint problems at all—in fact, the human body *wants* to be strong. The problem lies in the type of exercises used—they are *unnatural* to the human body. If we can replace them with natural, *authentic* movements, the pain will go away. The human body is like a well-designed machine. If you use it for the wrong purpose, it starts to break down. If you use it properly—if you ask it to do what it is *supposed* to do—no damage occurs.

Let's take a moment to examine the two worst offenders when it comes to shoulder pain and injuries; shoulder presses (military presses, press-behind-neck, jerks, etc) and the bench press. (In this category, I would also include the plethora of machine movements which mimic these exercises. They're just as bad.) "Proper" form on these movements requires that the elbows are kept out to the side—to activate the major muscles. On shoulder presses in particular, the elbows are supposed to be kept out to the side, supposedly to activate the side head of the deltoids. This is why the press-behind-neck was invented—the path of the bar behind the neck literally *forces* the elbows out to the side. It's actually quite hard not to keep the elbows flared out when pressing a straight bar, particularly if you are using a wide grip—which is one of the reason wide grips are favored for shoulder presses. The bench press is no better. The action of the weight coming down on the chest inevitably forces the elbows away from the body. In a bodybuilding context, it is usually considered "perfect" form to keep the elbows right out from the torso, nearly in line with the collarbones. This is supposed to activate the pectorals more. In all presses, a "full range of motion" is normally advised. This means that the bar touches the body, before being pushed away until the arms are extended, or nearly so.

These movements and their variants are totally unnatural. In particular, these two major elements of "good" form are incredibly artificial in terms of human biomechanics:

i.   the elbows flaring out to the side of the torso, and;
ii.   the bar being brought into contact with the body in the bottom position.

How do I justify the statement that these two respects are unnatural? Perhaps the best way to understand how the human body is *naturally* meant to move is to look at how humans *instinctively* move. Let's try to find an everyday movement similar to the shoulder press. Look at a father picking up his child. You'll notice that in instinctive upwards-pushing movements, the elbows are not splayed out—they are kept *forwards*. In fact, if you ask anybody to hold something up overhead, if their positioning allows it, they will *always* keep their elbows forwards. Splaying the elbows out to the side is totally unnatural. So is pushing from the point of contact. Think of an instinctive movement similar to the bench press; perhaps pushing a broken-down car, or shoving an attacker away. In neither instance would you bring the object you are pushing to your chest first. You'd begin the movement with your elbows only bent about *halfway*. The body naturally understands that its own structure has more strength and stability that way.

If we lifted weights as we instinctively moved, there would be virtually no chronic injuries in the gym. But we are too "smart" for that. We force our bodies into artificial positions they never evolved to accommodate; certainly not progressively and with heavy poundages. And then we wonder why we have to live with pain!

The above discussion of *natural*, authentic pressing movements as opposed to *artificial* pressing (the shoulder press and bench press) relates to the earlier passage describing the rotator cuff. On page 222, I stated that the rotator cuff is particularly vulnerable to injury when it is placed under load while the humerus is strongly twisted. I also wrote that exaggerated movements cause the humerus to twist in its socket. Both these major elements of barbell pressing—keeping the elbows out to the side of the body, and bringing the bar down to the chest, neck or shoulders—are exaggerated movements. They cause the humerus to twist. The humerus is attached to the rotator cuff, which bears the full brunt of the heavy bar being pressed. If you remove these two elements of pressing, you would remove virtually all chronic shoulder problems.

The Solution

If you have ever tried to press a barbell when you've suffered an inflamed, strained or torn rotator cuff yourself, you'll have noticed (agonizingly!) that all or most of the pain occurs in the bottom position; when the bar is near the chest on the bench press, near the shoulders on shoulder presses. As soon as somebody has a shoulder problem in the gym, they will immediately gain relief by reducing their range of motion by about half—by only doing the top half of the exercise, the portion nearest lockout.

Many have also noticed that their shoulder pain improves when they switch from barbells to dumbbells—even if they continue using heavy weights. Some coaches will tell you that this is because the shoulders and arms are free to move more "naturally," but very few understand what they really mean by this. What actually happens when you start pressing with dumbbells is twofold. Firstly, because they are not angled out to the side by following the path of the straight bar, the elbows are free to move *forwards* during the pressing motion. Doing this, even just a little, immediately alleviates pain. The single dumbbell press—with either one or two arms—is even better because the elbows are practically encouraged to travel forwards. The second reason is that—despite what some "experts" say—your range of motion is actually *reduced* when you use dumbbells compared to using a barbell. When you bench press or shoulder press with a barbell, you can keep lowering the bar until it touches your body. When you lower dumbbells, you can only keep lowering until the edges of the plates—not the dumbbell bars—touch your body. Since these stand out from the bars, the range of motion is reduced by a few inches. This is often enough to decrease some of the irritation caused by barbell pressing.

If you are addicted to the weights, you can try some of these methods to reduce your pain. But if your shoulders are really important to you, I'd advise you to drop them altogether, and replace them with the most natural shoulder movement in the history of exercise—*the handstand pushup*.

The Mighty Handstand Pushup

During the handstand pushup, the body instinctively positions itself in a position healthiest to the shoulders. The elbows are invariably kept *inside* the torso, opposite the chest muscles—pushing them out to the side feels very strange and makes balancing almost impossible, because the body wants to fall forwards in this position. An example of the natural elbows-forwards position can be seen in the handstand on the opposite page. Compare this to the elbows-out position of the classic barbell press shown below to it. In addition, very deep motions—which would twist the humerus and irritate the rotator cuff—are impossible during handstand pushups. You can't lower yourself until the floor is on your shoulders—the inverted equivalent of a shoulder press—for the simple reason that the *head* gets in the way. Even advanced handstanders who descend until their chins touch the floor can't really lower themselves to the point where the rotator cuff muscles are mechanically disadvantaged. Plus, the flat hand position is safer than the barbell grip; the flat hands distribute pressure evenly, allowing the forearms to strengthen in a healthy, harmonious way. Gripping the bar during presses is what causes forearm and elbow problems like tennis elbow. (This is as true for the standard pushup as it is for the handstand variety.) Handstand pushups—done properly—are incredibly safe.

The handstand pushup would be an important technique in the pantheon of training exercises, provided it simply trained the shoulders without causing injury. But it gives so much more, it's almost beyond belief. Let's start with *strength*. In effect, performing handstand pushups is the equivalent of shoulder pressing your bodyweight. It may take years (and many injuries) to get to this level of strength with a barbell—in fact, many athletes just never get there. But the average person can learn to do handstand pushups in a matter of months. The result is *incredibly* powerful, muscularized shoulders in a short span of time.

The handstand pushup also teaches advanced balance and total-body coordination skills that just can't be replicated with weights. The act of stabilizing yourself upside-down causes the *vestibular system*—the balance organ in the inner ear—to adapt and become more efficient. This translates into a sense of heightened equilibrium and kinesthetic awareness in all your other movements throughout the day, whether you are upside-down or not.

The simple act of adopting the inverse posture—being upside-down—also has major benefits. The blood supply is reversed—the veins and arteries work against gravity in the opposite direction and become more supple, stronger and healthier. The same principle applies to the digestive organs. When you're upside-down, the head becomes flushed with fresh blood. This is a tonic for the brain, and you will find that you feel refreshed and alert after finishing your exercises.

Strength, muscle, agility, and health—all in one exercise. What more could you possibly ask for?

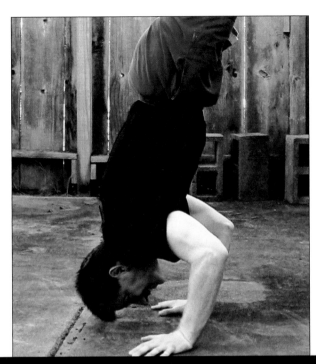
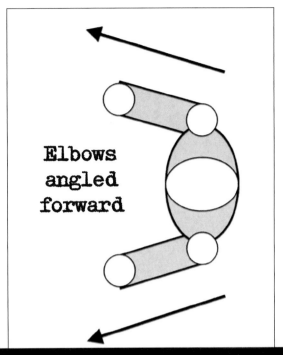

The above images display the elbow position during a handstand pushup. Notice how the elbows automatically angle forwards; this is the most natural and safest position for the rotator cuff musculature.

Elbows angled forward

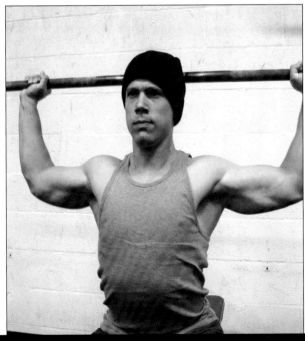
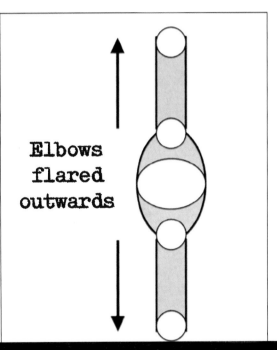

The above images display the elbow position during a barbell press. Notice how the elbows are forced to flare outwards, placing the rotator cuff in a hazardous and vulnerable position.

Elbows flared outwards

Perfect Form = Perfect Strength

Handstand pushups are a difficult movement. You will inevitably develop your own unique style. The best way to learn is to slowly progress through the ten steps, milking each exercise of everything it can teach you by way of balance, muscle control, coordination and power output. Here are some technical pointers that will help you perfect your technique during your journey:

- Handstand pushups can be done either with the back against the wall, or "free"—without support. The latter style requires that the athlete expend as much energy on *balance* as on *strength*. The main goal of *Convict Conditioning* is the development of muscle and might, so this system focuses on the wall-supported variety. If you are interested in the non-supported version, master the early steps against the wall first; this will give you more than enough power to tackle the non-supported version.

- The first few steps will gradually train your body and brain to adapt to balancing and turning upside-down. They'll also teach you to kick up against the wall and get down again safely. Resist the urge to race towards more glamorous steps, and master these preliminaries first.

- When kicking up, don't keep the hands too close to the wall. A position of six to ten inches away—sometimes more—will be much more stable. The hands should be approximately shoulder width apart. Weight-trained men may be tempted to place the hands wider than this, but doing so will make you less stable and render your motion less efficient.

- During the handstand pushup, don't force your elbows apart as you would in a military press. They will naturally angle inwards; either straight out in front of the chest, or diagonally out. Either is fine. Do what your body wants!

- Don't keep the body straight. It will want to curve somewhat, with the feet ending up a little farther back than the head (see fig. 112). This is due to the natural equilibrium of the inverse body, and represents good technique. Don't arch your back excessively, but don't try to iron your body straight. Retain a gentle curve.

- At first, there will be the tendency to crash the back flat against the wall with the full body-weight. This is a bad habit. Eventually, you want to get to the stage where only your *heels* are touching the wall. If you have followed the pointers above, and your hands are a short distance away from the wall with your body displaying a gentle curve, the heels will automatically become the point of contact with the wall as a consequence. You won't need to force yourself into any weird postures.

- Over time, your feet should only touch the wall with a few pounds of pressure—just enough to retain balance. If you slowly try to use less pressure over time, you will be able to move towards non-supported handstand pushups with very little effort if you wish to.

- Some guys find that there is some friction between their heels and the wall during wall work. This makes the pushups harder. You can alleviate any friction by wearing thick socks, and doing the exercises against smooth walls. I've seen athletes tape duct tape against the brick walls where they practice, to help their heels glide up and down. You might need this tip, you might not. See how you go.

The Handstand Pushup Series

Training on a bodyweight skill like handstand pushups is a real challenge and success provides a heck of a lot of satisfaction that can't be got from a barbell—not to mention the excitement of learning to master your body. Being able to flip up against a wall and start doing handstand pushups is cool. Without a doubt, it will look impressive to others. But don't expect to just hop on your hands and start doing reps. The handstand pushup is a very advanced, demanding exercise, particularly if you've experienced shoulder problems in the past. Beginners are advised to master *close pushups*, Step 6 of the regular pushup series (see chapter 5) before even *beginning* Step 1 of the handstand pushup series. Doing so will condition your hands, forearms and shoulder girdle to the rigors of supporting the entire bodyweight. Mastering *uneven pushups* (Step 7) will also strengthen your rotator cuffs and help to iron out any pre-existing shoulder problems before you attempt to support your entire bodyweight in the inverse position.

You will begin the handstand pushup series with an exercise that teaches you to get used to being upside-down. Step 2 will help you translate your strength into balance. Further steps will build muscle and strength in the handstand. From there, your muscles will be progressively tested, until you reach the ultimate goal—the *one-arm handstand pushup*.

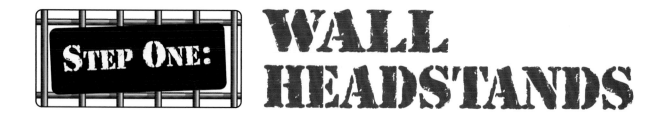

STEP ONE: WALL HEADSTANDS

Performance

Find a solid wall. Place a pillow, cushion or folded towel down by the base of the wall. This will be for your head. Get on your hands and knees, and place the top of your head on the cushion. Your skull should be between six and ten inches from the wall. Set your palms down securely on either side of your head, about shoulder width apart. Bring your strongest knee up close to your corresponding elbow, and straighten out your other leg so the knee is off the ground (fig. 107). Now, push down hard with your strongest leg, as you simultaneously kick your other leg up in the air so that both legs dynamically move up towards the wall. Once you have "found" the wall, slowly straighten your legs so that the body is aligned (fig. 108). Keep the mouth closed and breath smoothly though the nose. After you have remained up for the required time, bend the legs and bring them down under control.

Exercise X-Ray

For anybody who wishes to approach the *handstand pushup*, the first specific skill which must be mastered is the inverse position—being upside-down. *Wall headstands* are the perfect introduction to this skill. With just a small amount of practice, the blood vessels and organs of the torso and head become accustomed to the sudden reversal of gravity. During headstands, the entire body is above the head, which means that the balance is tested. The shoulders also receive some work as stabilizers.

Training Goals

- Beginner standard: 30 seconds
- Intermediate standard: 1 minute
- Progression standard: 2 minutes

Perfecting Your Technique

Most people can stay in the *wall headstand* for a few seconds—the major problem is getting up there in the first place! The difficulty is in learning the right level of pushing/kicking strength required to find the wall. If you find this difficult, ask a friend to help guide your legs up until you get it.

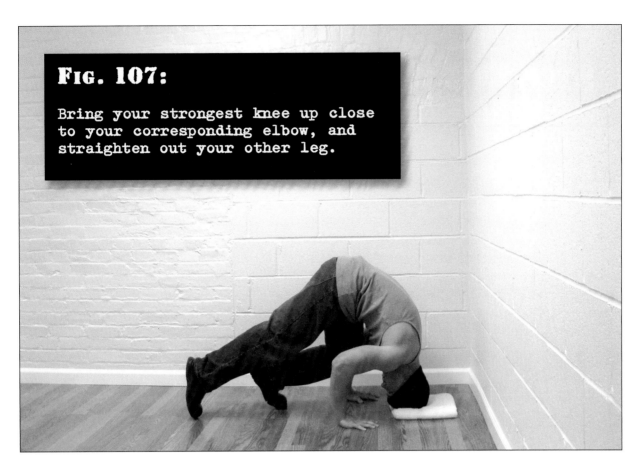

FIG. 107:

Bring your strongest knee up close to your corresponding elbow, and straighten out your other leg.

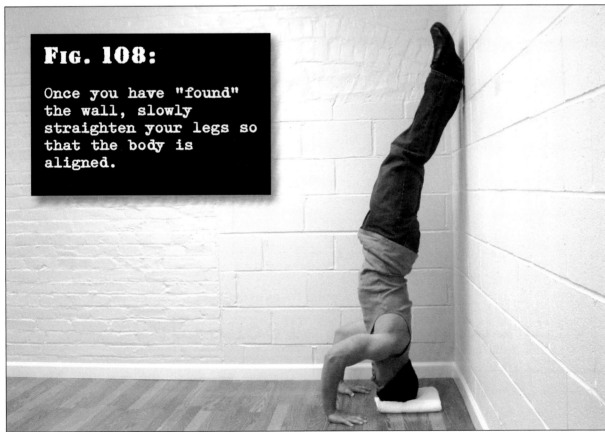

FIG. 108:

Once you have "found" the wall, slowly straighten your legs so that the body is aligned.

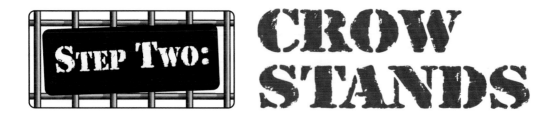

STEP TWO: CROW STANDS

Performance

Sit down on your haunches with your knees apart. Place your palms on the floor in front of you, at approximately shoulder width distance apart. Your arms should be bent a little. Lean forwards, placing your knees securely on the outside of your elbows (fig. 109). Now gradually continue tipping yourself forward, placing more and more weight through your palms and correspondingly less through your feet. Eventually the point of balance will shift, and your feet will lose contact with the ground. Hoist the legs up tight and balance for the required time, breathing steadily (fig. 110). When you are finished, reverse the movement by gently tipping your weight backwards until your toes come into contact with the floor again.

Exercise X-Ray

Crow stands will teach you to combine arm and shoulder strength with balance. They are an essential step in moving towards *handstand pushups* because you are supporting the entire bodyweight by balancing with the arms. The first step will have helped you become comfortable in balancing upside down. This posture will take you further by helping you develop basic "stabilizer" strength in your shoulders, wrists and fingers. Since this is not an inverse posture, always follow this exercise with *wall headstands* to combine the full effect of both strength-building and inverse balancing.

Training Goals

- Beginner standard: 10 seconds
- Intermediate standard: 30 seconds
- Progression standard: 1 minute

Perfecting Your Technique

The key to this technique is appreciating the unique leverage point. The art to holding the balance in this exercise—as with more advanced hand-balancing exercises—lies in the use of sensitive finger strength to stop you from tipping forwards. If you start falling forwards, press hard with your fingers. Lift the legs nice and high to prevent yourself falling backwards.

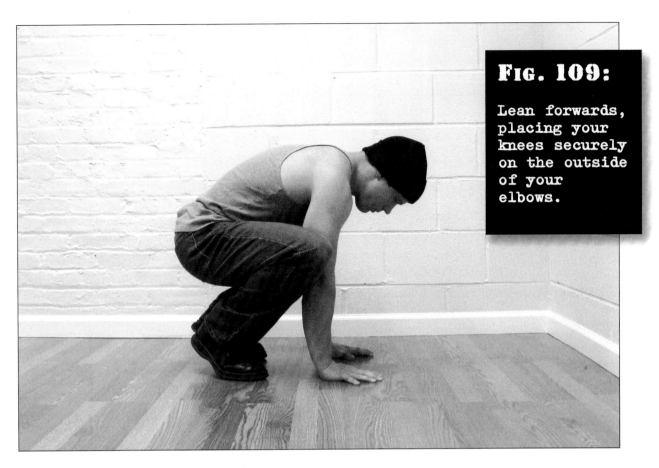

FIG. 109:

Lean forwards, placing your knees securely on the outside of your elbows.

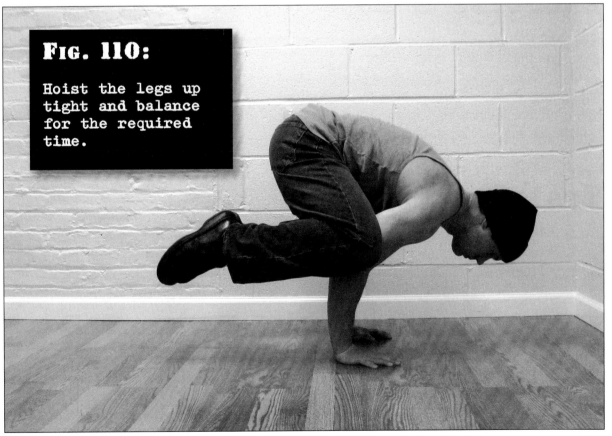

FIG. 110:

Hoist the legs up tight and balance for the required time.

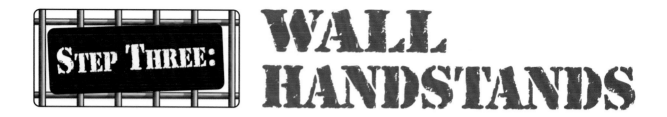

Performance

Approach a solid wall. Place your palms flat on the floor six to ten inches from the base of the wall, at about shoulder width apart. Your arms should be straight, or nearly so. Bend at the knees, bracing the whole body. Bring the knee of your strongest leg up towards the corresponding elbow (fig. 111) and push down hard with that leg, kicking back and up with the other leg. As you rise, allow the foot of your strongest leg to leave the floor and follow your other leg as it approaches the wall. Keep your arms extended. The heels of both your feet should touch the wall at the same time. At first your back and butt may also slam into the wall as you overestimate the power required to kick up, but over time you'll learn the art of finding the wall perfectly. At this point your arms should be straight and your body aligned with a slight arch towards the wall. This is the position for the *wall handstand* technique (fig. 112). Hold this position for the required time, breathing normally.

Exercise X-Ray

Wall headstands will have taught you to get used to being upside-down. *Crow stands* will have given you the arm and wrist strength to safely balance your entire bodyweight through your hands. Once you have mastered these postures, the next thing you need to learn is the art of kicking up into a full handstand against the wall, which is somewhat more difficult than kicking up into a headstand due to the extension of the arms. *Wall handstands* will teach you this important skill. It also increases basic shoulder strength.

Training Goals

- Beginner standard: 30 seconds
- Intermediate standard: 1 minute
- Progression standard: 2 minutes

Perfecting Your Technique

If you have been practicing the kick up into a *wall headstand* (Step 1), this technique shouldn't be too difficult. You do have to kick harder, however. If this is too tricky at first, try kicking off something, like a box or a chair.

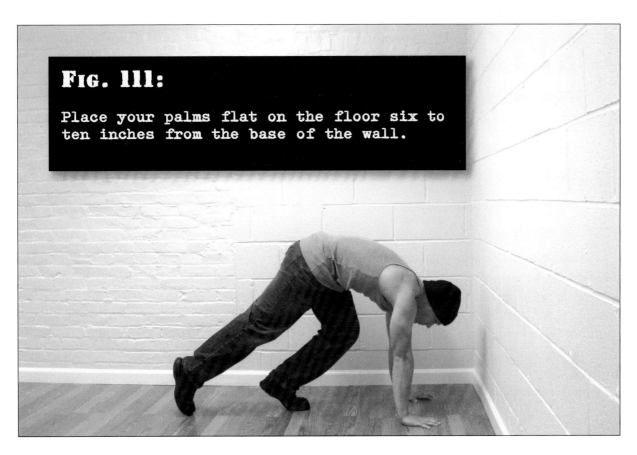

FIG. 111:

Place your palms flat on the floor six to ten inches from the base of the wall.

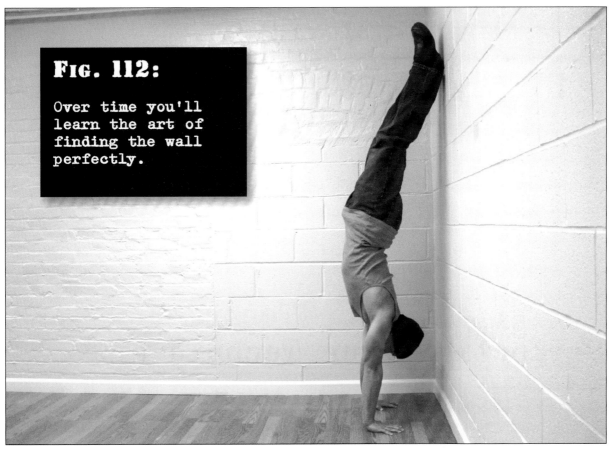

FIG. 112:

Over time you'll learn the art of finding the wall perfectly.

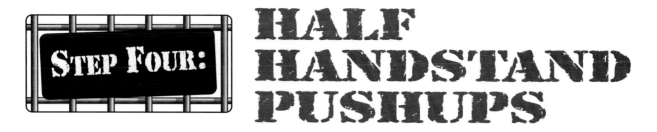

Performance

Approach a solid wall. Place your palms flat on the floor six to ten inches from the base of the wall, at about shoulder width apart. Keeping your arms as straight as possible, assume the position and kick up into a *wall handstand* (Step 3). You should now be in the classic wall handstand starting posture; your torso should be braced, your arms straight, and your body should curve backwards slightly to the point where your heels make a gentle contact with the wall. This is the start position for the *half handstand pushup* (fig. 113). Now bend at the shoulders and elbows until the top of your head is halfway towards touching the ground. This is the finish position (fig. 114). Pause briefly, before pushing firmly back up to the start position. The full range of motion for this technique will only be about six inches; at first, try not to overestimate and go too low. Breathe smoothly throughout the set.

Exercise X-Ray

Your shoulders, arms and torso will have gained some strength simply by holding the static posture of *wall handstands* (Step 3). This exercise is much more intense. It will add muscle and heft to the entire shoulder girdle, and help build powerful elbows and thick triceps. The upper pectorals also benefit.

Training Goals

- Beginner standard: 1 set of 5
- Intermediate standard: 2 sets of 10
- Progression standard: 2 sets of 20

Perfecting Your Technique

Previous steps will have taught you how to kick up into a handstand against the wall without a problem. The movement required in *half handstand pushups* requires significant upper body strength, however. If the technique described above is too strenuous, simply reduce your range of motion. Begin by bending your arms and shoulders a short way—even if only a fraction of an inch. Build up your repetitions, and gradually add depth over time until your head reaches halfway towards the ground. You'll get there, given time.

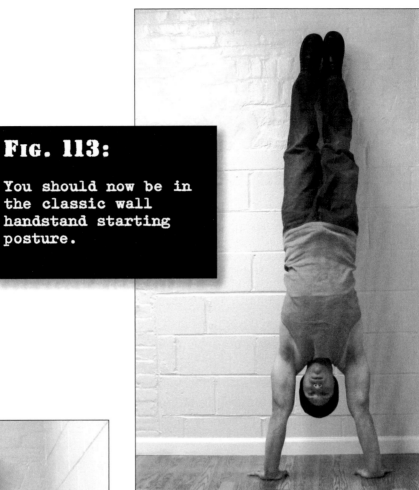

FIG. 113:

You should now be in the classic wall handstand starting posture.

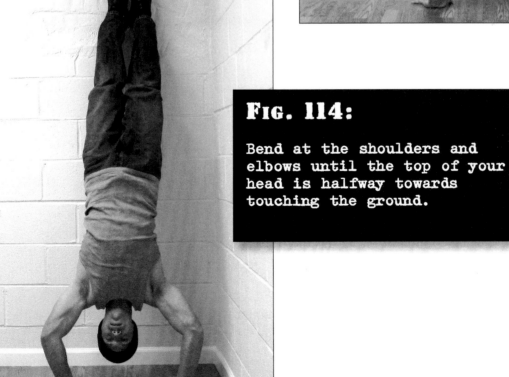

FIG. 114:

Bend at the shoulders and elbows until the top of your head is halfway towards touching the ground.

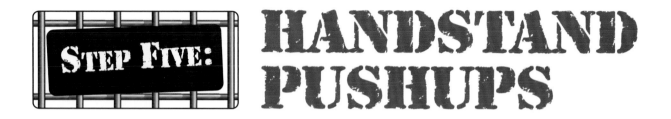

Performance

Approach a solid wall and place your palms flat on the ground approximately shoulder width apart and about six to ten inches from the wall. Bend at the knees and kick up against the wall into a handstand position. If you have worked through the steps so far you will now be pretty expert at this. If you have developed your own technique, that's fine; calisthenics isn't gymnastics—it's the muscle-building portion of the exercise that's of importance, not how you get there. Once you have found the wall, keep contact with it through your heels, maintaining a slight backwards arch in your body. Your arms should be straight. This is the start position (fig. 115). Bend at the shoulders and elbows until the top of your head gently makes contact with the floor. This is the finish position (fig. 116). Use "kiss-the-baby" pressure to protect your head (see pages 43—44). Pause briefly for a second, before pushing yourself back up to the start position. Apply muscular control and concentration in all inverse movements to ensure safety. Breathe as smoothly and evenly as possible.

Exercise X-Ray

This is the full *Convict Conditioning handstand pushup*, which develops and strengthens the shoulders, triceps, elbows, trapezius, pectorals and hands—in fact it has a power-building effect on the entire upper body. A lot of athletes feel the handstand pushup should be *free*—that is, clear of the wall. But this is a test of balance as much as strength. All the old school hand-balancers believed that if you want balance, you should build strength *first*.

Training Goals

- Beginner standard: 1 set of 5
- Intermediate standard: 2 sets of 10
- Progression standard: 2 sets of 15

Perfecting Your Technique

The bottom position is the most difficult due to leverage. If you can't do five full reps, don't go all the way down at first. Add depth as you get stronger.

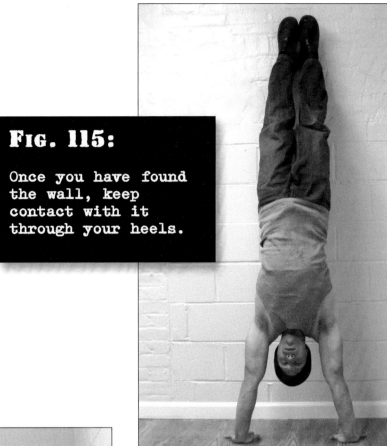

FIG. 115:

Once you have found the wall, keep contact with it through your heels.

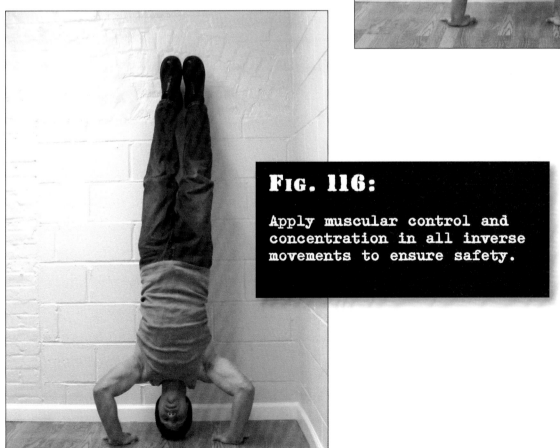

FIG. 116:

Apply muscular control and concentration in all inverse movements to ensure safety.

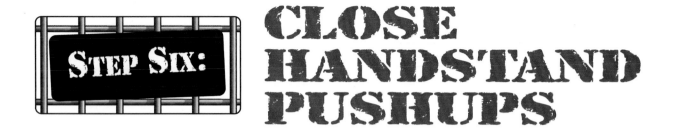

STEP SIX: CLOSE HANDSTAND PUSHUPS

Performance

Locate a solid wall and place your hands on the ground six to ten inches out from it. Your hands—specifically the index fingers—should be touching. Kick up into a handstand with straight arms and a lightly curved body tapering back to where the heels make contact with the wall. This is the start position (fig. 117). Keeping the elbows well out in front, bend at the shoulders and elbows until the head gently kisses the floor (fig. 118). Pause briefly—under full control—before pressing back up to the start position.

Exercise X-Ray

The *full handstand pushup* is an excellent basic exercise. It will teach you to use your strongest pressing muscles powerfully and with coordination. But if you want to move to very advanced unilateral handstand work you will need extremely powerful tendons, particularly around the elbows, forearms and wrists. *Close handstand pushups* develop that tendon strength. The close hand position makes it more difficult for the shoulder girdle to contribute to the movement, which in turn forces the elbows to become much stronger.

Training Goals

- • Beginner standard: 1 set of 5
- • Intermediate standard: 2 sets of 9
- • Progression standard: 2 sets of 12

Perfecting Your Technique

If you are strong enough you can usually jump from the progression standard of a step straight to the beginner standard of the next step without too many problems. In moving from *handstand pushups* to *close handstand pushups* however it's best to take things slowly to allow the tendons to properly adapt to the full bodyweight. Once you have mastered the handstand pushup, gradually move your hands an inch closer every time you workout, or whenever you feel able to. Use floor markings if it helps. If your handstand pushup hand position is about eighteen inches apart, you should take eighteen weeks *minimum* to get to this step—more if you need it.

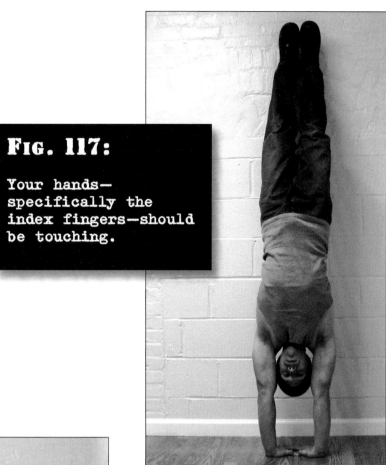

FIG. 117:

Your hands—specifically the index fingers—should be touching.

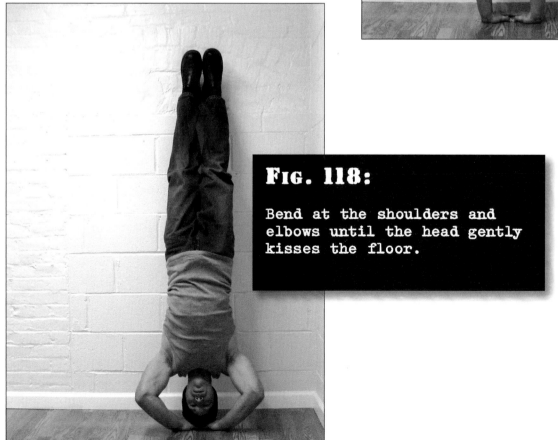

FIG. 118:

Bend at the shoulders and elbows until the head gently kisses the floor.

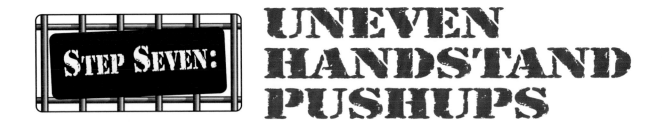

Performance

Place a basketball by the base of a wall. Kick up into a *wall handstand* next to the basketball using whichever technique you find easiest, then reach out and place one of your palms on the basketball. This motion sounds simple but is in fact very difficult; it will require supporting your body-weight on one locked arm for a fraction of a second, or as long as it takes to find the ball. Once your palm is secured on the basketball, position it so that your hands are about shoulder width apart. The arm of the hand which is on the floor should be straight, but your other arm will be bent. Apply your weight as evenly as you can through both hands, breathing smoothly. Your triceps, biceps and shoulders need to work very hard at this point, or you may lose control of the ball and crash down. This is the start position (fig. 119). Now bend at the elbows and shoulders until the head gently touches the floor. This is the finish position (fig. 120). Pause, and press back up.

Exercise X-Ray

In order to press yourself up, the basketball must be stabilized—it will tend to shoot outwards if not isometrically controlled. This will require huge arm and shoulder power, as well as Olympian rotator cuff muscles. The master of this exercise will earn shoulders like a gorilla and super-tough joints.

Training Goals

- Beginner standard: 1 set of 5   (both sides)
- Intermediate standard: 2 sets of 8   (both sides)
- Progression standard: 2 sets of 10   (both sides)

Perfecting Your Technique

Using the ball requires a high degree of strength and balance, combined with quick reflexes. I would advise all athletes to begin this exercise using stable objects rather than a ball. Perhaps start with a flat brick and over build up to using three stacked flat, or a cinderblock. In the pen a lot of guys use slim books in a pile, adding a book whenever they can. When the pile is as high as a basketball, *then* experiment with a basketball. Always play it safe!

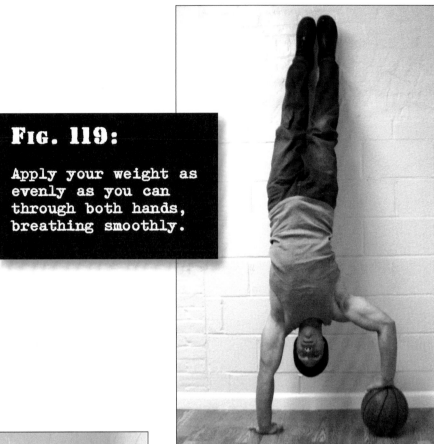

FIG. 119:

Apply your weight as evenly as you can through both hands, breathing smoothly.

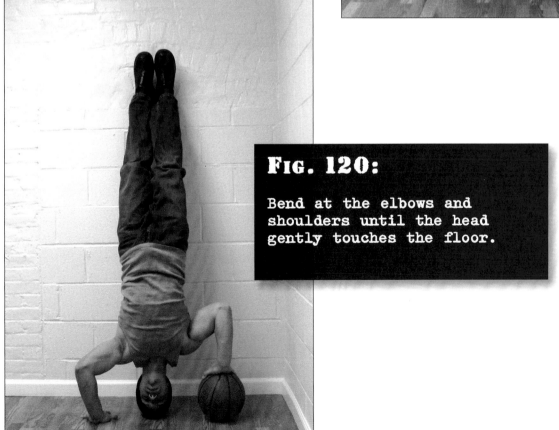

FIG. 120:

Bend at the elbows and shoulders until the head gently touches the floor.

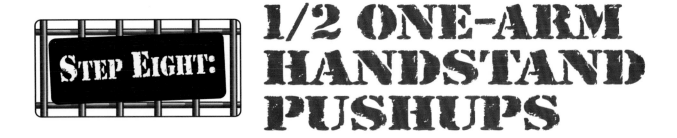

Performance

Kick up into a handstand against a wall. Your body should be slightly arched, with your heels in contact with the wall. Your hands should be six to ten inches from the base of the wall, and shoulder width apart. Keep your arms straight. Now gradually press off with one palm, so that your center of gravity shifts towards the other side of the body. This will put more of your body-weight through the opposite palm. Continue this transition over the course of a few seconds until there are only a few pounds of pressure left in the pushing palm. Now gently lift that palm away from the floor altogether, and hold it away from your body for balance. You will now be sup-porting yourself on one straight arm. This is the start position (fig. 121). Bend at the elbow and shoulder of your supporting arm until your head is halfway towards the floor. This is the finish position (fig. 122). Pause and press up.

Exercise X-Ray

This is the first technique in the series where you are pressing your entire bodyweight up with just one arm. This requires not only massive muscular strength in the shoulders and arms but extremely strong joints, total body coordination, excellent balance and an expert familiarity with inverse pressing techniques. To benefit from the *half one-arm handstand pushup* it's *essential* that you have invested a lot of time milking the earlier exercises for all they are worth—for at least six months, maybe even longer. Don't even attempt it otherwise, or you are only likely to injure yourself.

Training Goals

- Beginner standard: 1 set of 4   (both sides)
- Intermediate standard: 2 sets of 6   (both sides)
- Progression standard: 2 sets of 8   (both sides)

Perfecting Your Technique

This is a hard exercise which can only be gradually mastered by increasing your range of motion over time. Trying to push the weight though the *palm* rather than the *fingers* will help align the pressing muscles properly.

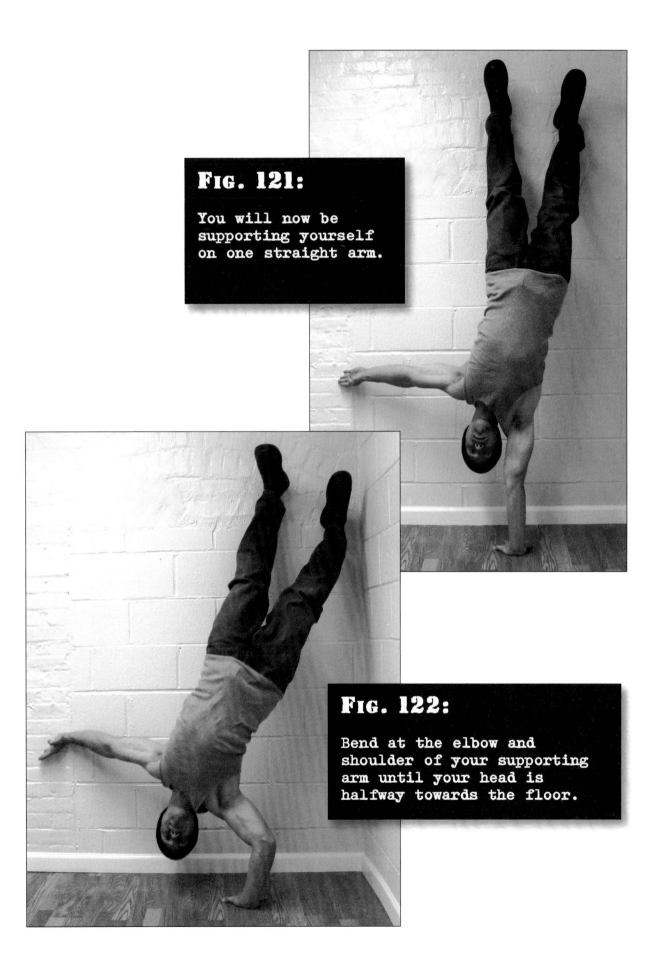

FIG. 121:

You will now be supporting yourself on one straight arm.

FIG. 122:

Bend at the elbow and shoulder of your supporting arm until your head is halfway towards the floor.

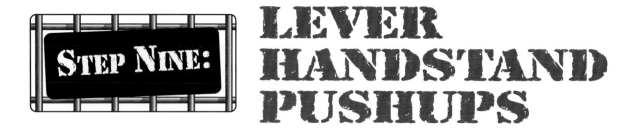

Performance

Kick up into a handstand against a sturdy wall. As usual, your arms should be shoulder width apart and your fingers should be six to ten inches from the wall with only your feet touching the surface. This will leave a slight natural curve in your body. As with Step 8, slowly transfer the majority of your weight—approximately ninety percent—onto one palm. Now flip your other palm over, so that the back of hand is flat on the floor with the fingers pointing away from you. Straighten out your arm in front of you, maintaining contact with the floor as you go. Some pressure should still be flowing through the digits of this hand. This is the start position (fig. 123). Keeping the arm of the upturned hand extended, bend at the shoulder and elbow of your other arm, with full muscular control—don't just allow your body to drop or you will hurt your head and possibly even crick your neck in the process. Pause as the top of your skull softly touches the floor. This is the finish position (fig. 124). Now, press back up to the start position, pushing through your palm and the back of your hand simultaneously.

Exercise X-Ray

This advanced exercise perfectly picks up where *half one-arm handstand pushups* leave off. The last step will have trained you to complete the top half of the motion, and *lever handstand pushups* help you master the more challenging bottom half. The position of the upturned hand makes it tough to apply much force with the assisting arm, ensuring you have just enough help to get you out of the bottom position with maximum muscular benefit.

Training Goals

- Beginner standard: 1 set of 3   (both sides)
- Intermediate standard: 2 sets of 4   (both sides)
- Progression standard: 2 sets of 6   (both sides)

Perfecting Your Technique

Bending the assisting (i.e., palm up) arm and bringing it closer to the body will allow you to apply greater leverage. Extend the arm as you get stronger.

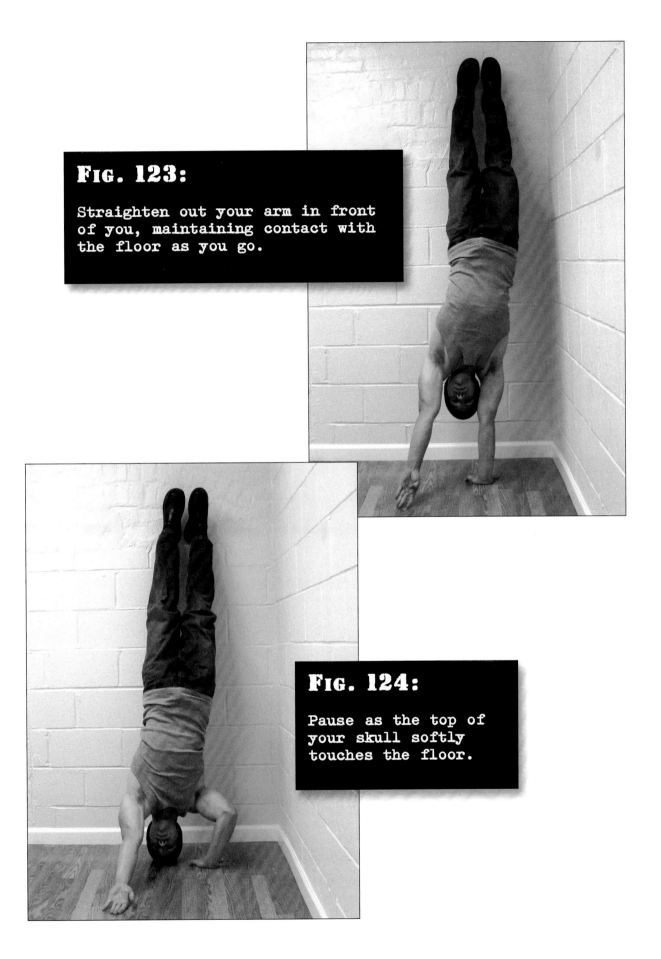

FIG. 123:

Straighten out your arm in front of you, maintaining contact with the floor as you go.

FIG. 124:

Pause as the top of your skull softly touches the floor.

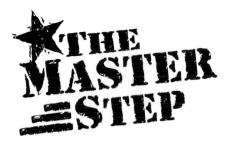

ONE-ARM HANDSTAND PUSHUPS

Performance

Kick up into a handstand against a wall, and lean out to the side until you are supporting yourself with one arm, as in *half one-arm handstand pushups* (Step 8). Keep your body gently arched with the heels against the wall. This is the start position (fig. 125). Bend at the elbow and shoulder of your supporting arm until the top of your skull very gently touches the floor. Keep your non-supporting hand ready in case you make a mistake and it has to help out. This is the finish position (fig. 126). In pressing back up to the start position, some explosiveness may be needed. To help you get out of the bottom position, a kick up with the legs is permissible. Bend the knees with the feet still against the wall, and straighten them quickly to add some thrust.

Exercise X-Ray

The *one-arm handstand pushup* is the ultimate shoulder and arm exercise. Forget bench presses—all they cause is injury and grief. Work your way carefully through the handstand pushup series right up to this Master Step and you will be stronger—in terms of pure, functional, *pick someone up and throw them* power—than any bench presser you meet. In terms of weights, it's the equivalent (for a two hundred pound man) of a one-arm two hundred pound press—that's four hundred pounds on a bar! How many guys do you know who can even *pick up* four hundred pounds, let alone shoulder press it? And calisthenics will give you this power *safely*—with healthy shoulders.

Training Goals

- Beginner standard: 1 set of 1   (both sides)
- Intermediate standard: 2 sets of 2   (both sides)
- Elite standard: 1 set of 5   (both sides)

Perfecting Your Technique

You will have to work into this exercise by gradually increasing depth. In truth, the only way to *really* master this exercise is to spend years—maybe three years or more—working on it. But you were planning on getting three years older anyway, right? So why not be super-strong when you get there?

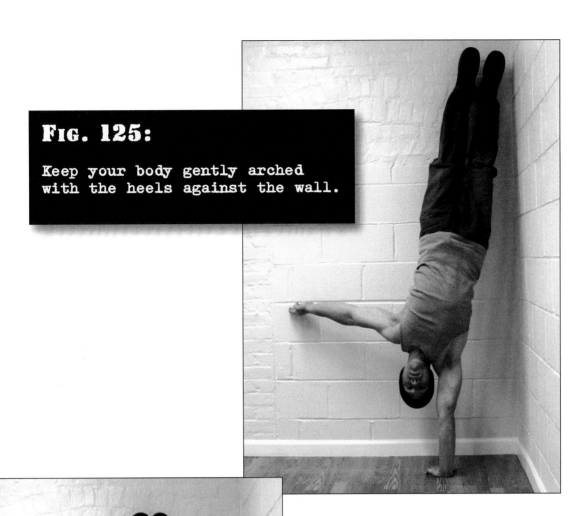

FIG. 125:

Keep your body gently arched with the heels against the wall.

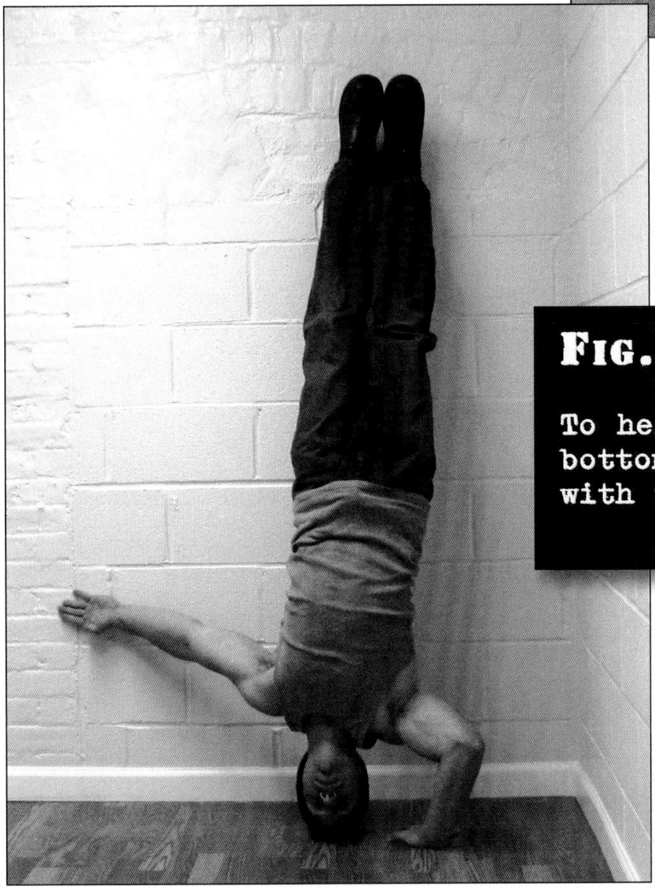

FIG. 126:

To help you get out of the bottom position, a kick up with the legs is permissible.

HANDSTAND PUSHUP SERIES PROGRESSSION CHART

STEP ONE	WALL HEADSTANDS Pages 230-231	WORK UP TO: 2 MINUTES Then Begin Step Two
STEP TWO	CROW STANDS Pages 232-233	WORK UP TO: 1 MINUTE Then Begin Step Three
STEP THREE	WALL HANDSTANDS Pages 234-235	WORK UP TO: 2 MINUTES Then Begin Step Four
STEP FOUR	HALF HANDSTAND PUSHUPS Pages 236-237	WORK UP TO: 2 SETS OF 20 Then Begin Step Five
STEP FIVE	HANDSTAND PUSHUPS Pages 238-239	WORK UP TO: 2 SETS OF 15 Then Begin Step Six

Handstand Pushup Series Progresssion Chart

STEP SIX	CLOSE HANDSTAND PUSHUPS — Pages 240-242	WORK UP TO: 2 SETS OF 12 — Then Begin Step Seven
STEP SEVEN	UNEVEN HANDSTAND PUSHUPS — Pages 242-243	WORK UP TO: 2 SETS OF 10 — Then Begin Step Eight
STEP EIGHT	1/2 ONE-ARM HANDSTAND PUSHUPS — Pages 244-245	WORK UP TO: 2 SETS OF 8 — Then Begin Step Nine
STEP NINE	LEVER HANDSTAND PUSHUPS — Pages 246-247	WORK UP TO: 2 SETS OF 6 — Then Begin Step Ten
MASTER STEP TEN	ONE-ARM HANDSTAND PUSHUPS — Pages 248-249	ULTIMATE POWER: 2 SETS OF 5

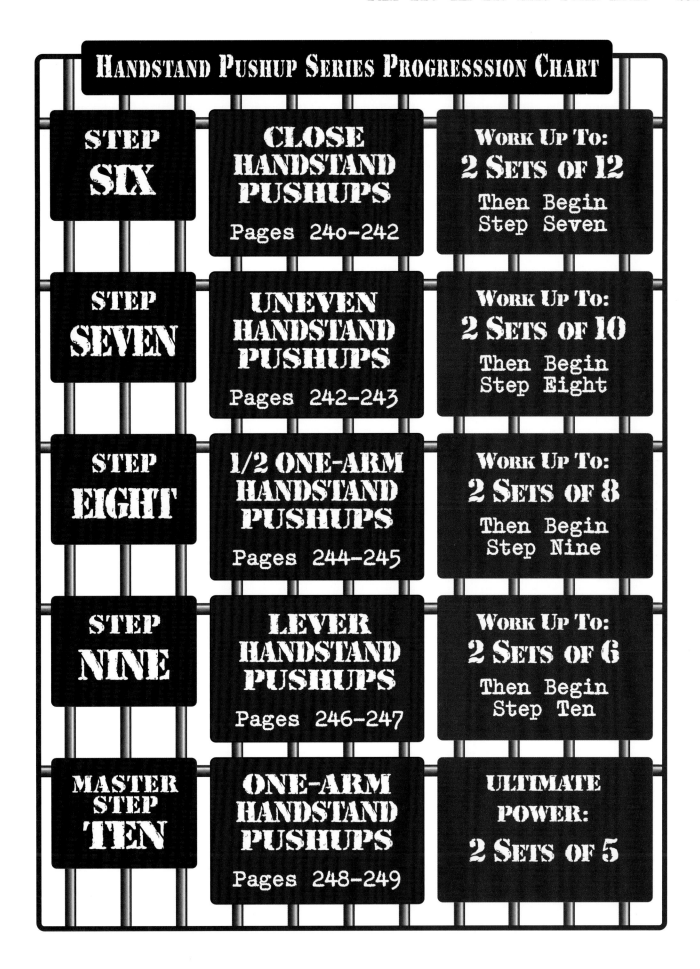

Going Beyond

Despite its age, the handstand pushup series is an incredibly advanced system of training for the shoulders and upper body pushing musculature. It's for this reason I advise that an athlete shouldn't even *begin* the handstand pushup series until his shoulders, chest and elbows are at least strong enough to perform *uneven pushups* (see pages 58—59). Once you have progressed to the point where you can do a few repetitions of the Master Step of this series—*one-arm handstand pushups*—your shoulders and triceps will be just about as strong as the human system will allow. You will have awesome strength, and this will be accompanied by the maximum natural muscle size for your frame.

For this reason, there's not much to suggest in the way of training for strength "beyond" this series; it's already highly advanced. You won't require any further strength exercises. However if you are gifted enough to progress all the way up to the one-arm work and you still want to explore further skills, I would suggest working on *coordination*. Learn the art of "free" hand-balancing, away from the guiding plane of a wall.

In you have properly mastered the *crow stand* (Step 2 of this series), starting "free" hand-balancing will be pretty easy. Just tip forwards from the top position (fig.110), and slowly extend your legs into the air. From there, straighten your arms fully and you'll be in a handstand. You will have the strength to push up into a handstand, provided you have (at least) progressed to Step 4 of this series, although the art of balancing your body without support will require some getting used to. The key lies in harmonizing the forwards arch of the body with the downwards pressure through the fingers; the arch will tend to topple you *forwards*, while the finger pressure will determine how far your center of gravity tilts *backwards*. At first these two elements will be out of sync, and you'll have to relocate your hands—essentially by walking on your palms—to prevent yourself from losing the inverse position. But once you have become expert in bringing these two types of forces into equilibrium, you will be able to balance on your hands for long periods of time.

Before long, you'll be able to do your handstand pushups without the wall—an impressive sight. They can be made even harder by using parallel bars (see photo opposite), which allow you to descend further than normal. Alternatively, you can work towards unilateral hand balancing and free unilateral one-arm pushups by using uneven objects (like chairs or steps). Hand-balancing is a beautiful and satisfying artform which is infinitely more rewarding than just heaving up heavy barbells.

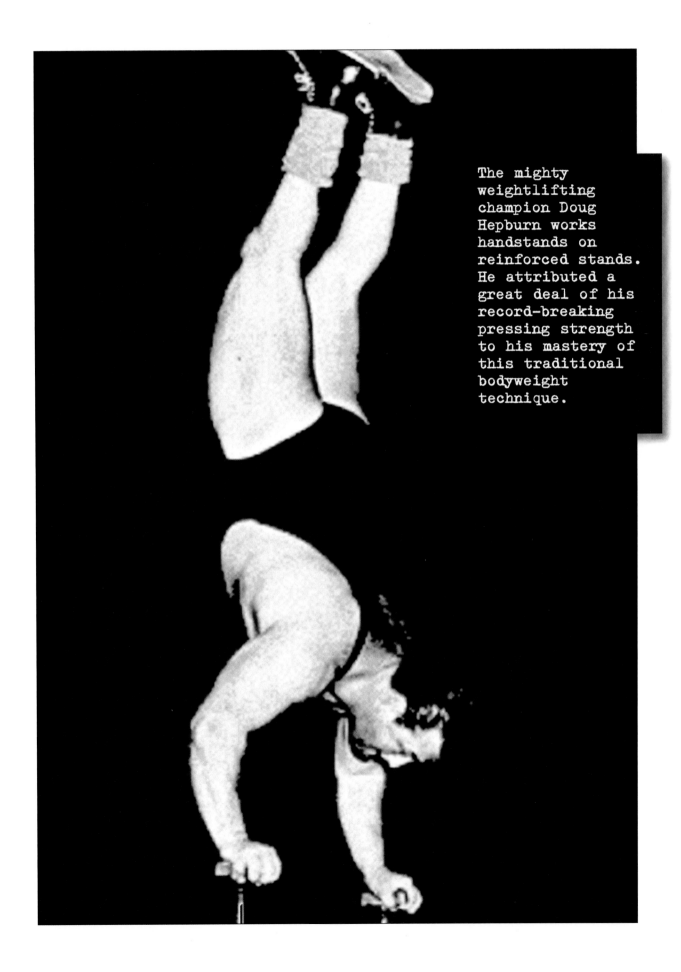

The mighty weightlifting champion Doug Hepburn works handstands on reinforced stands. He attributed a great deal of his record-breaking pressing strength to his mastery of this traditional bodyweight technique.

Variants

There are relatively few good bodyweight shoulder exercises, because the shoulders usually function by pushing vertically up against gravity. This is easy to do if you have weights like barbells and dumbbells—you just press them upwards, as in the case of shoulder presses, press-behind-neck, push presses, jerks, etc. But if you wish to work your shoulders *hard* and you don't have weights, you are largely limited to inverse positions; you turn your whole body upside-down, and push vertically up that way. Fortunately the lack of calisthenics-based shoulder exercises is more than compensated for by the fact that the few variants which exist are truly excellent for shoulder health.

Marion Pushups

Marion pushups are an intense, progressive form of *decline pushup* I learned in Marion Pen. Decline pushups are just pushups with your feet elevated—lifted up on something. If you lift your feet high enough, the pushups stop working the chest as much and start working the muscles at the front of the shoulders. In Marion these were a very popular cell exercise, and because the ten steps weren't well known, guys used to use decline pushups as a transitional method to work up to handstand pushups. The popular system involved starting with fifty pushups. When a con could do fifty flat pushups, he put his feet on his bunk and built up to forty pushups. When he could do this, he put his feet up on the john—which is a little higher than a bunk—and did thirty pushups. Then he put his feet on the basin and did twenty pushups. Finally he jammed his feet up on the wall above the basin and did ten pushups. The cons left a little mark or smudge on the wall where there feet were, and every time they trained they tried to go a little higher, still doing ten pushups. Eventually the cons would be pretty much in a handstand position against the wall, doing ten full handstand pushups. Marion pushups are an interesting approach to inverse work, but in my experience they just don't work as well as combining regular pushups and handstand pushups in a program using the ten steps. Use the ten steps and you'll get powerful shoulders faster and more easily.

Isometric Presses

Stand up straight with your open hands either side of your shoulders and your bent arms out wide, stretching your chest. Push your elbows as far back as you can; as if you were trying to crack a nut between your shoulder blades. Now powerfully tense all the muscles in your arms and torso. Exhale as you slowly push upwards, making your hands into tight fists as you go. Pause as your arms become straight, and contract as hard as possible for a count of two. Inhale as you reverse the movement of the way down, and repeat. Although this exercise uses a wide elbow position, it's still quite safe because of the lack of external forces. It's obviously difficult to quantify and measure progress in this exercise, although in a sense it *is* progressive because as your shoulders and their antagonistic structures become stronger over time, the opposing muscle groups are able to contract with increasing force. The same principle holds true for all isometric exercise. Isometric presses shouldn't be the mainstay of your delt workout, but they certainly serve as an excellent toning technique and are good for the rotator cuffs. This technique also really burns the muscles up and gets a good sweat on when done slowly and for high reps.

Windmills

Almost everybody has tried this great warm up exercise. Simply hold your arms out to the side and begin to make circles. This exercise is dynamic and requires more flexibility than most people realize, so don't just start wildly swinging or you might tweak cold muscles. Start with small circles—no larger than a Frisbee—and as your shoulders begin to loosen gradually expand your rotations to the maximum of your range of motion. One set of fifty reps (i.e., fifty full circles) will warm up even the tightest upper body, but don't forget to repeat the exercise for the same number of reps, circling in the opposite direction. A slightly harder variation is *alternate windmills*, which involves the arms circling in different directions before switching.

Hand Walking

Once you are comfortable in free handstands, you'll inevitably want to try walking around on your hands. Hand walking is difficult at first, but if you've gained good strength in the handstand position, all it requires is a little re-orientation to do it. Once you've got this "trick," you'll find you can walk around on your hands for extended periods without much effort. As a result, this exercise won't build much strength. If you really want to try a grueling variation, try walking on your hands down some steps (use short stairs or start part way up so you won't hurt yourself if you fall). When you can do this safely, walk *up* the stairs on your hands. That builds good strength.

Tiger Bends

These are a classic upper body feat favored by the old-time strongmen because it displays balance and coordination as well as enormous strength. Get into a free handstand, away from the wall. Drop down flat onto your forearms, and hold for a moment. In this position your arms will resemble the forepaws of a big cat—hence the name (see photo next page). Now if you are strong enough, you can kick your legs up and hop back into the full handstand position, although this second part of the movement requires massive power. Tiger bends give the shoulder girdle a vigorous workout, but their primary effect is on the triceps, elbows and outer forearms. The master of this old technique will have elbows strong as titanium axles.

You won't see it in today's gyms, but mega-strength feats like the tiger bend were well known to old school masters of bodyweight training. Here the exercise is performed by the famous twenties strongman Sig Klein. Klein's arms were so powerful that he could hold the average man overhead with one arm, and easily see-saw press 1oo lbs. dumbbells—and all at a bodyweight of barely 154 lbs.

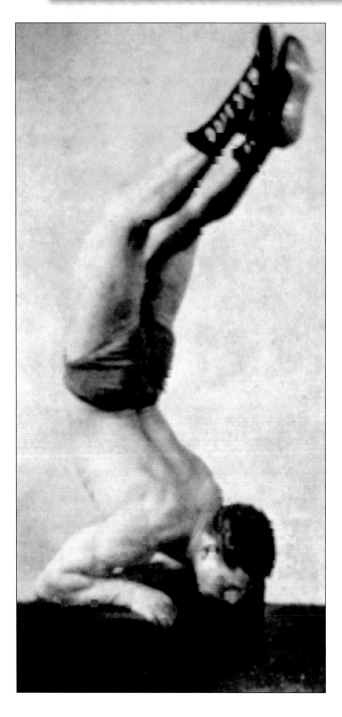
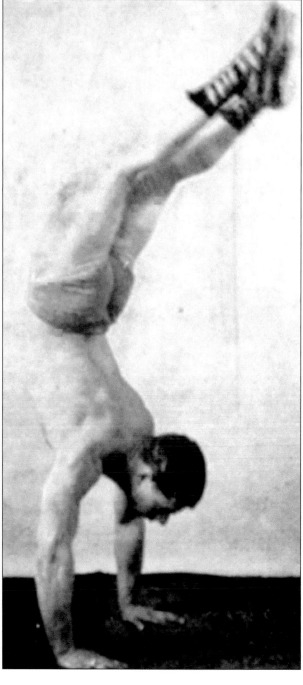

– Part III –

Self-Coaching

The previous section will have taught you everything you need to know about the most productive old school calisthenics techniques—enough to last a lifetime. But effective training is about a lot more than correctly performed exercises, no matter how productive those exercises may be.

In prison, you have to depend on yourself. You need to learn to coach yourself. To do this successfully, knowledge of exercise performance *must* be combined with body wisdom, an understanding of the principles of hardcore training, and an insight into how to structure a routine. The final two chapters will go a long way to teaching you everything you need to know.

11: BODY WISDOM

CAST IRON PRINCIPLES

O ver the last six chapters I've outlined all the exercises you need to start training in The Big Six:. Virtually every prison athlete has used these exercises—or at least some of them—at one point or another during their training.

But I've learned from my experience as a coach that it's no good just giving wannabe calisthenics experts a list of exercises—no matter how good those exercises are. Even if you combine those exercises with a fantastic training program, perfectly tailored to an individual's needs, there's *still* something missing.

What's missing is the "x factor" of training success. It's an innate understanding of the essentials underlying any given conditioning experience; like knowing how to warm up perfectly, how to progress at the ideal pace, or how hard to push your training, and when to cut back.

These matters are never black and white. They are more of an art than a science. You really can't just write these things down on a piece of paper and hand them to an athlete, because they are not simple objects of knowledge. They are about subjective inner understanding gained through experience. It's more a matter of *body wisdom* than conceptual memorization.

I do have a lot of experience, and a big ol' chunk of that experience has come from screwing up. It takes time to learn body wisdom, and it would be foolish of me to think that I could take all the useful training smarts in my head and put them into yours. It doesn't work that way. But I can at least try to point you in the right direction to get your own.

Let's start at the beginning.

Warming Up

Imagine taking a thick slice of mozzarella cheese out of the refrigerator and pulling on it. It crumbles to bits, right? But if you took that same slice and put it in the microwave for a few seconds before pulling on it, it would be all soft and stretchy—it wouldn't break. Your muscle cells are a lot like this. When they are cold, they are more delicate and vulnerable to trauma on a cellular level. When they are nice and warm, they are elastic and flexible. This is why all sensible athletes warm up before exertion. Warming up not only reduces the risk of injury, it also prepares the nervous system for action, sends fresh, shock-absorbing synovial fluid around the joints, and focuses the mind for the harder work to come.

The degree to which you need to warm up varies on factors like the external temperature, your conditioning and your age—senior athletes need to warm up a little longer than the young punks. I'm not a fan of long, extended warm ups. I prefer to get into the action. A lot of guys I've seen training like to warm up over several stages; a cardio warm up to get the heart pumping, some stretches, then some light sets of muscular warm ups before getting into the exercises they plan to do. Some guys warm up for nearly an hour before they start their training!

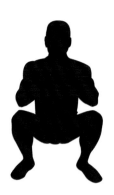

For me, this is way too much. You really don't need all this. The most efficient way to warm up is with two to four progressively harder higher rep sets of the movement you are going to be performing for your work sets. Do two warm up sets if you are young with no joint problems, three or even four if you are older, in poor shape or in a cold climate. Any more than this and you are just spinning your wheels. The only exception would be if you have an injury, in which case I'd advise an extra mini-warm up for that area; a pain-free higher rep (thirty or more) set, followed by some gentle stretching. That's all. Do this before your workout proper, just get some blood into the injured area and protect it.

It's difficult to give exact warm up protocols, because ability levels differ so widely. A good rule of thumb is to start with a twenty rep set, then follow it with a fifteen rep set of the movement you are doing. Then you should be good to go. In terms of effort, don't start too hard. Aim at about fifty percent of your maximum on both warm up sets. In other words, pick an exercise you could do at least forty reps on (if pushed) for the first warm up, and an exercise you could probably do thirty reps on for your second. The second set will necessarily seem *heavier* because you are using a lower rep range. The first warm up set should pump up the muscles you will be working. During the second set they should begin to burn a little as your strength kicks in. Following both sets you should feel stimulated and ready for more—not exhausted.

The techniques you choose to warm up with should be drawn from the earlier steps of the series of whichever movement you'll be working on. For example, let's say you are working on pushups. You are currently working on Step 6, *close pushups* for your work sets. For your first warm up, you might do twenty reps of Step 2, *incline pushups*, then for your second warm up, fifteen reps of Step 3, *kneeling pushups*. Your pushup workout might look like this:

SET NO:	EXERCISE:	REPS PER SET:
1. Warm up 1:	*Incline pushups*	*Twenty reps*
2. Warm up 2:	*Kneeling pushups*	*Fifteen reps*
3. Work set 1:	*Close pushups*	*Fourteen reps*
4. Work set 2:	*Close pushups*	*Twelve reps*

Obviously, if you are working on the earlier steps, you won't be able to warm up precisely using this rule. You'll just do a couple of sets of the exercise you are working on as a warm up. Use your discretion. If—due to age, climate, etc.—you require more warm ups, just repeat the second warm up exercise for twelve reps for another two sets *at the most*.

Some trainers also recommend a warm down/cool down. Historically, the idea of a cool down comes from Victorian exercise ideologists. They believed that if the heartbeat slowed too rapidly it would cause the body internal damage. We now know that this isn't true at all. Some people also believe that a cool down prevents or alleviates soreness the next day, although I've never found this and I don't believe it. All a cool down involves is more work for the muscles—how can *more* work possibly reduce damage? For this reason, I don't do systematic cool downs. Following a hard training session, I used to pace my cell, or sit on my bunk and do some deep breathing exercises. I found this helped me relax and regain equilibrium quickly. If you do like doing physical cool downs for psychological reasons though, you can. Just repeat your warm up procedure in reverse.

Starting Slow

A lot of guys are eager to start training as hard as possible. Hard training is important, but patience is important too. I always advise people new to calisthenics—no matter how strong they are—to begin with the first exercise. That's right. *Start your training with Step 1 of every single movement of The Big Six.* Resist the urge to jump in at Step 3, 4, 5 or even 6. Start with the easiest possible exercise, and gradually pick up the intensity. Give yourself at least four weeks until you are working hard, and perhaps *two months* until you are going nearly full bore.

Many people will think this is too slow. They will be sure that the earlier exercises are just too easy. But starting at the very beginning will bring greater benefits in the long run. It will strengthen the joints, teach coordination, balance, timing and cadence. It will develop good core strength and kick-start the motivation for harder exercises.

Getting really strong through calisthenics is not a fad for teenagers. It should be something you benefit from for your whole life. Devoting a few short weeks to mastering the basic, easy exercises doesn't seem like much time in that context, does it?

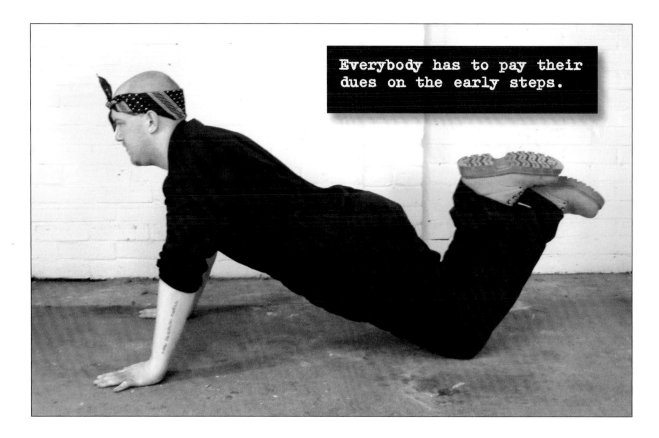

Everybody has to pay their
dues on the early steps.

Training Momentum

There is a damn good reason why you should proceed slowly and methodically through any training program. The reason has to do with generating *training momentum*. Basically put, this means that if you build a head of steam by moving forwards more slowly, you'll actually reach your goals much faster than if you proceeded with haste. This sounds like a paradox, but it's true.

The old-timers of the iron game understood this principle only too well. They used to talk in terms of "milking" a program, and "putting strength in the bank." One of the old sayings wise weightlifting coaches used force down the throats of eager young trainees was the phrase; *the heavy weight isn't going anywhere.*

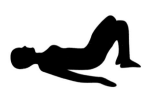

Unfortunately, modern athletes don't understand this approach at all. When people start training, they normally throw themselves in at the deep end. This is partly for cultural reasons. We live in "want it now" society; kids today don't see patience as a virtue. Nor do adults. (That's why our nation is in as much debt as it is—we want what we want *now*. We don't want to have to wait until we have really *earned* it.) Steroids are another reason why modern people expect to see results tomorrow. Steroids bring such fast—albeit *temporary* and *unhealthy*—results, that the older art of gradually building training momentum has largely been lost or forgotten.

Put Strength in the Bank

Maybe you have heard the old-fashioned (but unbelievably important) term "milking" being applied to a training cycle or routine, or you have read about "putting strength in the bank." If you've heard these phrases and wondered what they mean, here's how it works.

Putting it as simply as possible, the harder you train, the better your results. Because of this, a lot of trainees assume that the quickest way to get big and strong is to work as hard as they possibly can. Unfortunately—particularly for the average natural athlete—training *super*-hard has its drawbacks. It drains the system, eats up training motivation, and it can be rough on the joints. When you train as hard as possible, you will probably get a spurt of good gains—for a few weeks or a couple of months at the most—but then those gains will grind to a halt as the body rebels. Our bodies only have so much energy in them to build muscle and strength, and if you are training really hard, drug-free, that energy gets used up pretty quick.

When you train more moderately you don't get the same results you do when you train at your limit, but you do get *some* results, and you can keep coaxing those results out of your body for much longer periods of time. As the months pass, these moderate gains add up to much more total muscle and strength than the big initial gains made by the athlete who worked super-hard but burned himself out.

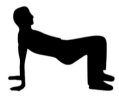

Here's an example of what I mean. I've taught lots of enthusiastic new fish about The Big Six and the ten steps. Imagine I teach two different inmates the ten steps of the pushup series. Both of them have the same genetic potential, but they have different levels of *patience*.

The Dumb Way

One guy—fickle and only interested in immediate results—looks at the ten steps and figures he's strong enough to do Step 5, *full pushups*. So he launches into his pushups straight away. He pushes as hard as he can, and manages to meet the progression standard in only two weeks. Great, huh?

Now he tackles Step 6, *close pushups*. These seem a lot harder than they should, because he hasn't invested the time building his strength base. But, fired up by his success on the pushups, he keeps pushing himself as hard as he can—too hard. He wobbles and strains because he hasn't allowed his body the time to build the energy it needs, but he still forces out more reps every week even though his form is gradually getting worse. After four weeks of trying, he has nearly met the progression standard of two sets of twenty reps. Determined to make progress, he forces out an *abysmal* extra rep—barely a rep at all—and convinces himself that he has met the progression standard. He is pretty pleased with his "achievement," despite the fact that in real terms he's not much stronger. He also has nagging pains in his joints, because he never allowed them the time to adapt to all that hard work. His shocking exercise technique doesn't help his achyness, either.

The next week—week seven of his training program—he psychs himself up and shoots for Step 7 of the series, *uneven pushups*. To his shock and disappointment, he can't even manage a single rep. He struggles and pushes on tired muscles, but no matter how hard he tries, he just can't do it. His body seems to weigh a ton, and the exercise, even just one rep, seems like an insurmountable mountain peak. He becomes depressed, because—at least in his mind—he's been making incredible progress, which has suddenly just stopped for no reason. He's confused, and at this point he either blames the training program or figures that he's just not cut out for calisthenics. So he embarks on some new method—which he will inevitably screw up too—or he quits altogether. His program lasted a mere seven weeks, and gave him very little beyond sore shoulders and disappointment.

The Smart Way

The second guy is also hungry for results. But he's got a smart enough head on his shoulders to temper that hunger with a little patience. Like the first guy, he is also pretty sure he could pump out some *full pushups* (Step 5). But he doesn't. Instead, he begins with Step 1—*wall pushups*. These seem incredibly easy to him, but he does them anyway. His joints begin adapting from day one. He sticks with wall pushups for a month, slowly adding reps until he meets the progression standard. Then he moves to Step 2, *incline pushups*. These are a little more challenging, and he begins to "feel" the technique. He sticks with them for the required time, slowly building muscle condition and tendon strength without even really realizing it. One month later, he progresses to Step 3, *kneeling pushups*. After all the patient work he's put in, these still seem as easy as Step 1 did, despite the fact that they are a significantly harder exercise.

Three months in and he hits the floor for Step 4, *half pushups*. By now he is beginning to feel that his pressing muscles are tighter, more toned, and he knows damn well he could ace Step 5 right away. But he holds himself back, faithfully putting his energy into half pushups. One month later, he finally begins working on Step 5, *full pushups*. By now his motivation has built up to the point where it's practically bubbling over. The exercise doesn't even seem difficult—it almost feels like he's doing pushups underwater. But he devotes himself to pushups, and because they don't cause him any strain, he can really cherish every rep, cultivating picture-perfect form. Our man doesn't realize it, but this makes him even stronger.

Five months in and he effortlessly glides to Step 6, *close pushups*. Whereas they seemed pretty tough to the guy who did it the dumb way, our smart trainee can't understand what the fuss was about. Perhaps they seem slightly more challenging, but not much. By now he's used to slowly taking his time and increasing his reps with textbook form. Before long, he's worked his way up to Step 7, *uneven pushups*. Whereas the guy in the above example couldn't even do a single rep, our hero does all the reps required in the beginner standard, and he does them easily. He's left feeling that if he pushed, he could actually meet the progression standard if he wanted. But he doesn't—he keeps a little something in the bank for next time.

The months pass, and so does Step 8, *half one-arm pushups*. By now, things are getting a little more challenging, but not enormously so. He's having to work hard, but things aren't *grueling*, and he's confident. Plus, he's noticed a real change in his body; his pectorals are thicker, and there is a dense horseshoe of muscle hanging off his upper arm that wasn't there before. His shoulders are rounder, and cool veins have appeared on his delts.

By the time he gets to Step 9, *lever pushups*, he has a little difficulty with his reps, so he regroups, focuses on his form and gradually begins to improve by adding a rep here and there when he feels ready. Even as he approaches the progression standard, he's not working all-out—sometimes he feels as though he couldn't do one more perfect rep. So he doesn't. Rather than throwing out a sloppy rep, he saves that next *perfect* rep for one week, two weeks down the line. And you know what? He gets there.

Whereas the guy trying to achieve this the dumb way short-circuited his gains and crashed out of his program like a failure after only seven weeks, this guy—who has identical genetic potential—has stayed the course for nearly a year. During that time, he's aced the coveted Master Step of the pushup series, gained a ton of strength, and has gone up a shirt size due to the prime beef added to his upper body. Not to mention that his pride and confidence are through the roof. Next year, he decides, he's going to master the *one-arm handstand pushup*. Will he manage it? You bet. Training like this, how can he fail?

This is the real way to get genuine, lasting gains. Forget books that promise size and strength tomorrow. They are all smoke and mirrors, and will only wind up helping you towards failure and frustration.

Intensity

Just because I don't recommend training like an idiot—beyond your safe capabilities, and using undisciplined form—it doesn't mean you shouldn't train *hard*. You should. Once your joints and muscles are ready for it, you should always train hard.

Working hard is the key to achieving your goals. But "hard" in the context of bodyweight training doesn't mean just pushing until you can't move. Once you have worked up to it, pour your effort into the most difficult exercises you can do, but when your exercise technique starts to deteriorate significantly it's time to terminate a set. When you are advanced, you can extend a set beyond normal by using partial movements or doing "rest-pause" reps—which is simply performing another rep or two after a brief rest. But always use common sense and be safe. Training to total "failure" is a bad idea in calisthenics—you should always leave a little energy in your limbs so you can control your body. Training to failure, especially on inverse exercises (like handstand pushups), or when you are hanging above the ground (as in leg raises and pullups) is totally unsafe. Always leave something in the tank.

Most bodybuilding and strength training programs contain the concepts of "cycling" or "periodization." These are just ways of varying intensity throughout the training year—meaning that training is sometimes easy, sometimes moderate, sometimes hard. This is often necessary in bodybuilding and powerlifting, because weight-training irritates the joints and depletes the body's hormonal-immune system in a way that proper bodyweight work does not. Bodybuilders *need* to back off from their hardest weights, or they'd cripple themselves and become sick or exhausted. This constant "backing off" is unnecessary for a calisthenics expert. Instead of varying intensity, *you should always aim at performing the hardest versions of the ten steps possible*—providing that:

- You have followed the advice given in *starting slow* on page 261
- Your form is perfect
- You are not sick or ill
- You are not injured or experiencing the precursors of injury
- You can meet the desired number of repetitions given for an exercise in the *beginner standard*

If you are sick—perhaps with a virus or infection—hard training will deplete your immune system and may prolong the illness. If you are well enough to train, back off from your hardest movements and exercise some *discretion*. If you have an injury or the beginnings of an injury, you can often still train—in fact in most cases you *should* still train. But you need to do so in a way that brings more blood to the injured are and heals it. This is an art in itself.

The *beginner standard* is given opposite the pictures of the exercises in Part Two of this book. It's usually about five repetitions. If you can't do this many repetitions in good form, you are liable to start struggling and that's when injury happens. If you don't meet the *beginner standard* on a given step, go back to the former step and keep working on it, perfecting your form, increasing your reps and finding ways to make that particular exercise harder. When you feel ready, try the next step again.

Making Progress

This raises another issue; of how to make progress from step to step, along the ten steps. Generally speaking, this is simple—start by meeting the *beginner standard* and simply aim to add another repetition to the exercise you are working on every week or two (or three or four perhaps, for harder exercises). If you continue doing this consistently, you will very quickly be able to do one set of ten reps in any given exercise. When you can do this, begin doing two work sets.

Keep adding reps to both your work sets over time, and you will quickly reach the *intermediate standard* (also given on the pages opposite the exercise photos). When you reach that level, add a third work set—but only if the exercise's *progression standard* demands it (most exercises don't). Continue adding to your reps—using perfect form—over time until you meet the *progression standard*, and then move to the next step in the series.

If you follow this simple method of progression, you will ultimately reach the tenth step of each movement—the highly coveted *Master Step*. When you do, pat yourself on the back—you are one hell of an impressive athlete. But even this is not the peak of mountain. The road to greater strength goes on and on. When you get to this stage, check out the advice in the *Going Beyond* section of the Big Six chapters for some ideas on how to continue improving further and further.

Troubleshooting

Making progress sounds simple. Many things in this world *sound* simple! But in reality, life is not so simple. Things get in the way. On occasion you will find that your progress plateaus. From time to time you may be unable to add reps to your exercises, but plateaus most often happen when an athlete has met the *progression standard* to move up to the next step in the series. Despite this achievement, sometimes they just can't make the jump from one exercise to the next. If this happens to you, here are four helpful ideas to get things moving again:

1. **Drop bodyweight.** The more advanced the exercises become, the more they depend upon a good level of *proportionate* strength. Muscular bodyweight is no barrier to success. Body fat is. If you are having trouble moving up in your exercises, focus on losing flab over a few months.

2. **Rest more.** Motivation and effort are to be admired. But if you are overworking a body part, an exercise or an entire routine, your performance will suffer. Try adding more rest days. Usually if over-trained athletes go back to a routine like *Good Behavior* or *Veterano* (on pages 279 and 280) they find that they start making gains again.

3. **Be patient.** This is a common problem. Often athletes get addicted to progress. They push themselves to add too many reps in one shot, to move up the steps too quickly. Their form suffers. They get sloppy and start using momentum instead of strength. Pretty soon they are attempting movements that are way out of their league and they can't understand why their progress has come to a crashing halt. If this is you, go back a few steps and start over. Double check that your form is perfect, and build up s-l-o-w-l-y. The body will adapt, I promise. But it will do so at its *own* pace—not necessarily *yours*!

4. **Live clean.** One way to help your body adapt is to treat it right. Get plenty of sleep. Don't fill your body with booze and drugs. Don't get it all beat up. Respect it.

Above all, *have faith*. Don't get despondent, depressed or angry. Stick to your training long enough to get used to it, to feel the benefits. Trust in your body. Follow the above advice, and you'll keep making progress in your training for years to come.

Consolidation Training

If you are really having a problem getting just a handful of reps on a particular exercise, try *consolidation training*. Consolidation training is a handy little trick I learnt from a fellow prison athlete. Most of the time, you should focus on moderate to high repetitions, somewhere in the ten to twenty-five range. This is good for building strength, muscle, and joint integrity. Higher reps also mean that when you move to harder exercises, they will seem easier by contrast.

But there is an exception to this rule. When you have been working a movement series for a prolonged period, sometimes it can be tough to move from one step to the next. For example, you might be able to do nine reps in the *uneven pullup*, but once you switch to the *half one-arm pullup*, you can barely get one or two good reps. This is not uncommon as you become increasingly advanced.

Consolidation training is an excellent way of coping with this situation. Instead of working the new exercise once or twice a week and struggling to improve your reps every time, try working the new exercise every day—sometimes even twice or three times a day. Loosen up, then instead of doing as many reps as possible, only do one—two at the very most. Maybe do one rep of a half one-arm pullup when you wake up; another one after lunch; another before lights out, and so on. Use good form, but *don't* strain. The name of the game is to spread your effort by performing lots of reps over a period of several days, not to push your muscles hard in any single attempt. If you get excessively sore, back off for a couple of days.

Follow this unique protocol for a week or two. As the days pass, the once nearly-impossible technique will gradually seem easier. When you go back to your regular training, you will find that multiple reps are much, much more attainable.

I don't know why consolidation training works, but it definitely does work. I've been told that it works because the multiple mini-sessions "teach" the nervous system how to manage the technique in a more efficient way than just one prolonged session can. Don't use it for exercises where you can already get multiple reps—keep it for those occasions when you move up to a new, advanced technique which you find a real struggle.

How Many Work Sets?

A work set is any set that's not a warm up—any set where you're having to *push* to perform your target reps in good style.

I can't deny that in the past I've done a lot of high volume training. This was partly just because it distracted me from prison life. But you really don't need hours and hours of training, particularly if you are looking for strength. These days I usually advise very few work sets—and this often confuses trainees who see calisthenics as *endurance exercise*. I see it as a *strength training method*. Getting stronger requires *intensity*, not volume. Certainly, it's possible to gently build up your conditioning levels so that you can perform harder work over longer periods, but despite what some cocky trainees may claim, intensity and volume are mutually exclusive qualities. This basically just means that they don't go together. If you are pushing to do the hardest exercises—the highest of the ten steps—that you can, you'll only be able to do them for a brief period before you are pretty much ready to collapse on the floor. If you can do them for hours and hours, it stands to reason that the movements you are doing are not the hardest ones you can potentially do. You should be trying harder movements!

If you want to see a good example of how volume and intensity are mutually exclusive, look at a 100-meter sprinter. He is much stronger and has a far more muscular body than a marathon runner, despite the fact that his event lasts only a fraction of the time. This is because the sprint is more *intense* than a marathon. The marathon has much more *volume* in terms of energy expenditure, but far from adding strength and muscle it strips these qualities away.

To adapt, you only really need to do a couple of work sets. A lot of guys get nervous about doing so little—especially ex-bodybuilders who are used to being totally exhausted and sore after a gym workout. Bodyweight work is more authentic; it works the human body in the way it *evolved* to work. For this reason there is less microtrauma, and less of a sense of systemic depletion. You don't need to be totally shattered after a bodyweight workout. If you want to get strong doing calisthenics, think like a sprinter—not a marathon runner. Warm up, then BOOM! Give it your all over a small number of sets. Don't keep working on and on, adding sets for no reason.

Rest Between Sets

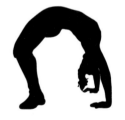

How long you rest between sets depends upon your goals. If you're looking for maximum stamina, rest as briefly as possible. Some guys use a stopwatch to allow them to gradually decrease their time between sets workout by workout. Another way to monitor your time in-between sets is to count your breaths. This is only semi-accurate compared with the stopwatch method, but it has the added benefit of helping the athlete get in touch with their respiration pattern, the first step towards breath control.

If you are training for strength and muscle, you must rest as long as it takes for you to get ready to tackle the next set and give it your all. No guidelines can be given for this—it entirely depends on how fit you are. Some people feel the need to rush between sets of bodyweight exercises; perhaps because they were taught this at school, or perhaps because they don't take bodyweight strength work as seriously as heavy weight-training. Whatever the reason, this is a mistake. Calisthenics performed for strength depletes internal muscle sugars and fatigues the body. Respect the techniques of the Big Six. If you find you need to rest for five minutes between sets to get most of your strength back, do so. Just be aware that if you need to rest for more than five minutes, the body will start to get cold. Pace the room, and stretch out the muscles you are working to keep the blood circulating in them.

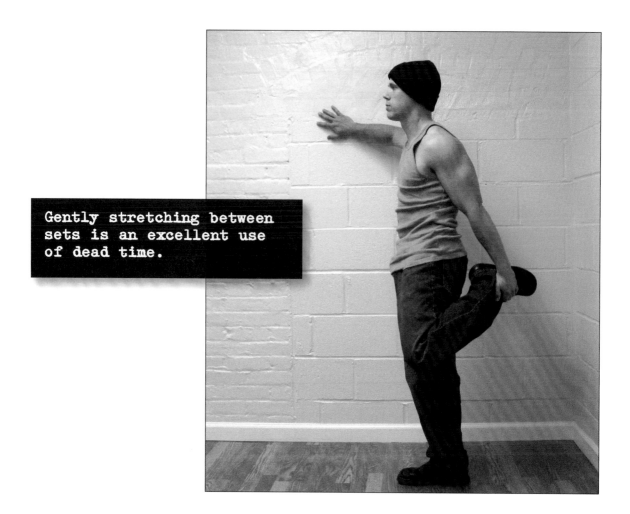

Gently stretching between sets is an excellent use of dead time.

Recording Your Training

If you can directly apply the above principles of body wisdom to your own training, then you are on the path to making excellent progress on a regular basis, with a minimum by way of plateaus or injuries. Making progress simply means beating what you've done in the past—but this requires a good knowledge of your performance in previous workouts.

Unfortunately, the mind of man is a fragile, partial thing. When you're new to training, it can be real hard to remember recent workouts; when you've been working out for a while—maybe years—the workouts can blend together. Often, memory can be infected by factors such as time, emotion, exhaustion, or motivation; as a result, an athlete's recall of performance levels from workout to workout may often be unreliable. This is a problem, because you need a good working knowledge of your performance to know what you need to beat next time, and to analyze your recent progress.

Luckily, a form of technology has been developed that can help athletes completely overcome this potential problem.

The miracle technology I'm about to reveal to you is so astonishing, so unbelievably helpful, that I'd like to invest a few lines in selling it to you. As a platform, it seamlessly integrates text and images at the user's whim, facilitating maximum freedom and creativity in note-taking. It isn't dependent upon an external power source or an internal battery; it cannot become corrupted by viruses, Trojan horses or an EMP; it can't be "hacked" from a remote location; and its format never becomes obsolete and unusable when new advances are made. Plus, it's easy to use—I guarantee that every person reading this right now has been successfully training in the use of this technology for *years*. Perhaps best of all, this incredible, versatile technology is available pretty much everywhere, and it costs only a few cents.

You already know what this astonishing development is though, right? You got it; *pen and paper*.

When you finish your training—or a soon as possible afterwards—*write down what you did*. Before the next session, briefly review your notes, so you'll know what you need to match or beat this time.

Don't write on loose sheets of paper as they easily become disordered or lost. Get yourself a cheap lined A4 or A5 hard-backed journal from a stationary store. You don't need to buy anything flashy or pretty—training journals tend to get knocked around, anyway. Just get something plain and solid.

Benefits of Recording Your Training

Athletes have been writing down their training sessions for centuries now, and for damn good reasons:

* Since the birth of our species, human beings have recorded the things in life that are important to them. Setting down your training career—with its struggles and achievements—is a rewarding activity in itself. A training journal is a document of personal history, and reading your journals back in years to come will be enormously gratifying.

* Writing your workouts down allows you to analyze the efficacy of your conditioning methods, in both the short and long term. I've been keeping training journals for over twenty years, and whenever I've felt my training heading in the wrong direction I look at what I was doing years ago when my training was going well. Often I'm quite shocked by what I read—my *memory* of the workouts I did back in the day can be quite different from the *reality*.

* Writing about your exercise sessions is an act of education in *self-coaching*. It forces you to think about the structure of your own workouts, teaching you a great deal about exercise theory in general.

* The very act of recalling a training session to write about it develops the area of the brain that remembers training routines. After a while, your memory of your training becomes much quicker, much more accurate if you keep a journal.

• Recording your workouts allows you to accurately gauge your performance; which in turn allows you to set progression goals for future training sessions.

This last reason is of more importance than most casual athletes realize. Training *must* be progressive, and keeping track of workouts in black-and-white definitely helps the athlete maintain a progressive edge. You don't need to improve your performance *every* time you train—this becomes impossible as you get more advanced—but your sessions should display a general line of progression through the months and years, or you've just been spinning your wheels.

Writing in Your Training Journal

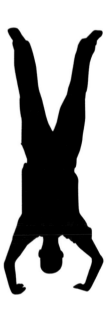

The practice of recording your training should be *quick* and it should be *efficient*. If it turns into some protracted, drawn-out hassle, the less likely it is that you'll continue with it.

When recording your training, all you really need to set down is the *date* of your workout, a list of the *exercises* you utilized, and details of the *sets and reps* you performed. If you feel the need, you can follow the description of your training session with any *comments* that seem relevant to you, although this is optional.

You'll find a good example of a journal entry on the opposite page.

If you want, you can make your entries even easier; you can write "1 x 20" instead "SET 1: 20 REPS." Use whatever simple notation that makes sense to you, and that you can easily understand and remember.

Some guys really get a kick out of writing in their training journal; they set down everything from ideas about exercise techniques, to new theories, details on their intensity levels, psychological feedback and information about the effects of their diet. I must admit, my training journal entries have sometimes looked more like chapters from *The Lord of the Rings* than succinct Zen stanzas. This was partly because writing about training was a welcome distraction from the endless stretches of dead cell time. You don't need to waste this much ink, if you don't want to. Keep your entries short, neat and accurate and you'll do fine.

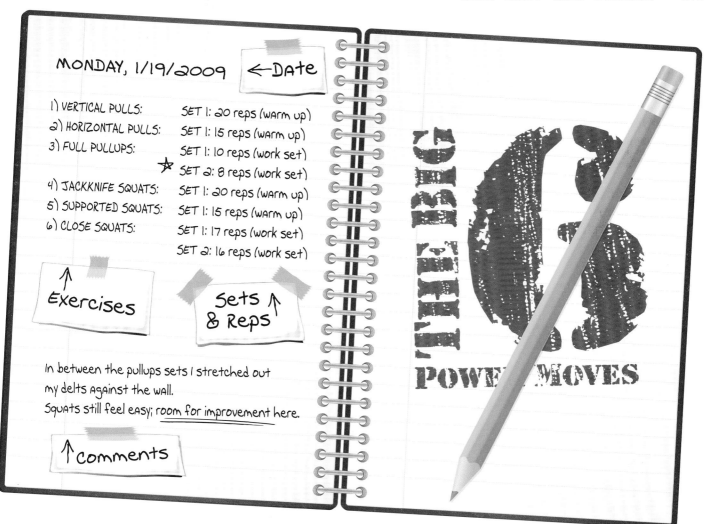

MONDAY, 1/19/2009   ←Date

1) VERTICAL PULLS: SET 1: 20 reps (warm up)
2) HORIZONTAL PULLS: SET 1: 15 reps (warm up)
3) FULL PULLUPS: SET 1: 10 reps (work set)
                      ☆ SET 2: 8 reps (work set)
4) JACKKNIFE SQUATS: SET 1: 20 reps (warm up)
5) SUPPORTED SQUATS: SET 1: 15 reps (warm up)
6) CLOSE SQUATS: SET 1: 17 reps (work set)
                          SET 2: 16 reps (work set)

↑ Exercises   Sets ↑ & Reps

In between the pullups sets I stretched out
my delts against the wall.
Squats still feel easy; room for improvement here.

↑ Comments

THE BIG 6 POWER MOVES

Lights Out!

Believe it or not, and despite what you may have heard, the very finest prison athletes *don't* train like wild beasts. Yes, they train hard, and yes, they drive themselves. But many of them fill their days with training, and if they didn't pace themselves—or if they got a dumb injury—it would seriously hamper their efforts to get stronger and tougher. In hopping around that razor-thin line between not pushing enough and pushing too much, they apply as much body wisdom as their experience has allowed them to garner.

You can profit from their example. *Walk the line*, like the man Johnny Cash said. Start slow, and get to know the movements you are using. Become an expert of every little nuance—grow to love them. Once your joints are ready, train hard—damn hard—but don't let your desire to improve outstrip your body's inherent potential to acclimatize to all that work. Focus on form, and most importantly, give your muscles and soft tissues the precious time they need to develop. Train progressively, and train intelligently; keep track of your improvements in a training journal. Warm up well, don't burn yourself out with too many sets, and rest plenty if you want to get stronger.

If you can put these age-old general principles in place—and apply them to the Big Six—you will gain long-term success beyond your wildest dreams. All you need to add to the mix are some specific *routines* to get you there. That's up next.

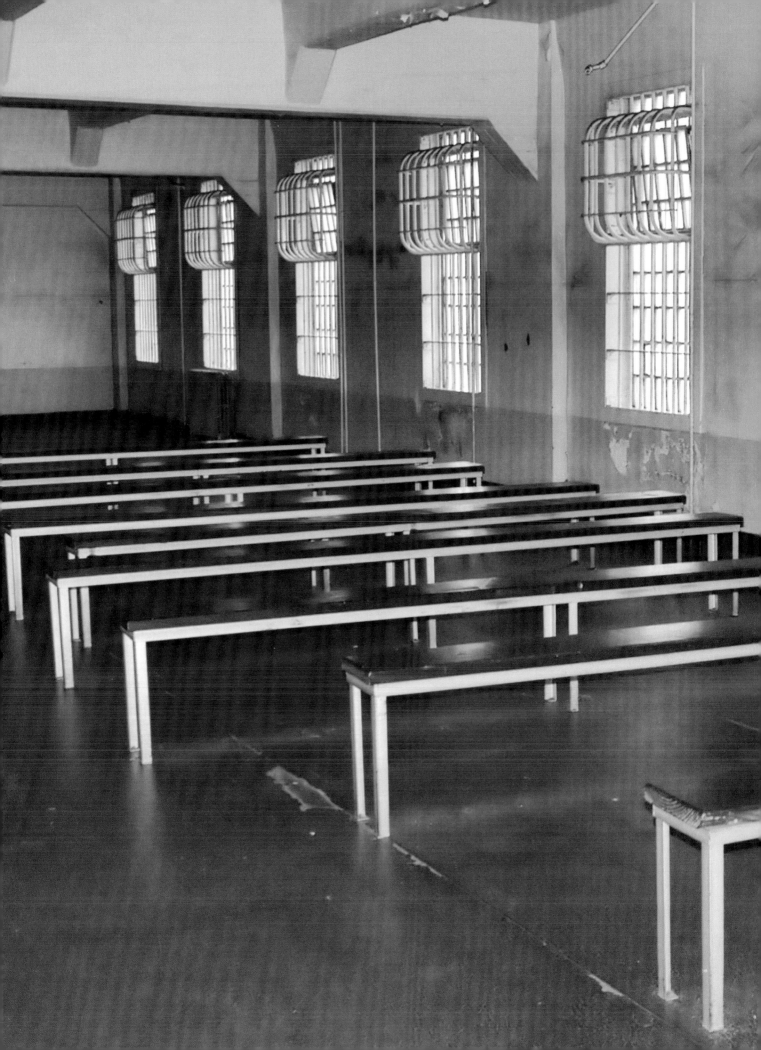

12: Routines

WORKOUT PROGRAMS

Some of you may be tempted to just launch into your training by scanning the exercises in this book, maybe discovering the hardest techniques you can do, or just attempting whatever catches your eye and looks cool. This is not training. This is *playing*.

Training requires discipline and focus. It requires the discrimination to know where to start, the knowledge of what to do, the insight into when to really push, and the wisdom to understand when to stop. It requires *regime*.

Living by the Buzzer

Living in prison, you learn all about regime. There's a time for you to eat, a time for you to sleep, a time for you to socialize, a time for you to get inspected, and a time for you to do your duties. Everything is done according to the clock, and very little is left to your control. In some places they called this *living by the buzzer*, because a buzzer sounds when a certain period of the day begins or ends.

Living like this—with an enforced timetable—for so many years has taught me to appreciate the value of *time*. After a while, the body and mind thrive on a set routine—which is one of the reasons veteran cons tend to become so institutionalized. If they get out, they miss that timetable. There's nobody to tell them what to do and when to do it, and they become *lost*, in a deep, deep way. The smart ones have the brains to create their *own* timetables to stick to on the outside. This helps many survive and stops them going off the rails.

The prison athletes who are most successful are also smart enough to develop timetables. They don't just do their calisthenics when they *feel* like it, or when they're bored or lonely. Far from it. They look at their prison routine, and purposefully insert training times within that routine. Doing this gave us a sense of control in a world where we had very little control. It also gave us something of our own, something we *owned* to look forwards to. Sometimes—maybe after a hard day, or just through laziness—you don't always want to work out when your allotted training time comes around. This happens to the best of us from time to time. But you get down to the work anyway, get done what you need to get done. Afterwards, you get that corresponding hit of accomplishment, a mental and physical high that would have otherwise been replaced by long, dull, wasted minutes or hours. A solid, well thought-through training timetable is invaluable in cultivating motivation and discipline.

Training in the Outside World

If you are going to get the most out of yourself and the methods in this book, you need to think like a prison athlete. You need to work out a training timetable, and stick to it.

In some ways, this can be harder when you're living on the outside. In the joint, your daily routine—from the time you get woken up until lights out when you go to sleep—is very firmly fixed, and doesn't really change from day to day or week to week. This usually isn't true for guys on the outside. For civilians, there is variation between weekdays and weekends; people have different commitments on different days; work schedules may vary, as in the case of shift work. In addition, there are less distractions in prison. Buddies don't call up or come to visit. You don't get to spend time with your girlfriend. During free time, there's not the lure of nightclubs, bars, cinema trips, etc. All in all, things are less complex for athletes on the inside.

But just because your daily routine is less simple on the outside, it doesn't mean you can't thrive on a good exercise program. It just means you need to be more organized. Before selecting a program, really think about how you spend your time; what days or nights are best to train? How much time can you spare? Which chores or tasks can be juggled to make room for training? If we think ahead and look hard enough, *everybody* can find time for training. People who really believe that they can't afford the time to train don't have their priorities right. Given the benefits to your health, strength and life in general, you need to ask yourself whether you can afford *not* to train!

Training Programs

Okay, time for the nitty-gritty. How long should you train, and how often? It depends mostly upon three factors; your available time, your conditioning levels, and your goals. The issue of available time is a no-brainer. I knew a lot of guys in the joint who built up to training several hours a day. If you work long shifts or have a lot of schoolwork, this is hard to squeeze in. If you are a husband and father with a lot of other domestic commitments, it's impossible. Your conditioning levels are also important. Long, frequent training sessions are only productive if you have built up to them. If you aren't in good shape, excessive training will exceed your body's recovery ability and wear you down rather than build you up—no matter how motivated you might be. Perhaps goals play the biggest role in deciding how long and often you train. Prolonged training sessions with lots of exercise volume will build stamina and endurance, *but they won't build muscle and strength*. True brawn and power are developed by *hard* training sessions, not by *long* training sessions. *Quality over quantity* is an excellent motto for strength.

Power is the motivating factor of my training nowadays, and it's the reason I generally frown on long, drawn-out training sessions. I advise a good warm up (see pages 260—261), followed by two or three "work" sets—sets where you are really putting a lot of effort into a single exercise. If it's strength you want, any more than two or three work sets is a waste of time—you're just covering the same ground and exhausting yourself. Once you've really given your all, doing any more just eats into your recovery ability and makes you sorer for longer—meaning you have to wait longer until you train on that particular technique again.

With these three factors in mind, I've outlined five basic training programs on the following pages. The first, *New Blood*, is a two-day a week routine ideal for beginners. The second, *Good Behavior*, is a three-day per week program that will help practically everybody gain strength and muscle. The third, *Veterano*, is a six-day per week protocol, and will work excellently for those who are in good shape. The fourth routine is called *Solitary Confinement*, and is only for advanced athletes with plenty of recovery ability. The fifth and final routine is *Supermax*. It's designed for elite trainees who wish to specialize in endurance rather than strength.

NEW BLOOD

This is an excellent routine for anybody new to calisthenics training or muscular exercise in general. I'd strongly advise it for all trainees who wish to build up a good base and become very advanced in *Convict Conditioning* over a long period of time. It only involves four of the most basic exercises performed over two sessions a week.

MONDAY:	Pushups	2-3 work sets
	Leg raises	2-3 work sets
TUESDAY:	Off	
WEDNESDAY:	Off	
THURSDAY:	Off	
FRIDAY:	Pullups	2-3 work sets
	Squats	2-3 work sets
SATURDAY:	Off	
SUNDAY:	Off	

• When you first start training, conditioning is poor and muscular soreness can be really debilitating. This program provides plenty of recovery time.

• This early routine features only four of the Big Six. *Bridges* and *handstand pushups* require greater levels of contractile strength and joint integrity than these four, and should only be attempted when the athlete is well versed in these basics.

• Muscles adapt quicker than joints. This routine gives the soft tissues—which are new to this type of work—enough time off to catch up.

• Practice this program, or a similar routine, during your early work on the ten steps. Once you get past Step 6 *on all four* of the exercises mentioned, it's time to move to the next program.

GOOD BEHAVIOR

This is perhaps the best basic bodyweight training program that exists. It involves all of the Big Six movements, performed over three sessions a week. It represents a step up in volume from *New Blood*, but also provides the average athlete with plenty of rest to grow and get stronger. As such, this program is good for intermediate athletes, but it's also productive for advanced athletes to practice over long periods of time. If you are really dedicated to bodyweight training, you should always return to a program like *Good Behavior* every once in a while, just to keep your feet in contact with the ground and get back to basics—no matter how advanced you are.

MONDAY:	Pushups	2 work sets
	Leg raises	2 work sets
TUESDAY:	Off	
WEDNESDAY:	Pullups	2 work sets
	Squats	2 work sets
THURSDAY:	Off	
FRIDAY:	Handstand pushups	2 work sets
	Bridges	2 work sets
SATURDAY:	Off	
SUNDAY:	Off	

• *Good Behavior* can be worked into almost anybody's busy schedule.

• This program can (and should) be used by *any* athlete to achieve solid strength gains—no matter how advanced they are.

• For those trainees with good recovery abilities, this program will err on the side of caution. The extra rest can be useful for cross-trainers who wish to indulge in other physical activities—running, boxing, martial arts, etc.

VETERANO

This is a tasty, intelligent little routine which can be used by anybody who has been practicing *Convict Conditioning* for several months or more. Instead of working out two or three days a week, the athlete works out six days per week—but he only focuses on one of the Big Six movements per session. The seventh day is a day of rest.

MONDAY:	Pullups	2-3 work sets
TUESDAY:	Bridges	2-3 work sets
WEDNESDAY:	Handstand pushups	2-3 work sets
THURSDAY:	Leg raises	2-3 work sets
FRIDAY:	Squats	2-3 work sets
SATURDAY:	Pushups	2-3 work sets
SUNDAY:	Off	

- This workout is good for those with limited time on their hands. Sessions can often be completed in under six or seven minutes per day!

- Recovery is actually pretty fast during this program because the athlete never works the upper or lower body two days in a row. The exercises alternate in the most efficient manner possible.

- For athletes looking to gain strength and work their way up through the ten steps, this routine can be very productive. Because only one exercise is performed on a given day, the athlete can really focus and give his all.

- This routine is a good template for experimentation. If it proves too much for you, add the odd rest day whenever you need it. Don't feel constrained by the arbitrary concept of a seven-day week. Just remember that however fit you are, a regimented day off is always advisable during whatever routine you're working on, to ensure systemic rest.

SOLITARY CONFINEMENT

Solitary Confinement is a brutal routine. It will give awesome total-body conditioning and fitness benefits to the dedicated, although strength development will be compromised somewhat by the lack of rest built into the program—more is not better where strength is concerned. It involves the Big Six performed over a three-day cycle, repeated twice over seven days. To this dense routine, ancillary work is added for masochists. It should only be attempted by individuals with excellent recovery ability who have been in hard calisthenics training for over a year. You'll need at least six or seven hours free per week to finish this program. Don't abuse it all year-round.

MONDAY:	Pullups	3-5 work sets
	Squats	3-5 work sets
	Grip work	Various
TUESDAY:	Pushups	3-5 work sets
	Leg raises	3-5 work sets
	Calf work	3-5 work sets
WEDNESDAY:	Handstand pushups	3-5 work sets
	Bridges	3-5 work sets
	Neck work	2-4 work sets
THURSDAY:	Pullups	3-5 work sets
	Squats	3-5 work sets
	Grip work	Various
FRIDAY:	Pushups	3-5 work sets
	Leg raises	3-5 work sets
	Calf work	3-5 work sets
SATURDAY:	Handstand pushups	3-5 work sets
	Bridges	3-5 work sets
	Neck work	2-4 work sets
SUNDAY:	Off	

• This program includes ancillary work—for the grip, neck, and calves. If you like the idea of trying these extras, but can't take the daily workload, add a day's rest between training sessions, or whenever you feel the need.

• This program is *mean*. Unless you are in good shape and living clean—regular meals, plenty of sleep, etc.—be prepared to get bullied, big time.

SUPERMAX

Supermax is an example of the kind of volume training routine I used for prolonged periods, particularly during my stay in Angola Penitentiary. In order to survive a routine like this, you need to be as serious as cancer—and have about as many friends. Provided you have built up to it using more basic conditioning programs—like the four listed earlier—it can give the right athlete inhuman endurance and stamina. It does zero for your strength or power however, so make sure you have worked up through then ten steps before you devote a chunk of your life to this program. Don't even attempt such a routine unless you have been in hard training for several years.

MONDAY:	Pullups	10-50 work sets
	Squats	10-50 work sets
TUESDAY:	Pushups	10-50 work sets
	Leg raises	10-50 work sets
WEDNESDAY:	Handstand pushups	10-50 work sets
	Bridges	10-50 work sets
THURSDAY:	Pullups	10-50 work sets
	Squats	10-50 work sets
FRIDAY:	Pushups	10-50 work sets
	Leg raises	10-50 work sets
SATURDAY:	Handstand pushups	10-50 work sets
	Bridges	10-50 work sets
SUNDAY:	Off	

- Do the sets throughout the day, however you wish. All in one go is an option, but spread throughout the day in mini-sessions is more tolerable. Alternating the two exercises set-by-set is another way to survive.

- To get through a lot of sets quickly, I often used to rest between sets by just pausing to take a few breaths. This sometimes squashed twenty or thirty sets into a single staggered set!

- Start with ten sets of ten reps per exercise and aim to build up to fifty sets per exercise, per day. If you are doing two exercises per day, this equals one hundred sets per day—nearly *two and a half thousand* sets per month. If you want even more work than this, increase your reps.

Hybrid Programs

Throughout this book I've pushed the idea of bodyweight training as an alternative to weight-training, machine work and other forms of resistance training. This is because I love old school calisthenics, and I know from experience—in my own career, and through training others—that it truly is the greatest form of strength training. Ever. Hands down. Nothing else is required.

But I'm not a dummy. I know a lot of you guys reading this book are already in love with the various forms of weight-training—bodybuilding, powerlifting, Olympic weightlifting, kettlebell work, etc. Many of you will have no desire to quit hitting the weights, and are just looking for something new to add to your repertoire.

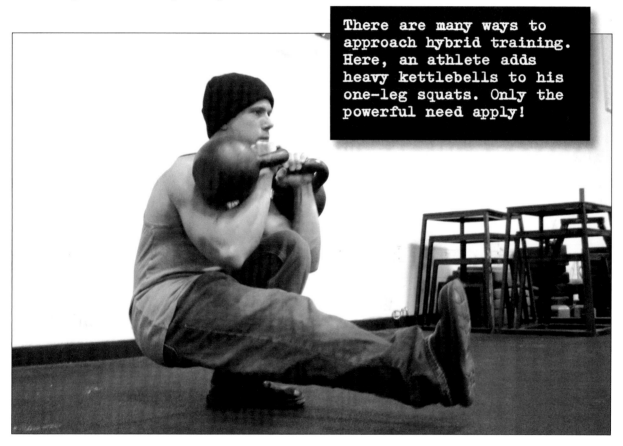

There are many ways to approach hybrid training. Here, an athlete adds heavy kettlebells to his one-leg squats. Only the powerful need apply!

I'm not a Nazi—I'll try and work with you. If I must. (See what a nice guy I am?) With a little creativity, there are literally dozens of ways you can apply bodyweight training to your chosen discipline. Here are three examples to get you thinking:

HYBRID TRAINING ROUTINES

The Three-Day Split:

In the gym three days per week? Most gyms now have mats or stretching areas where you can do bodyweight exercises between weights work. Why not add one of the more conventional Big Six movements to each gym/weights day, completing the other three on a weekend? For example:

MONDAY:	<u>Pushups</u>, chest work, shoulder work, triceps
WEDNESDAY:	<u>Leg raises</u>, leg work, hamstring work, calves
FRIDAY:	<u>Pullups</u>, back work, biceps, forearms
SATURDAY:	<u>Squats</u>*, <u>bridges</u>, <u>handstand pushups</u>

The Home Training Day:

Instead of going to the gym three times per week to split the body three ways, how about splitting the body over two days while focusing on the major muscle groups, and training the smaller muscles on the third day at home using bodyweight exercises? Such a split might look like this:

MONDAY: (Gym)	Squats, deadlifts, leg curls, leg press, etc.
WEDNESDAY: (Home)	<u>Leg raises</u>, <u>bridges</u>, <u>calf raises</u>, <u>handstand pushups</u>
FRIDAY: (Gym)	Bench press, bent-over row, curls triceps, etc.

Bodyweight as a Plateau-Busting Tool:

Reached a plateau with a certain muscle group? Continue with your weight-training, but add a bodyweight exercise for the lagging bodypart: one-leg squats for quads, pullups for back, pushups for chest, etc.

---

*Bodyweight squats, not barbell squats.

Flexibility and Freedom

At the beginning of this chapter I spoke about the powerful benefits of *regime*. But routines should always exist for the individual who uses them. Once it becomes the other way round—once the individual exists only for the routine—things have gone badly wrong.

By all means apply discipline, and once you have constructed a training timetable try to stick to it. But you should also give yourself room for personal freedom. Boundaries which are too rigid lead to boredom, staleness and burnout. If this is happening to you, get creative. Experiment. Try some variation. You don't have to adhere rigidly to the programs given earlier. Mix and match. Invent your own routines. Throw in some of the *variant* exercises once in a while. Experiment with different rep ranges. Try different hand or foot spacings on your favorite exercises. Add some volume and decrease intensity for a few weeks. Explore different training speeds—from super-slow reps to more explosive work. Try different angles. Play with doing partial sections of each movement. For a challenge, add a "killer" set to the end of each workout—pick a movement that's easy (for you) and do as many reps as you can. Enjoy your body and its newfound strength and skill through cross-training; try some sports like running, boxing, walking, martial arts, yoga.

On the inside, I never felt the need to stop my training because there was very little else available to distract me. On the outside there are a million and one things to lead people astray, even from basic practices that are *enormously* valuable. Please don't quit. There are dozens of ways to spice up your training if you feel things starting to flag.

Lights Out!

Training is a serious business in prison. It certainly helped me stay sane, and I know a lot of other guys who would say exactly the same thing. It was something *real*, something we could look forwards to. No matter how insane the rest of the day got, training was like a rock, a stable place in a crazy world. Whatever else we might have *lost* being on the inside, training sessions were a time when we could *gain* something very significant—not just health and fitness, but *self-respect*. You add a rep here; improve your technique there; move up to a harder exercise. It's logical. Meaningful. It makes sense. You're always moving forwards, always in control. For me, that's a very special, powerful thing. You have to be really into it to understand what I mean. A lot of you who are also into exercise will probably be nodding your heads. You'll understand.

So take your training seriously. Treat your training time with respect, wherever you are. The second that session starts, you need to change your attitude, shift gears into a new mentality. The humor and screwing around have to stop. Put your training head on; bring your goals—one more rep, better technique or whatever—into your mind's eye and get psyched up to achieve those targets. A psycho, screaming, grunting attitude, like many gym bodybuilders have, is not what you want. It just wastes energy. Be aggressive, yes. But master it—learn to *channel* it. You need to cultivate a focused, controlled aggression. Really work on this. You will reap serious rewards if you can develop this attitude.

Find some space where you can be alone—or at least not disturbed—and get your workout done. Most people now advise working out with friends or training partners. I don't. I believe in training alone—it develops better focus, reduces distraction and is good for the soul.

This opinion may not be very popular or New Age, but I certainly prefer training over spending time with people. Any day. My exercises have done more for me than any of my "friends." In my life, I've met hundreds—thousands—of people who wanted to attack me, steal from me, bully me, humiliate me, or even kill me. But my training has given me nothing but benefits. It gives far more than it takes. I've wasted great chunks of my time on human beings who I now wish I'd never even met. But training? I don't regret a *single second* of the time I spent working out.

Every moment of effort, every drop of sweat was worthwhile.

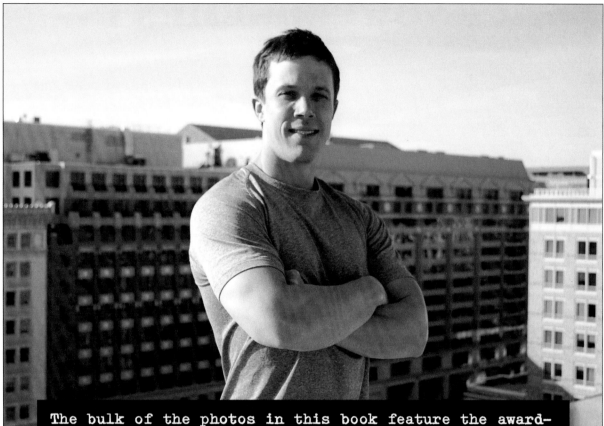

The bulk of the photos in this book feature the award-winning athlete Jim Bathurst. Jim has been studying acrobatics for well over a decade. He has taken that passion and experience and started *BeastSkills.com*, a website that teaches bodyweight feats of strength. BeastSkills.com has been well-received by the fitness community and Jim has been invited to host seminars internationally. He holds a CSCS from the NSCA and currently resides in Washington DC, where he works as a personal trainer.

ACKNOWLEDGEMENTS

This book wouldn't have seen the light of day without the endless understanding and support of John Du Cane. Thanks John!

Many of the methods and techniques in this volume, and in all my teaching, were given to me freely by Joe Hartigen. RIP, Joe.

A massive thank you has to go out to the main model for this manual, Jim Bathurst. Jim has dedicated an enormous amount of time to getting these photos perfect for students of *Convict Conditioning*, and the book wouldn't be half as good without his input.

I was amazingly lucky to have the help of the mighty Brett Jones (Master RKC) in the technical editing of my manuscript. Brett's knowledge is *incredible*. All the mistakes in this book are my own. Anything that sounds clever or cool comes from Brett! Check out Brett's cutting edge training blog at: *www.appliedstrength.com*.

Big respect also goes out to the book's designer, Derek Brigham—"Big D." Derek took my huge stack of heartfelt scribbles and a pile of photos, and turned them into a thing of beauty. He also tolerated my crotchety attitude (and the hundreds of sticky notes I forced on him) with competence and good grace.
Check his work at *www.dbrigham.com*. Thanks bro.

The image of the perfect free handstand pushup on page 227 was generously contributed by the athlete, gymnastics expert Roger Harrell. Roger can be found at *www.crossfitmarin.com*. He also maintains the website *www.drillsandskills.com*, a great gymnastics training resource.

Most of the prison images in this book were created by the US government, as were the images which appear on pages 220 and 222.
All public domain images are used with my gratitude.

The majority of the photos in *Convict Conditioning* were shot in and around Balance Gym, which is located in the Kalorama neighborhood of Washington DC. We thank them for the generous use of their facility.

INDEX

V

W

X

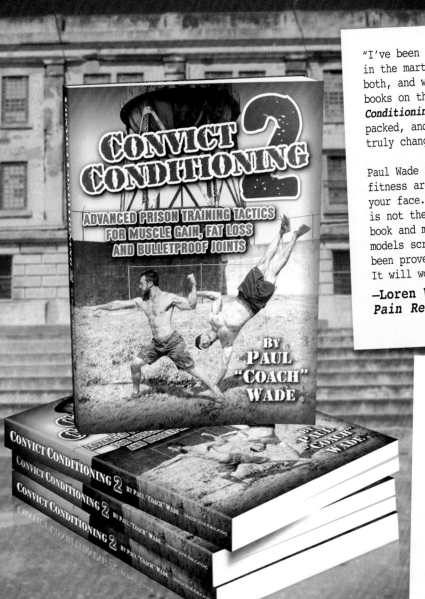

"I've been lifting weights for over 50 years and training in the martial arts since 1965. I've read voraciously on both, and written dozens of magazine articles and many books on the subjects. This book and Wade's first, *Convict Conditioning*, are by far the most commonsense, information-packed, and result producing I've read. These books will truly change your life.

Paul Wade is a new and powerful voice in the strength and fitness arena, one that is commonsense, inspiring, and in your face. His approach to maximizing your body's potential is not the same old hackneyed material you find in every book and magazine piece that pictures steroid-bloated models screaming as they curl weights. Wade's stuff has been proven effective by hard men who don't tolerate fluff. It will work for you, too—guaranteed."

—Loren W. Christensen, author of *Fighting the Pain Resistant Attacker*, and many others

"Coach Paul Wade has outdone himself. His first book *Convict Conditioning* is to my mind THE BEST book ever written on bodyweight conditioning. Hands down. Now, with the sequel *Convict Conditioning 2* Coach Wade takes us even deeper into the subtle nuances of training with the ultimate resistance tool: our bodies.

This book is, as was his first, an amazing journey into the history of physical culture disguised as a book on calisthenics. But the thing that Coach Wade does better than any before him is his unbelievable progressions on EVERY EXERCISE and stretch! He breaks things down and tells us EXACTLY how to proceed to get to whatever level of strength and development we want. AND gives us the exact metrics we need to know when to go to the next level.

Add in completely practical and immediately useful insights into nutrition and the mind set necessary to deal not only with training but with life this book is a classic that will stand the test of time. Bravo Coach Wade, Bravo."

—Mark Reifkind, Master RKC

"I can say without a doubt that this is one of the best books about productive strength training ever written. I urge *all* readers of *Muscles of Iron* to buy a copy of this book. It doesn't matter whether you are a wrestler, a weightlifter, a powerlifter, a bodybuilder, a martial artist, a gymnast, a boxer, a bodyweight purebred, or some other kind of strength athlete, you owe it to yourself to read this book. It offers insights about training and health that you won't find anywhere else, and the perspectives which Paul Wade provides will positively challenge your thinking."

—Robert Drucker, Musclesofiron.com

"I didn't expect to like this book, but I come away from it practically insisting that everyone read it. It is a strongman book mixed with yoga mixed with street smarts. I wanted to hate it, but I love it."

—Dan John, Senior RKC, National Masters Weightlifting Champion, author of *Never Let Go*

Convict Conditioning 2
Advanced Prison Training Tactics for Muscle Gain, Fat Loss and Bulletproof Joints
By Paul "Coach" Wade   *$39.95*

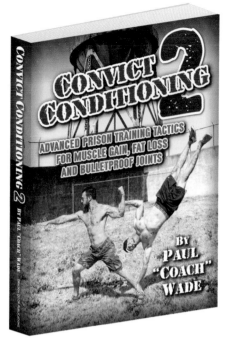

CONVICT CONDITIONING 2

ADVANCED PRISON TRAINING TACTICS FOR MUSCLE GAIN, FAT LOSS AND BULLETPROOF JOINTS

TABLE OF CONTENTS

Serious About Your Bodyweight Training? Then You'll Also Want to Invest in a Hard Copy of Convict Conditioning

A Strength Training Guide That Will Never Be Duplicated!

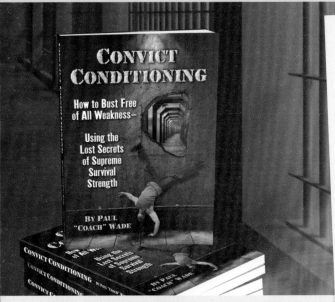

Brutal Elegance.

"I have been training and reading about training since I first joined the US Navy in the 1960s. I thought I'd seen everything the fitness world had to offer. Sometimes twice. But I was wrong. This book is utterly iconoclastic.

The author breaks down all conceivable body weight exercises into six basic movements, each designed to stimulate different vectors of the muscular system. These six are then elegantly and very intelligently broken into ten progressive techniques. You master one technique, and move on to the next.

The simplicity of this method belies a very powerful and complex training paradigm, reduced into an abstraction that obviously took many years of sweat and toil to develop.

Trust me. Nobody else worked this out. This approach is completely unique and fresh.

I have read virtually every calisthenics book printed in America over the last 40 years, and instruction like this can't be found anywhere, in any one of them. *Convict Conditioning* is head and shoulders above them all. In years to come, trainers and coaches will all be talking about 'progressions' and 'progressive calisthenics' and claim they've been doing it all along. But the truth is that Dragon Door bought it to you first. As with kettlebells, they were the trail blazers.

Who should purchase this volume? Everyone who craves fitness and strength should. Even if you don't plan to follow the routines, the book will make you think about your physical prowess, and will give even world class experts food for thought. At the very least if you find yourself on vacation or away on business without your barbells, this book will turn your hotel into a fully equipped gym.

I'd advise any athlete to obtain this work as soon as possible."
—*Bill Oliver - Albany, NY, United States*

"I knew within the first chapter of reading this book that I was in for something special and unique. The last time I felt this same feeling was when reading *Power to the People!* To me this is the Body Weight equivalent to Pavel's masterpiece.

Books like this can never be duplicated. Paul Wade went through a unique set of circumstances of doing time in prison with an 'old time' master of calisthenics. Paul took these lessons from this 70 year old strong man and mastered them over a period of 20 years while 'doing time'. He then taught these methods to countless prisoners and honed his teaching to perfection.

I believe that extreme circumstances like this are what it takes to create a true masterpiece. I know that 'masterpiece' is a strong word, but this is as close as it gets. No other body weight book I have read (and I have a huge fitness library)...comes close to this as far as gaining incredible strength from body weight exercise.

Just like Power to the People, I am sure I will read this over and over again...mastering the principles that Paul Wade took 20 years to master.

Outstanding Book!"—*Rusty Moore - Fitness Black Book - Seattle, WA*

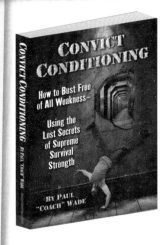

Convict Conditioning
How to Bust Free of All Weakness—Using the Lost Secrets of Supreme Survival Strength
By Paul "Coach" Wade

#B41 $39.95
Paperback 8.5 x 11 320 pages
191 photos, charts and illustrations

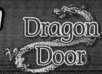

How to Instantly Increase Your Upper Body Strength With the *Irradiation* Technique

Hit the deck and give me five pushups, Comrade! Only five, but of a challenging variety, for instance with your feet up or on one arm. When you are done with five you should be able to grind out another couple but no more than that.

Note the difficulty of your first set. Rest briefly. Do another fiver but with one difference: on the way up grip the deck hard with your fingertips. Don't go up on your fingertips; just grip the floor so your fingertips turn white. Only on the way up. All the way up or just at the sticking point. You will have to experiment whether you will get the best results by gripping throughout the lift or just at the sticking point.

You cannot help noticing that your arms have suddenly gotten a jolt of extra energy, as if your tensing forearms have sent some juice up into your triceps. Which is exactly what has happened. Whenever a muscle contracts, it irradiates "nerve force" around it and increases the intensity of the neighborhood muscles' contraction. The effect is strongest in your hands.

Make a fist. A tight fist. A white-knuckle fist! Note that as you grip harder the tension in your forearm overflows into your upper arm, and even your shoulder and armpit. You will increase your strength in any upper body exertion, bodyweight or not, by strongly gripping the floor, the bar, etc.

Power to you, Naked Warrior! Anywhere, anytime.

41 yr old mom using GTG to do something she has never done

"My wife has been using GTG (greasing the grove) for a couple of weeks to learn how to do chin ups. She started with 2 assisted chins 3 or four times a day four a week then doing 1 unassisted chin then one more a few minutes later 4 or 5 times a day. **2 weeks later she is doing 3 unassisted chins without leaving the bar and yesterday's total was 15 unassisted chins for the day.** This stuff really works, it is pure science for pure results!!!"
—Rick Giese - Casper, WY

Pavel has done a fantastic job on this book, a must read for all

"I briefly want to say that I will be forever grateful to Pavel and his real world views and knowledge of the body and what it takes to really get in shape. I'm a 53 year old two tour former Marine Sgt. Listen, I had knee surgery a little over a year ago and have tried everything to get my strength back and nothing has worked -- until now! Pavel, man you have blown me away with this program. **Not just my knees but my whole body are stronger by the week** -- and the side effect for me, from reading this book and following the program as it is written is; I know I am going to lose some weight and get back into fighting shape again. If you are ready to suck it up, forget the health clubs, do like I did, order a appropriate size kettlebell& DVD and get busy!! Pavel can put you back in the game!"
—Gene Simmons - New Jersey

Any time, any place

"When I first purchased Naked Warrior and began using GTG, I saw immediate results. **I GTG'd military presses with a 65 lb. dumbbell and when I first got my 70 lb. KB, I was able to press it 13 times at a bodyweight of 175 lbs.** When I demonstrate the one arm, one leg pushup, people look at me in amazement. I am convinced that anyone using the techniques outlined in this book will be able to perform them in time. Being a law enforcement officer, I am often in need of strength training, but have little time or equipment. I am able to maintain or build strength, flexibility and balance with only my body. When I finish a GTG set, I feel powerful and energized. The secondary effects of hypertrophy are an added bonus. For those of you who are concerned that there are few exercises outlined here, you should know that the principles in this book can be applied to any lift and to many athletic endeavors. It is a powerful system for physical culture. Get this book."
—Douglas Moore – Bangor, Maine

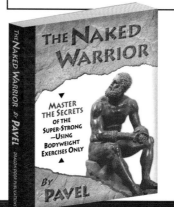

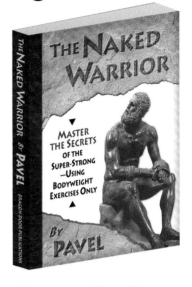
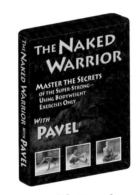
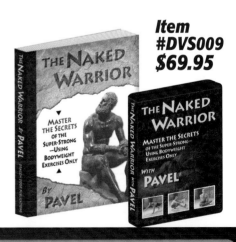

Discover New Keys to Superior Athletic Achievement

In his strength books Pavel emphasizes the importance of learning to maximally tense the muscles. Because tension IS strength. But strength/ tension is only half of the total performance package. The other half is relaxation. The body of a karate expert will freeze in total tension at the moment of impact, but will remain totally loose before and after.

Mastery of relaxation is the hallmark of an elite athlete. Soviet scientists discovered that the higher the athlete's level, the quicker he can relax his muscles. The Soviets observed an 800% difference between novices and Olympians. Their conclusion: total control of tension = elite performance.

If you can master your muscular tension, a new dimension of athletic excellence opens to you. New achievements. New heights of performance. Some genetically-endowed superstars seem to possess this ability from birth. But according to former Soviet Special Forces trainer, Pavel, a SKILL–SET is available that can transform *anyone's* current physical limitations.

Now, for the first time, Pavel reveals these little known Soviet performance secrets, so you too can become the master of your body — not its victim. From years of research and experience, Pavel has selected these *Fast & Loose* techniques as the best-of-the-best for practical and quick results.

Mandatory for the serious fighter "I've spent the last couple of years desperately trying to recover the speed I've been losing by inches. Before I'd even finished watching this DVD, it became clear what I'd really lost. Years ago, I used to 'snap' strikes in. As I've become a more serious fighter, I've succumbed to trying to 'drive' them in (karateka can read this as misunderstanding what it really means to train "with kime"). It's ironic that the fact that I'm trying so much harder is what has been slowing me down all along. I credit Pavel for explaining this so clearly & demonstrating drills that deliver rapid results. If you're a serious competitor looking for that extra edge, you *must* add these drills to your routine. Thank you, Pavel, for another excellent product. OSU!!" —B, Boston – MA

Fast and Loose + Rough and Tough = Deadly Force

Invest in the "Deadly Force" set of Pavel's *Fast and Loose* DVD with Pavel's *The Naked Warrior* DVD and book— and SAVE...

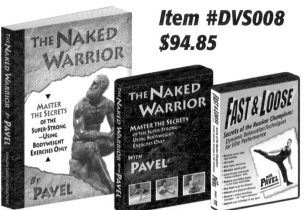

Item #DVS008
$94.85

Fast & Loose
Secrets of the Russian Champions: Dynamic Relaxation Techniques for Elite Performance
with Pavel
#DV021 $29.95
DVD Running time: 27 minutes

- **Recover sooner after hard** training
- **Kick higher and faster**
- **Hit harder**
- **Minimize muscle pulls**
- **Stay loose to go the** distance
- **Improve your technique in** any sport
- **Enhance your physical** efficiency
- **Remove your hidden** brakes — to run faster and further
- **Learn Russian commando** "instant readiness" drills
- **Discover a unique** breathing technique — for "super-relaxation"

"*Fast & Loose* is another amazing tool from Pavel... Everyone knows that once you really start pushing the envelope on your current abilities, you need those subtle yet all-important tools to move from average to elite performance. They can seem insignificant to the untrained observer, but are better than gold to those who have the faculties to incorporate them. Pavel delivers as always."—Mark Hanington, Huntington Beach, CA.

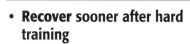

Instantly Amplify Your Power and Strength!

Can you easily and instantly turn yourself into a coiled steel spring — ready to burst into action and leap past your previous athletic best? Or are you more like an overstretched rubber band — no longer capable of suddenly generating performance-busting power? Now, for the first time in the West, Russian strength master Pavel reveals the Soviet secret of *Loaded Stretching* — guaranteed within MINUTES of its application to have you:

- PULLING HEAVIER
- SQUATTING MORE
- JUMPING HIGHER
- KICKING AND PUNCHING HARDER
- THROWING FARTHER
- PRESSING BIGGER!

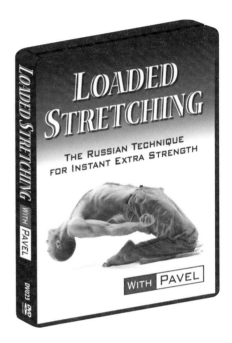

In the glory days of the Soviet empire a team of researchers lead by weightlifting world champion and scientist A. Vorobyev devised a special instant strength technique. Immediately after its application experienced lifters pulled their barbells more than two inches higher! Further research determined that the unique *Loaded Stretching* (LS) technique — unlike any other type of stretching you have seen — not only increased immediate performance but also delivered long term strength gains.

Finally, you too can take advantage of this powerful technique — and watch your athletic performance soar to new heights. Take the *Loaded Stretching* challenge today: perform the exact LS technique Pavel specifies for your chosen strength-skill — and see immediate, measurable gains... be it deadlift, squat, vertical jump, kicks, throws or presses.

Loaded Stretching

The Russian Technique for Instant Extra Strength
with Pavel
#DV023 $24.95
DVD Running time: 20 minutes

Instant Results

"The dvd presents thought provoking material concerning preloading muscles prior to performance of a lift. I immediately began to practice a few of the stretches prior to my squats, deadlifts and overhead presses with spectacular results. The performance of each lift was enhanced significantly along with an increase of control. I wish Pavel was in our country years ago to re-introduce strength training to America."
—TOM GELVELES Brightwaters, NY

It's gonna hurt, deal with it

"The high end concept of controlled strain, when applied to various movements, have demonstrated ability to improve sport performance in the short and long run and can be used by everyone. The loaded hip stretch using a box, the loaded Russian twist, the loaded RKC clean stretch, and the KB loaded triceps stretch are very powerful tools that I have put in my bag of tricks. The loaded RKC clean stretch has been a real blessing to my football and powerlifting ravaged shoulders. There is a lot more here too for every athlete."
—JACK REAPE, *Armed Forces Powerlifting Champion*

"It is interesting that we have all these great minds in America, and a tremendous amount of info from the Easter Bloc, but never really entered that special door of duplicating elite performance. It took someone from the Eastern Bloc, to show where the door was. Now he has given the key to that all-important first door to creating elite performance. Pavel's *Loaded Stretching* DVD is that key. Thank You Pavel!"
—JAY SCHROEDER, arpprogram.com

LOADED STRETCHING

"It's not about flexibility. It's about STRENGTH!"

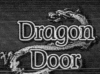

"The Do-It-Now, Fast-Start, Get-Up-and-Go, Jump-into-Action Bible for HIGH PERFORMANCE and LONGER LIFE"

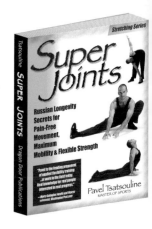

You have a choice in life. You can sputter and stumble and creak your way along in a process of painful, slow decline—or you can take charge of your health and become a human dynamo.

And there is no better way to insure a long, pain-free life than performing the right daily combination of joint mobility and strength-flexibility exercises.

In *Super Joints*, Russian fitness expert Pavel Tsatsouline shows you exactly how to quickly achieve and maintain peak joint health—and then use it to improve every aspect of your physical performance.

Only the foolish would deliberately ignore the life-saving and life-enhancing advice Pavel offers in *Super Joints*. Why would anyone willingly subject themselves to a life of increasing pain, degeneration and decrepitude? But for an athlete, a dancer, a martial artist or any serious performer, *Super Joints* could spell the difference between greatness and mediocrity.

Super Joints

Russian Longevity Secrets for Pain-Free Movement, Maximum Mobility & Flexible Strength

Book By Pavel Tsatsouline
Paperback 130 pages 8.5" x 11"
Over 100 photos and illustrations
#B16 $34.95

Super Joints
DVD

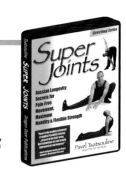

With Pavel Tsatsouline
Running Time 33 minutes
DVD **#DV003 $24.95**

Discover:

- The twenty-eight most valuable drills for youthful joints and a stronger stretch
- How to save your joints and prevent or reduce arthritis
- The one-stop care-shop for your inner Tin Man—how to give your nervous system a tune up, your joints a lube-job and your energy a recharge
- What it takes to go from cruise control to full throttle: The One Thousand Moves Morning Recharge—Amosov's "bigger bang" calisthenics complex for achieving heaven-on earth in 25 minutes
- How to make your body feel better than you can remember—active flexibility fosporting prowess and fewer injuries
- The amazing Pink Panther technique that may add a couple of feet to your stretch the first time you do it

Purchase Pavel's *Super Joints* book and DVD as a set and SAVE...

Item #DVS006
$54.90

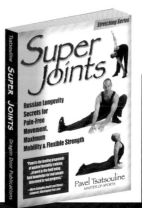

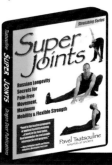

www.dragondoor.com
1·800·899·5111
Dragon Door

Buy Now at www.DragonDoor.com

"Injuries Flee the Scene of the Crime— When Attacked by Pavel's Fast-Response, Rescue-Your-Own-Body *Super Joints* System

Super Joints

"The "Super Joints" by Pavel Tsatsouline was excellent. After 30 years of practicing and teaching martial arts (Uechi/Shohei Ryu, and Ju Jitsu), and the natural "break down" of the joints with age, the "Super Joints" has helped to restore the flexibility and strength of my joints especially an arthritic shoulder. I have incorporated the "Super Joints" into my Russian kettlebell and functional training workouts."
—Dr. Dan Rinchuse, DMD, MS, MDS, PhD, 6th Degree Black Belt-Uechi/Shohei Ryu, 2n Degree Black Belt - Ju Jitsu-Greensburg, PA

Joints of a teen again...

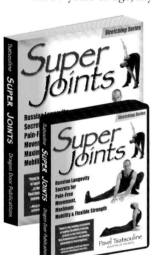

"At 37 years of age, my joints had already been cracking and hurting in the morning. I sustained an injury parachuting in the Air Force in 1989 and since, have had many back pains. I ordered Super Joints figuring it would be good, as all of Pavel's dvd's and books have been excellent. The first day I went through the dvd and did all the joint mobility drills. I felt better that day and over the course of the following week noticed that in the morning, my back wasn't as stiff and my elbows didn't hurt. I would highly recommend this dvd to anyone that cares about their joints."
—Jim Lavelle – NY

DON'T BE A FOOL

"There are two reasons for not doing Super Joints. #1 You don't know about it. #2 You are a damn FOOL. I'm 49 and have had knee trouble all my life. I have done those big squats in my 20's and 30's (500lb+). I gave up squatting at 39 and for the last 9 years I suffered with aching knees and was afraid to squat. I have been doing Super Joints for the last 6 months (have not missed a day). <u>No more pain, no discomfort</u>. This is my second copy. I love the way it makes all my joints feel. Thanks Pavel." —Scott G. - cedar point , NC

An Owners Manual for Your Aging Joints

"If you're over 40, this is must-read material. If you ever wondered how to warmup before strenuous exercise, the routines you need are right here. My body works better than it did 20 years ago and I thank Pavel and Super Joints for that. The older we get, the more important preventative maintenance of our bodies becomes. Performing the movements in Super Joints is like giving your engine an oil change - if you do it right, you won't notice, but neglect it and it might cause serious damage.

Super Joints is vintage Pavel - enough explanation to let you understand the thinking behind the exercises, but mostly short, to the point, no-nonsense instructions that you know will work for you. I cannot recommend Super Joints highly enough ."
—Steve Freides - New Jersey

"As an older guy, I don't really care whether I can do the splits. I just want to walk around pain free all day. *Super Joints* does that job for me." —Tim Cahill, travel adventure writer and founding editor of *Outside*

Russian Army's Top Hand-to-Hand Combat Instructor Recommends a Unique Stretching Technique for High Kicks

An excerpt from Super Joints by Pavel ▶

Super Joints

DVD With Pavel Tsatsouline
Running Time 33 minutes **#DV003 $24.95**

Book By Pavel Tsatsouline
Paperback 8.5" x 11"   **#B16 $34.95**

Alexander Medvedev—not to be confused the weightlifting champion and expert Alexey Medvedev—is the hand-to-hand instructor of elite Frunze Post-graduate Army Academy and the chief subject matter expert to Spetsnaz magazine. He recommends the following technique for improving your kicks or splits.

Raise your leg as high as possible in the chosen direction and rest it atop a table or another piece of furniture that is

barely within your reach. Relax for a minute or as long as necessary, then lift your leg a little higher using only its muscles, no help from your hands or your partner. Have your training partner quickly slide a book between your ankle and the table. Repeat the sequence while it works. Medvedev promises that although this drill is quite painful and unpleasant in the beginning, it becomes quite enjoyable once you get a hang of it. More importantly, you will get more flexible for a change.

Stay informed of the latest advances in strength and conditioning by visiting:
WWW.DRAGONDOOR.COM

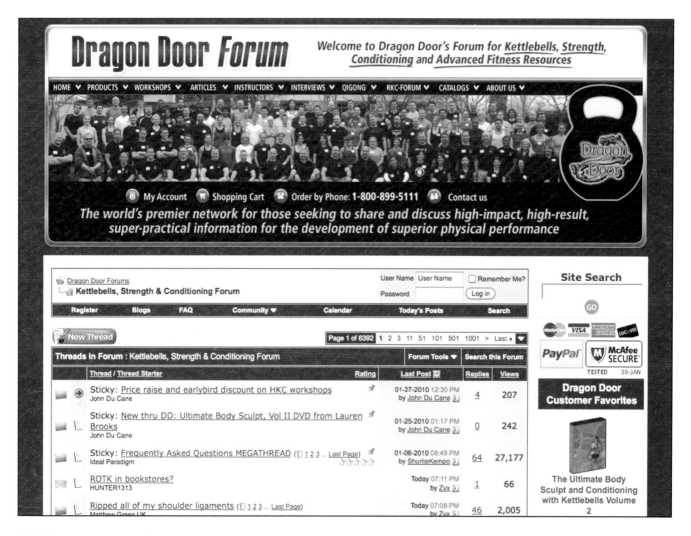

Visit www.dragondoor.com and sign up for Pavel Tsatsouline's free monthly e-newsletter, giving you late-breaking news and tips on how to stay ahead of the fitness pack.

Visit www.kbforum.dragondoor.com and participate in Dragon Door's stimulating and informative **Strength and Conditioning** Forum. Post your fitness questions or comments and get quick feedback from Pavel Tsatsouline and other leading fitness experts.

Visit www.dragondoor.com and browse the **Articles** section and other pages for groundbreaking theories and products for improving your health and well being.

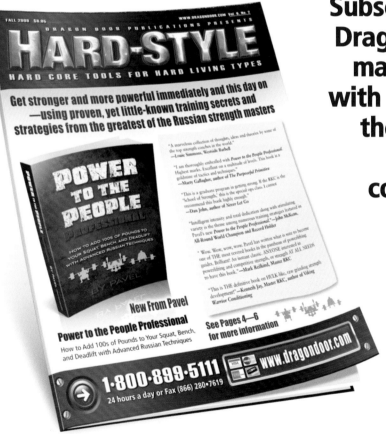

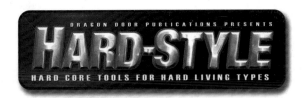

DRAGON DOOR PUBLICATIONS PRESENTS

HARD-STYLE

HARD CORE TOOLS FOR HARD LIVING TYPES

1·800·899·5111
24 HOURS A DAY
FAX YOUR ORDER (866) 280-7619

ORDERING INFORMATION

Customer Service Questions? Please call us between 9:00am– 11:00pm EST Monday to Friday at 1-800-899-5111. Local and foreign customers call 513-346-4160 for orders and customer service

100% One-Year Risk-Free Guarantee. If you are not completely satisfied with any product—we'll be happy to give you a prompt exchange, credit, or refund, as you wish. Simply return your purchase to us,

and please let us know why you were dissatisfied—it will help us to provide better products and services in the future. *Shipping and handling fees are non-refundable.*

Telephone Orders For faster service you may place your orders by calling Toll Free 24 hours a day, 7 days a week, 365 days per year. When you call, please have your credit card ready.

Complete and mail with full payment to: Dragon Door Publications, 5 East County Rd B, #3, Little Canada, MN 55117

Please print clearly
Sold To: A

Name_____

Street _____

City _____

State _____ Zip _____

Day phone*_____
* Important for clarifying questions on orders

Please print clearly
SHIP TO: *(Street address for delivery)*   B

Name_____

Street _____

City _____

State _____ Zip _____

Email _____

Warning to foreign customers:
The Customs in your country may or may not tax or otherwise charge you an additional fee for goods you receive. Dragon Door Publications is charging you only for U.S. handling and international shipping. Dragon Door Publications is in no way responsible for any additional fees levied by Customs, the carrier or any other entity.

Item #	Qty.	Item Description	Item Price	A or B	Total

HANDLING AND SHIPPING CHARGES · NO COD'S
Total Amount of Order Add (Excludes kettlebells and kettlebell kits):

$00.00 to 29.99	Add $6.00	$100.00 to 129.99	Add $14.00
$30.00 to 49.99	Add $7.00	$130.00 to 169.99	Add $16.00
$50.00 to 69.99	Add $8.00	$170.00 to 199.99	Add $18.00
$70.00 to 99.99	Add $11.00	$200.00 to 299.99	Add $20.00
		$300.00 and up	Add $24.00

Canada and Mexico add $6.00 to US charges. All other countries, flat rate, double US Charges. See Kettlebell section for Kettlebell Shipping and handling charges.

Total of Goods	
Shipping Charges	
Rush Charges	
Kettlebell Shipping Charges	
OH residents add 6.5% sales tax	
MN residents add 6.5% sales tax	
Total Enclosed	

METHOD OF PAYMENT p Check p M.O. p Mastercard p Visa p Discover p Amex

Account No. *(Please indicate all the numbers on your credit card)*   EXPIRATION DATE

☐☐☐☐ ☐☐☐☐ ☐☐☐☐ ☐☐☐☐   ☐☐/☐☐

Day Phone: (   )_____

Signature: _____ **Date:** _____

NOTE: *We ship best method available for your delivery address. Foreign orders are sent by air. Credit card or International M.O. only. For* **RUSH** *processing of your order, add an additional $10.00 per address. Available on money order & charge card orders only.*

Errors and omissions excepted. Prices subject to change without notice.